PROGRESS IN CLINICAL AND BIOLOGICAL RESEARCH

Please contact the publisher for information about previous titles in this series.

KAWASAKI DISEASE

KAWASAKI DISEASE

Proceedings of the Second International Kawasaki Disease Symposium held in Kauai, Hawaii, November 30 to December 3, 1986

Editor

Stanford T. Shulman, M.D.

Chief, Division of Infectious Diseases
Children's Memorial Hospital
Professor of Pediatrics
Northwestern University Medical School
Chicago, Illinois

ALAN R. LISS, INC. • NEW YORK

Library of Congress Cataloging-in-Publication Data

International Kawasaki Symposium (2nd : 1986 : Kauai)
    Kawasaki disease.

    (Progress in clinical and biological research ;
v. 250)
    Includes bibliographies and index.
    1. Mucocutaneous lymph node syndrome—Congresses.
I. Shulman, Stanford T.   II. Title III. Series.
RJ406.M83I58   1986   616.4'2   87-21443
ISBN 0-8451-5100-2

Contents

POSTER PRESENTATIONS

Yoo Sook Kim, Department of Mental Health, School of Health Sciences, Tokyo University, Tokyo, Japan **[531]**

Soichiro Kitamura, Department of Surgery, Division of Thoracic and Cardiovascular Surgery, Nara Medical College, Nara 634, Japan **[455]**

Kazuo Kitani, Division of Pediatrics, Heart Institute, Kurashiki Central Hospital, Kurashiki City, Japan **[515]**

Nobuyuki Kiyosawa, Department of Pediatrics, Kyoto Prefectural University of Medicine, Kyoto 602, Japan **[425,529]**

Noboru Kobayashi, The National Children's Medical Research Center, Tokyo 154, Japan **[571]**

Yohnosuke Kobayashi, Kansai Medical University, Osaka 570, Japan **[555]**

Yuko Koga, Department of Pediatrics and Child Health, Kurume University School of Medicine, Kurume 830, Japan **[73,209]**

M. Koike, Department of Microbiology, Kumamoto University Medical School, Japan **[569]**

Chisato Kondo, Department of Pediatric Cardiology, The Heart Institute of Japan, Tokyo Women's Medical College, Tokyo 162, Japan **[311]**

Mutsuko Konno, Kitami Red Cross Hospital, Kitami 090, Japan **[113]**

Shuzo Kono, Kansai Medical University, Osaka 570, Japan **[555]**

Gideon Koren, Division of Clinical Pharmacology, Research Institute and Department of Pediatrics, The Hospital for Sick Children, Toronto, Ontario, Canada M5G 1X8 **[415]**

Takao Kosaka, The National Children's Medical Research Center, Tokyo 154, Japan **[571]**

Shozo Kotani, Department of Microbiology and Oral Microbiology, Osaka University Dental School, Osaka 565, Japan and Osaka College of Medical Technology, Osaka 530, Japan **[101]**

Hitoshi Koyanagi, Department of Cardiovascular Surgery, Heart Institute of Japan, Tokyo Women's Medical College, Tokyo 162, Japan **[527]**

Nakako Kubo, Department of Epidemiology, The Institute of Public Health, Tokyo 108, Japan; present address: Department of Public Health, Nagoya City University Medical School, Nagoya 467, Japan **[549]**

J.D. Kugler, Department of Pediatrics, University of Nebraska Medical Center, Omaha, NE 68105 **[517]**

Tadatoshi Kuratsuji, The National Children's Medical Research Center, Tokyo 154, Japan **[571]**

Sanji Kusakawa, Department of Pediatrics, Tokyo Women's Medical College, Daini Hospital, Tokyo 116, Japan **[401,579]**

Masahisa Kyogoku, Department of Pathology, Tohoku University School of Medicine, Sendai 980, Japan **[257]**

L.A. Latson, Department of Pediatrics, University of Nebraska Medical Center, Omaha, NE 68105 **[517]**

Ronald M. Laxer, Department of Pediatrics, Division of Immunology/ Rheumatology, The Hospital for Sick Children, University of Toronto, Toronto, Ontario, Canada, M5G 1X8 **[175,567]**

Du Bong Lee, Department of Pediatrics, St. Mary's Hospital, Catholic Medical College, Seoul, Korea 150 **[55]**

Thomas J.A. Lehman, Department of Pediatrics, University of Southern California School of Medicine, and Rheumatology Research Laboratory, Division of Rheumatology, Children's Hospital of Los Angeles, Los Angeles, CA 90027 **[149]**

Donald Y.M. Leung, Department of Pediatrics, Harvard Medical School, Division of Allergy/Immunology, The Children's Hospital, Boston, MA 02115 **[125,159]**

Michael Levin, Departments of Immunology and Infectious Disease, Institute of Child Health, London, UK WC1N 1EH **[227]**

J.T. Lie, Department of Pathology, Mayo Clinic and Mayo Medical School, Rochester, MN 55905 **[521]**

Nancy E. Lightfoot, Division of Cardiology, The Hospital for Sick Children, Toronto, Ontario, Canada, M5G 1X8 **[45]**

Thomas Lint, Department of Immunology/Microbiology, Rush Presbyterian - St. Luke's Medical Center, Chicago, IL 60612 **[193]**

Noel Maclaren, Department of Pathology, University of Florida College of Medicine, Gainesville, FL 32610 **[475]**

Yutaka Manabe, Department of Pediatrics, Mimihara General Hospital, Sakai 590, Japan **[425]**

Nyven J. Marchette, Department of Tropical Medicine and Medical Microbiology, John A. Burns School of Medicine, University of Hawaii, Honolulu, HI 96816 **[87,131,545]**

Wilbert Mason, Department of Pediatrics, Division of Infectious Disease, Children's Hospital of Los Angeles, Los Angeles, CA 90027 **[219]**

Hirotake Masuda, Research Laboratory of Pathology, Toho University, Ohashi Hospital, Tokyo 153, Japan **[341,525]**

Shuzo Matsumoto, Department of Pediatrics, Cancer Institute, Hokkaido University School of Medicine, Sapporo 060, Japan **[113]**

Norio Matsuo, Department of Pediatrics, Toho University, School of Medicine, Japan **[559]**

Yoshiko Matsuoka, Department of Pediatrics, School of Medicine, Tokyo Medical and Dental University, Tokyo, Japan **[553]**

Hiroyuki Matsuura, Department of Pediatrics, Toho University, School of Medicine, Japan **[559]**

Marian E. Melish, Kapiolani-Children's Medical Center, and Department of Pediatrics, John A. Burns School of Medicine, University of Hawaii, Honolulu, HI 96816 **[87,131,545,547]**

A. Michael Michelson, Institute de Biologie Physico Chimique, 75005 Paris, France **[573]**

T. Minaga, Cutter Japan, Ltd. **[529]**

Masumi Minowa, Department of Epidemiology, The Institute of Public Health, Tokyo 108, Japan **[549]**

Hisahiro Mitomori, Division of Pediatrics, Heart Institute, Kurashiki Central Hospital, Kurashiki City, Japan **[515]**

Kazuyo Mitsudo, Division of Pediatrics, Heart Institute, Kurashiki Central Hospital, Kurashiki City, Japan **[515]**

Fumio Mizuno, Department of Virology, Cancer Institute, Hokkaido University School of Medicine, Sapporo 060, Japan **[113]**

Chuzo Mori, Department of Pediatrics, Shimane Medical College, Izumo 693, Japan **[425]**

Hiroko Mori, Department of Epidemiology, The Institute of Public Health, Tokyo 108, Japan **[549]**

D.C. Morrison, Division of Infectious Diseases, Children's Memorial Hospital, Department of Pediatrics, Northwestern University Medical School, Chicago, IL 60614 **[117]**

Hisao Murata, Department of Public Health and Research Laboratory of Pathology, Toho University School of Medicine, Tokyo 153, Japan **[523]**

Barry L. Myones, Division of Rheumatology, University of North Carolina, Chapel Hill, NC 27514 **[175]**

N. Nagamatsu, Department of Pathology, Aichi Medical University, Japan **[529]**

Yosikazu Nakamura, Department of Public Health, Jichi Medical School, Tochigi 329-04, Japan **[19]**

Toshio Nakanishi, Department of Pediatric Cardiology, The Heart Institute of Japan, Tokyo Women's Medical College, Tokyo 162, Japan **[311]**

Hiroyuki Nakano, Division of Pediatric Cardiology, Shizuoka Children's Hospital, Shizuoka 420, Japan **[287,425]**

Masao Nakano, Department of Pediatrics, Gifu Prefectural Tajimi Hospital, Japan **[535]**

Makoto Nakazawa, Department of Pediatric Cardiology, The Heart Institute of Japan, Tokyo Women's Medical College, Tokyo 162, Japan **[311]**

Shiro Naoe, Research Laboratory of Pathology, Toho University School of Medicine, Ohashi Hospital, Tokyo 153, Japan **[341,523,525]**

Jane W. Newburger, Department of Cardiology, The Children's Hospital, Boston, MA 02115 **[125,441]**

Hiroshi Nishida, Department of Cardiovascular Surgery, Heart Institute of Japan, Tokyo Women's Medical College, Tokyo 162, Japan **[527]**

Masaru Nishida, Kansai Medical University, Osaka 570, Japan **[555]**

Koichiro Niwa, Department of Pediatric Cardiology, The Heart Institute of Japan, Tokyo Women's Medical College, Tokyo 162, Japan **[311]**

Yukie Niwa, Niwa Institute for Immunology, Japan **[573]**

H. Nomura, Department of Pediatrics, Nagoya Daini Red Cross Hospital, Nagoya Higashi Shimin Hospital, and Nagoya City University Hospital, Japan **[543]**

Shigeaki Nonoyama, Department of Pediatrics, School of Medicine, Tokyo Medical and Dental University, Tokyo, Japan **[553]**

Valerio Novelli, Infectious Disease Unit, The Hospital for Sick Children, London, UK WC1N 1EH **[227]**

Minoru Ogawa, Kansai Medical University, Osaka 570, Japan **[555]**

Hirotaro Ogino, Department of Pediatrics, Kansai Medical University, Osaka 570, Japan **[555]**

Hidekazu Ohkuni, Kansai Medical University, Osaka 570, Japan **[555]**

Hisashi Ohnishi, Radiation Effects Research Foundation **[557]**

Hiromi Ohta, Hiroshima University, Hiroshima, Japan **[557]**

Motohiko Okano, Department of Virology and Pediatrics, Cancer Institute, Hokkaido University School of Medicine, Sapporo 060, Japan **[113]**

Tomio Okazaki, Hiroshima City Hospital, Hiroshima, Japan **[557]**

Ko Okumura, Department of Immunology, Juntendo University, School of Medicine, Tokyo 113, Japan **[167]**

Masahiko Okuni, Department of Pediatrics, Nihon University School of Medicine, Tokyo 173, Japan **[433,577]**

Kazuo Okuyama, Department of Pediatrics, Showa University, Japan **[531]**

Z. Onouchi, Department of Pediatrics, Aichi Medical University, Japan **[529]**

Toyoro Osato, Department of Virology, Cancer Institute, Hokkaido University School of Medicine, Sapporo 060, Japan **[113]**

Lauren M. Pachman, Department of Pediatrics, Division of Immunology/ Rheumatology, Northwestern University Medical School, Children's Memorial Hospital, Chicago, IL 60614 **[193]**

P. Pelkonen, Children's Hospital, Helsinki University Central Hospital, Helsinki, Finland SF-00290 **[563]**

Alan M. Rauch, Division of Viral Diseases, Center for Infectious Diseases, Centers for Disease Control, Public Health Service, U.S. Dept. of Health and, Human Services, Atlanta, GA 30333 **[33]**

Christian Rieger, Universitätskinderklinik, 3550 Marburg, Federal Republic of Germany **[61]**

Thomas L. Robertson, Cardiac Diseases Branch, Division of Heart and Vascular Diseases, National Heart, Lung, and Blood Institute, Bethesda, MD, 20892 **[325]**

Vera Rose, Division of Cardiology, The Hospital for Sick Children, Toronto, Ontario, Canada M5G 1X8 **[45]**

Richard D. Rowe, Departments of Pediatrics and Cardiology, The Hospital for Sick Children, University of Toronto, Toronto, Ontario, Canada, M5G 1X8 **[175, 299, 567]**

Anne H. Rowley, Department of Pediatrics, Division of Infectious Diseases, Northwestern University Medical School, Children's Memorial Hospital, Chicago, IL 60614 **[117,357]**

Laurence Rubin, Department of Rheumatology, Sunnybrook Hospital, University of Toronto, Toronto, Ontario, Canada, M4N 3M5 **[175]**

O. Ruuskanen, Department of Pediatrics, University of Turku, Finland **[563]**

David J. Sahn, Department of Pediatrics, University of California at San Diego, School of Medicine, La Jolla, CA 92093 **[379]**

Tsutomu Saji, Department of Pediatrics, Toho University, School of Medicine, Japan **[559]**

Y. Sakakibara, Department of Pediatrics, Aichi Medical University, Japan **[529]**

Tatsuichiro Sakatani, Fukushima Seikyo Hospital, Japan **[557]**

Eeva Salo, Children's Hospital, University of Helsinki, SF-00290 Helsinki, Finland **[67,563]**

Setsuko Sasa, Department of Mental Health, School of Health Sciences, Tokyo University, Tokyo, Japan **[531]**

Sumiko Sasagawa, Radiation Effects Research Foundation **[557]**

Keiko Sasai, Department of Pediatrics, Juntendo University School of Medicine, Tokyo 113, Japan **[565]**

Takehiko Sasazuki, Department of Genetics, Medical Institute of Bioregulation, Kyushu University, Fukuoka 812, Japan **[251]**

Gengi Satomi, Department of Pediatric Cardiology, The Heart Institute of Japan, Tokyo Women's Medical College, Tokyo 162, Japan **[311]**

Hiroshi Satomi, Department of Epidemiology, The Institute of Public Health, Tokyo 108, Japan **[549]**

Frederick M. Schaffer, Department of Pediatrics, Division of Immunology/ Rheumatology, The Hospital for Sick Children, University of Toronto, Toronto, Ontario, Canada M5G 1X8 **[175]**

Jane G. Schaller, Department of Pediatrics, Floating Hospital for Infants and Children, Boston, MA, 02111 **[193]**

S. Schuh, Department of Pediatrics, The Hospital for Sick Children, Toronto, Ontario, Canada, M5G 1X8 **[567]**

Shiro Seto, Department of Pediatrics, Kohga Public Hospital, Shiga 528, Japan **[425]**

T. Shimbo, Department of Pediatrics, Mizonokuchi Hospital, Teikyo University School of Medicine, Kawasaki, Japan **[539]**

K. Shinohara, Department of Pediatrics, Wakayama Medical College, Japan **[569]**

Keisuke Shinomiya, Department of Pediatrics, Kyoto University, Kyoto 606, Japan **[425]**

Noriaki Shinomiya, The National Children's Medical Research Center, Tokyo 154, Japan **[571]**

Akira Shirahata, Department of Pediatrics, University of Occupational and Environmental Health, Kitakyushu 807, Japan **[239]**

Toshikazu Shirai, Department of Pathology, Juntendo University School of Medicine, Tokyo 113, Japan **[185]**

Stanford T. Shulman, Department of Pediatrics, and Division of Infectious Diseases, Northwestern University Medical School, Children's Memorial Hospital, Chicago, IL 60614 **[117,193,357]**

Earl D. Silverman, Department of Pediatrics, Division of Immunology/ Rheumatology, The Hospital for Sick Children, University of Toronto, Toronto, Ontario, Canada M5G 1X8 **[175]**

Nicos Skordis, Department of Pathology, University of Florida College of Medicine, Gainesville, FL 32610 **[475]**

J. Smallhorn, Department of Pediatrics, The Hospital for Sick Children, Toronto, Ontario, Canada, M5G 1X8 **[567]**

Kyoichi Somiya, Department of Pediatrics, Hamamatsu Medical Center, Japan **[573]**

Tomoyoshi Sonobe, Department of Pediatrics, Japanese Red Cross Medical Center, Tokyo 150, Japan **[367,433]**

Leonard D. Stein, Department of Pediatrics, The Hospital for Sick Children, University of Toronto, Toronto, Ontario, Canada M5G 1X8 **[175]**

Toshiaki Sugawara, Department of Pediatrics, Juntendo University School of Medicine, Tokyo 113, Japan **[185]**

K. Sugiyama, Department of Pediatrics, Nagoya Daini Red Cross Hospital, Nagoya Higashi Shimin Hospital, and Nagoya City University Hospital, Japan **[543]**

Atsuko Suzuki, Department of Pediatrics, National Cardiovascular Center, Osaka 565, Japan **[347]**

Kazuo Suzuki, NIH/Japan, Hiroshima 730, Japan **[557]**

Kunihisa Takagi, The National Children's Medical Research Center, Tokyo 154, Japan **[571]**

Kei Takahashi, Research Laboratory of Pathology, Toho University, Ohashi Hospital, Tokyo 153, Japan **[341]**

Masato Takahashi, Division of Cardiology, Children's Hospital of Los Angeles, Los Angeles, CA 90027 **[493]**

Atsuyoshi Takao, Department of Pediatric Cardiology, The Heart Institute of Japan, Tokyo Women's Medical College, Tokyo 162, Japan **[311,527]**

Kozo Takase, Department of Pediatrics, School of Medicine, Tokyo Medical and Dental University, Tokyo, Japan **[553]**

Tae Takeda, The National Children's Medical Research Center, Tokyo 154, Japan **[571]**

H. Tamiya, Department of Pediatrics, Aichi Medical University, Japan **[529]**

Tokio Tamura, Division of Pediatric Cardiology, Tenri Hospital, Tenri 632, Japan **[425]**

Mutsuo Tanaka, Division of Pediatrics, Heart Institute, Kurashiki Central Hospital, Kurashiki City, Japan **[515]**

Noboru Tanaka, Research Laboratory of Pathology, Toho University, Ohashi Hospital, Tokyo 153, Japan **[341,525]**

Katsunori Tatara, Department of Pediatrics, Tokyo Women's Medical College, Daini Hospital, Tokyo 116, Japan **[401,579]**

Osamu Tatsuzawa, The National Children's Medical Research Center, Tokyo 154, Japan **[571]**

Shobun Tomita, Department of Pediatrics and Child Health, Kurume University School of Medicine, Kurume 830, Japan **[73,209]**

Takashi Tsurumizu, The Kitazato Research Institute, Tokyo, Japan **[571]**

Tetsuro Umezawa, Department of Pediatrics, Toho University, School of Medicine, Japan **[559]**

Hitoshi Usami, Department of Pediatrics, Nihon University School of Medicine, Japan **[577]**

M. Viander, Department of Microbiology, University of Turku, Finland **[563]**

Y. Wada, Department of Pediatrics, Nagoya Daini Red Cross Hospital, Nagoya Higashi Shimin Hospital, and Nagoya City University Hospital, Japan **[543]**

O. Wager, Laboratory of Clinical Immunology, Helsinki, Finland **[563]**

James W. Wiggins, Jr., Department of Pediatric Cardiology, University of Colorado Health Sciences Center, Denver, CO 80262 **[81]**

Keijiro Yabuta, Department of Pediatrics, Juntendo University School of Medicine, Tokyo 113, Japan **[185,565]**

Hyakuji Yabuuchi, Kansai Medical University, Osaka 570, Japan **[555]**

Kaneo Yamada, Department of Pediatrics, School of Medicine, St. Marianna University, Kanagawa 213, Japan **[239]**

Hideo Yamaguchi, Department of Pediatrics, Nihon University, Tokyo 173, Japan **[433]**

Hiroshi Yanagawa, Department of Public Health, Jichi Medical School, Tochigi 329-04, Japan **[5,19,433]**

Yoshio Yanase, Department of Pediatrics, Japanese Red Cross Medical Center, Tokyo 150, Japan **[167]**

Junichi Yata, Department of Pediatrics, School of Medicine, Tokyo Medical and Dental University, Tokyo, Japan **[553]**

Tatsuo Yokoyama, Department of Pediatric Cardiology, Kinki University School of Medicine, Osaka 589, Japan **[425]**

N. Yoshimura, Department of Immunology, Institute of Medical Science, University of Tokyo, Tokyo, Japan **[541]**

William J. Yount, University of North Carolina, Chapel Hill, NC 27514 **[175]**

Tomio Tada, Department of Immunology, University of Tokyo, Tokyo, Japan **[Chairman of Sessions]**

Fred Rosen, The Children's Hospital, Boston, Massachusetts **[Chairman of Sessions]**

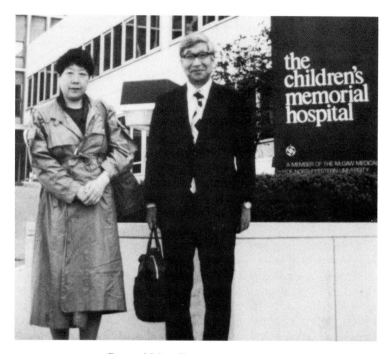

Dr. and Mrs. Tomisaku Kawasaki

Preface

"The beginning is the most important part of the work." Plato

It is now just about 20 years since Dr. Tomisaku Kawasaki published his classic 1967 report that clearly described the distinctive illness now known as Kawasaki Disease. This marked the real beginning of the efforts to solve the mysteries and secrets of this fascinating and increasingly important pediatric disorder. These efforts continue actively, as evidenced by the size of this volume.

These proceedings of the Second International Kawasaki Disease Symposium held November 30–December 3, 1986, on Kauai, Hawaii, include presentations by investigators from around the world regarding a wide variety of aspects of Kawasaki Disease. In addition, a number of outstanding scientists who had not previously devoted much time (if any) to thinking about Kawasaki Disease contributed fresh perspectives to the problems posed by this complex illness from their respective disciplines of vascular immunobiology, epidemiology, pathology, statistics, genetics, virology, and others.

I wish to acknowledge the outstanding efforts of the symposium organizing committee in the planning of this meeting. They include Dr. Tomisaku Kawasaki (Tokyo); Dr. Hirohisa Kato (Kurume); Dr. Noboru Kobayashi (Tokyo); Dr. Alan Rauch (Atlanta); Dr. Kay Chung (San Diego); Dr. Masato Takahashi (Los Angeles); Dr. Itsuzo Shigematsu (Hiroshima); and particularly, Dr. Marian Melish (Honolulu). Essential for the success of this symposium was the most generous support of the four separate non-commercial sponsors of the symposium, the Japan Heart Foundation, American Heart Association, Centers for Disease Control, and the National Heart, Lung, and Blood Institute of the National Institutes of Health. These organizations collaborated in an unprecedented fashion in this regard; I believe that this degree of cooperation serves as a tribute to the importance of Kawasaki Disease.

The organizers are also most grateful for additional symposium support from the following corporate sponsors: Immune Aktiengesellschaft fur Chemisch-Medizinische Produckte (Immuno AG) from Austria; Hyland

Therapeutics Division of Travenol Laboratories; Marion Laboratories; Mead Johnson Pharmaceuticals; Merrill Dow Pharmaceuticals; E.R. Squibb and Sons; and Sterling Incorporated.

Mr. Len Cook of the American Heart Association and Mr. Yasutaro Owaku and Mr. Takao Muramatsu of the Japan Heart Foundation were particularly instrumental behind the scenes in helping to organize the symposium, and they deserve particular credit. Dr. Mary Jane Jesse of the American Heart Association was also most helpful to the organizers.

The proceedings are organized in sections devoted to History and Epidemiology, Etiology, Pathogenesis, Cardiology, Therapy, and Future Directions. Each section includes a set of invited papers followed by an analysis by one or two invited discussants, generally from a discipline outside the immediate field of Kawasaki Disease, and then by a summary of the subsequent open discussion. It is my hope that these proceedings serve both to summarize the current state of knowledge regarding aspects of Kawasaki Disease as well to suggest future research directions that hold great promise for advancing our knowledge of this unique disorder.

This volume is dedicated to the memory of my parents, to my wife, Claire, to our children, Deborah, Elizabeth, and Edward, to Esther and Sam Levitt, and to the children around the world who have been afflicted by this remarkable disorder.

Stanford T. Shulman, M.D.
April 1, 1987

Kawasaki Disease, pages 1-4

HISTORICAL BACKGROUND AND CURRENT ISSUES

Tomisaku Kawasaki

Department of Pediatrics, Japanese Red Cross Medical Center, Tokyo, Japan 150

I feel that I am too young to speak about the history of MCLS and yet I also feel I have one foot in the grave. I would like to talk about some episodes that are footnotes to the history of MCLS and these episodes illustrate how bridges were built between the United States and Japan, the two sides of the Pacific.

Perhaps the first introduction of Kawasaki disease to the United States was in Dermatology in Practice, vol. 3, no. 2, March/April, 1970. As you know, my original paper in Japanese was in March, 1967 so this is three years after I had presented my paper. In 1969 the editor had asked me for my slides. I believe that although this paper was distributed among American pediatricians, very few doctors read it.

I next received a letter from a medical librarian. The letter was dated April 7, 1970 and stated that a doctor of Children's Hospital Medical Center of Northern California, Oakland, California, was very interested in this new clinical entity.

Two years later, I received a letter dated February 28, 1972. A pediatrician, assistant professor of State University Kings County Hospital Center in Brooklyn, New York had read a short description of the syndrome and requested reprints because she believed that she had seen several children who had a similar entity. Unfortunately, I never heard from her again but it may be that I never sent her the reprints. This was Dr. Elizabeth Smithwick.

The third communication, dated December 13, 1973, was from a pediatrician, Chief, Dept. of Pediatrics, Tripler Army Medical Center. He wrote that he had seen several cases at Children's Hospital in Honolulu as a pediatric infectious disease consultant and that he wanted copies of all the papers I had written. This was Dr. James Bass.

These letters show that there were pediatricians here and there in America who were experiencing the disease and interested in it but there was no one who pursued the disease.

My most memorable letter was the fourth letter which was from Dr. Marian E. Melish. It was dated March 15, 1974. She began her letter with, "We have seen 9 children with mucocutaneous lymph node syndrome." She said that until the eighth patient, she and her colleagues had not known that I had already categorized cases. She was preparing to give a paper on the results of her work to the Society for Pediatric Research held in Washington D. C. on May 2 and she wanted more information and the latest information even if it was in Japanese. She was kind enough to tell me to send her any information that I wished disseminated.

In this letter I was strongly impressed by the phrase: "We will, of course, give you full credit." This is almost never heard in Japan and I was deeply touched by this. I sent all the information that I had to Dr. Marian Melish.

There is another episode which helped to form a bridge across the Pacific. Dr. Benjamin Landing of Los Angeles came to Tokyo in June, 1972. At that time I was program chairman of the Tokyo Pediatric Society. I had a call from Dr. Noboru Kobayashi asking me to include Dr. Landing as a special lecturer in the meeting on June 17. I gladly did so and his title was "Neonatal hepatitis and congenital biliary atresia". I asked Dr. Kobayashi to ask Dr. Landing to make time for a discussion on MCLS. The reason why I wanted this meeting is that Dr. Kobayashi and his group at the University of Tokyo did not recognize MCLS as a new entity.

On June 19, Dr. Sanji Kusakawa, Dr. Takajiro Yamamoto, Dr. Kobayashi and his staff and I were able to have a special meeting with Dr. Landing on MCLS at the department of Pediatrics, Tokyo University Hospital. Dr. Landing showed a strong interest in MCLS and he was able to show us that the disease might be different from other similar diseases. This was an encouraging moral support.

The other doctor who met me in Japan was Dr. Se Mo Suh of Honolulu. In November, 1973, he came to Japan as an invited speaker of the Japan Neonatology Society's Annual Meeting held in Okayama City. I had a long discussion with him on MCLS at that time; he showed a strong interest in it and returned to Honolulu. After he returned to Hawaii, I received letters from a doctor at Tripler Army Hospital and from Dr. Melish. I imagine that Dr. Suh was one of the contributors to the bridge that was beginning to be built across the Pacific.

Opinion grew among our group that since this was definitely new clinical entity, we should publish a paper in English. Dr. Shigematsu and I wrote a manuscript on clinical features and epidemiology. In October, 1973, after attending a conference in Mexico, Dr. Shigematsu took our manuscript to Dr. Landing. He immediately submitted it to Pediatrics. In September, 1974, the paper was published and this episode shows the contribution of Dr. Landing (Kawasaki et al., 1974). I attended the XIV International Congress of Pediatrics held in Buenos Aires, Argentina, October 3-9, 1974. On my way back to Japan, I stopped off in Los Angeles and met Dr. Landing at the Children's Hospital of Los Angeles. At the Hospital I met Dr. Melish for the first time. She showed me slides of her patients, I showed her slides of mine and we were able to compare the cases that we had seen. We were able to confirm that we were seeing the same disease in the United States and in Japan. In the June, 1976 issue of the American Journal of Diseases of Children, Dr. Melish published the first paper on MCLS in America (Melish et al., 1976).

Subsequently, as you all know, Dr. Marian Melish has concentrated her efforts on this disease and has been an important contributor to general research on both sides of the Pacific. The Second International Symposium being held today is due to the efforts of Dr. Stanford Shulman but the efforts and tremendous contribution of Dr. Marian Melish lie behind the scenes and are a part of the history of this disease. I would like to pay tribute to Dr. Marian Melish and her immeasurable contribution toward research on this disease.

In Japan when the husband becomes a success, we praise the wife's behind-the-scene contribution. In this case, I would like to pay tribute also to the contribution of the man behind-the-scene, Dr. John Melish.

Discussion on current issues is another theme I have been asked to talk on but it will be freely covered this time so I will omit it from my presentation. I would only like to say a few words on the recent American retrovirus theory for the etiology of Kawasaki disease.

I have been doubtful about most of the theories that have been advanced so far about the etiology of Kawasaki disease. However, Dr. Stanford Shulman's paper in the Lancet (Shulman and Rowley, 1986), Dr. Jane Burns' paper in Nature (Burns et al., 1986) and discussions with Dr. Melish have persuaded me that the reliability of the theory is quite high. The 20 year race to make known the cause of the disease has made me quite excited but I have the feeling that the goal is near. Thus this symposium may be able to end the history of this disease. I am full of hope that this will be a fruitful symposium.

REFERENCES

Burns JC, Geha RS, Schneeberger EE, Rosen FS, Glezen LS, Huang AS, Natale J, Leung DYM (1986). Polymerase activity in lymphocyte culture supernatants from patients with Kawasaki disease. Nature 323: 814-816.
Kawasaki T, Kosaki F, Okawa S, Shigematsu I, Yanagawa H (1974). A new infantile acute febrile Mucocutaneous Lymph Node Syndrome (MLNS) prevailing in Japan. Pediatrics 54: 271-276.
Melish ME, Hicks RH, Larson EJ (1976). Mucocutaneous Lymph Node Syndrome in the United States. Am J Dis Child 130: 599-607.
Shulman ST, Rowley AH (1986). Does Kawasaki Disease Have a Retroviral Aetiology?. Lancet ii: 545-546.

Kawasaki Disease, pages 5–17
© 1987 Alan R. Liss, Inc.

EPIDEMIOLOGY OF KAWASAKI DISEASE IN JAPAN

Hiroshi Yanagawa
Department of Public Health, Jichi Medical School
Minami-kawachi-machi, Tochigi-ken, 329-04 Japan

INTRODUCTION

Since the Research Committee of Kawasaki Disease was first organized in Japan in 1970, a total of eight nationwide surveys have been conducted by the end of December 1984. The Committee collected 63,399 cases from pediatric departments of hospitals with more than 100 bed throughout Japan (Kawasaki et al., 1974; Yanagawa and Shigematsu, 1983; Yanagawa, 1986).

A nationwide epidemic of Kawasaki Disease was first recognized in Japan in April 1979, the number of cases reported in April–May of that year being twofold that observed in the preceding year. Three years after the first epidemic, an extraordinary pandemic attacked again in Japan in 1982, the number of cases reported then being at least 15,000. The epidemic began in January 1982 and the number of cases in May 1982 was more than six times that reported in the same month in 1981.

A detailed description of the epidemiological pictures of this disease entity has been made available through these studies. A summary of the epidemiological pictures revealed in Japan will be presented in this paper.

NATIONWIDE EPIDEMICS

The first topic of this paper is recent nationwide

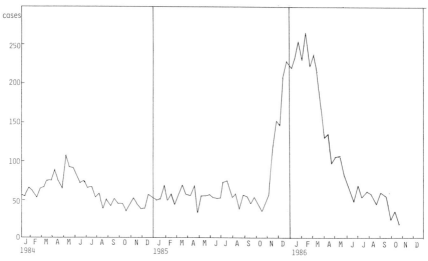

Figure 1. Number of reported cases in every 10-day period.

large scale epidemic of Kawasaki Disease in Japan. The epidemic came to light by the surveillance data reported from 148 representative hospitals which cover all the geographic areas in Japan. Since January 1984, the Japan Kawasaki Disease Research Committee has produced periodic estimates of Kawasaki Disease every month (Yanagawa et al., 1985).

The number of cases reported at 10-day intervals since January 1984 is plotted in Fig. 1. A sudden increase in the number of cases was seen in the 10-day interval of the 10th-19th of November 1985. The increase continued until the middle of February 1986 and then it sharply decreased to reach the normal level in July 1986. The peak number of cases observed in the 10-day interval from the 10th-19th of February was at least 4.5 times greater than that seen in the same period in 1985. An excess number of cases was seen for a period of six months since November 1985. A slight increase was seen in March-June 1985, but the increment was trivial.

Shown in Fig. 2 is the geographical distribution of the month showing a peak number of cases for the 47 prefectures in Japan, which illustrates how the epidemic waves reached almost all prefectures within four months

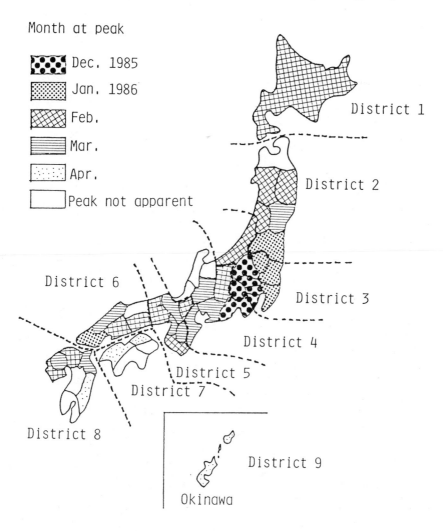

Figure 2. Geographical distribution of the month with peak
number of cases during the epidemic in 1985-86.

District No. is applicable to Fig. 3

except a few prefectures in the southern parts of two
southern islands.

Fig. 3 shows the time trend of the number of cases

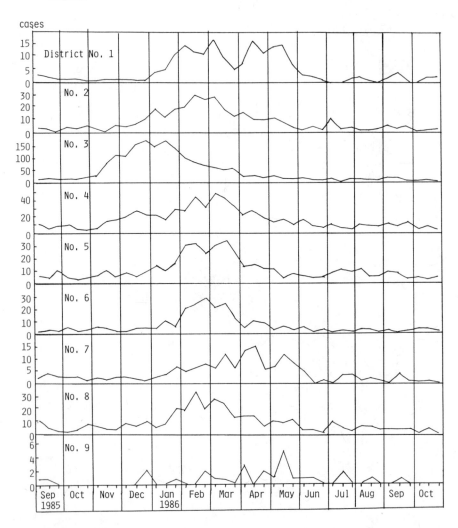

Figure 3. Number of reported cases in every 10-day period by district.

observed by 10-day intervals by nine geographical districts from the north to the south. The epidemic originated in District 3 which includes Tokyo and the metropolitan area. The increase began in December in northern Japan (Districts 1 and 2), whereas it appeared rather late in western Japan such as Districts 7 and 9.

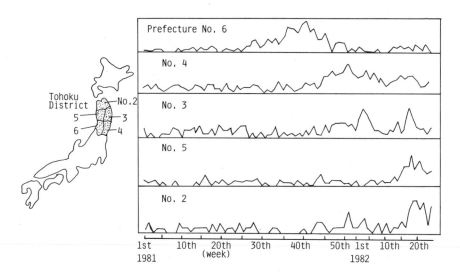

Figure 4. Propagation of epidemic waves in Tohoku District in Main island in Japan.

In contrast to the recent epidemic, the epidemic in 1979 broke out in western Japan and extended towards the west and the east. The propagation to the east reached the northernmost island in three months. The wave to the west extended to northern Kyushu island in two months. The epidemic did not reach southern Kyshu and Okinawa Islands.

The second epidemic observed in 1982 in Japan was characterized by a small peak in January and an extraordinary large peak in May and by its origin in four different areas from which the disease spread.

Fig. 4 is an example illustrating the movement of the epidemic waves in 1982 epidemic in north main island, Tohoku District. Prefecture No. 6 had its peak in 40th week of 1981 followed by Prefecture 4, Prefecture 3 and finally Prefectures 5 and 2. The time interval between the peaks of Prefecture No. 6 and No. 2 was 30 weeks. Such inter-prefectural progression were also observed in other districts.

Fig. 5 illustrates three epidemics in Japan as

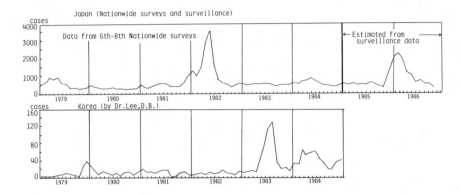

Figure 5. Monthly number of reported cases in Japan and Korea.

compared with the epidemics in Korea reported by Dr. Lee (Lee, 1985). While the peaks of three epidemics in Japan were seen in May 1979, in May 1982 and in February 1986, they were seen in December 1979 and August 1983 in Korea. The first peak appeared 7 months behind and the second peak appeared 15 month behind the Japanese ones.

Incidence rates during the 18 month period from January 1981 to July 1982 for 3,000 local governments were calculated. It should be noted that the areas with high incidence clustered in various parts in Japan. The boundaries of the aggregated areas are closely related to the network of public communication system and geographical ranges of daily life activities in the community.

FAMILIAL INCIDENCES OF KAWASAKI DISEASE

Another point of interest in the epidemiology of the disease is observation on the incidence among the family member of the cases.

Under the co-operation of the Association of the Parents with Children of Kawasaki Disease, a questionnaire survey on the incidence of secondary cases of Kawasaki Disease in a family during one year period after onset of the first cases was made (Fujita et al., 1986).

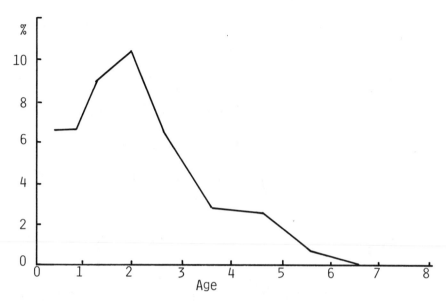

Figure 6. Secondary attack rate among siblings in one year after onset.

In 2,649 families responding to the survey, there were 4268 children including 2645 primary cases in these families.   In four families, the disease attacked two children at the same time.   Total number of children at risk of secondary attack was 1615, of whom 32 cases (2.0 %) were attacked within one year after the onset of primary cases.

The age distribution of the primary cases showed a peak at the 6-11 month and that for the secondary cases at latter half of age one.   However, the curve for the siblings who were not attacked had rather smooth and slow peak in age 3-5 years.   The age specific secondary attack rate during one year period after the onset of the primary cases among siblings are shown in Fig. 6.   The rate is more than 6 % in the age of less than one year 6 months. The highest is 10.2 % in the latter half of age one.   The rate decreased after 2 years of age.

The attack rate among family siblings are higher than that observed in general population in the epidemic of 1982.   The rate in Ishikawa Prefecture that showed the highest incidence rate in all the prefectures was 0.33 per

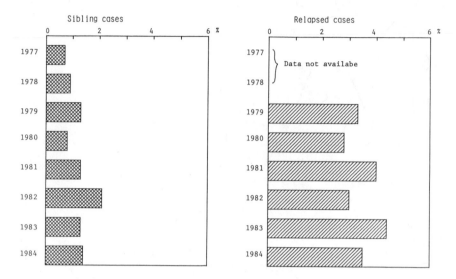

Figure 7. Proportion of sibling cases and relapsed cases among reported cases.

100 children of age 0-4 years.

Dr. Imada disclosed in the observation of 186 families with sibling cases of Kawasaki Disease that the interval from the onset of the primary cases to that of the secondary cases was a week or less in about 50 %. The onset was on the same day in 10 % (Imada, 1984).

Fig. 7 illustrates the proportion of sibling cases and relapsed cases among total reported cases in the nationwide surveys. The proportion of siblings are larger in the years when the incidence rates are high, but that of relapsed cases are not.

An epidemiological study on 467 sibling cases and 933 relapsed cases reported in 3-year-6-month period from January 1979 to June 1982 in the 6th and 7th nationwide surveys in Japan (Yanagawa et al., 1985) disclosed that:

(1) The male/female ratio of relapsed cases is 1.6 which is higher than that of total reported cases (1.4). However, the sex ratio of the risk of relapsing for the children with previous history of the disease is almost

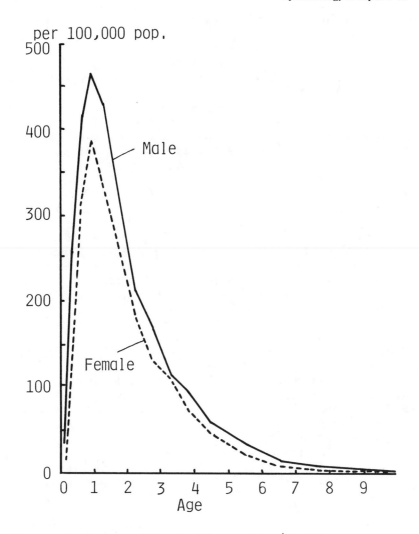

Figure 8. Age specific incidence rate by sex.
1982 (8th nationwide survey)

equal (1.1).

    (2)   The sex ratio of sibling cases is 1.1.

    (3)   The fatality rates are 0.9 % for relapsed cases
and 1.1 % for sibling cases. Both the rates are three

times higher than that of total cases reported in the survey (0.3 %).

(4) The proportion of sibling cases among relapsed cases is 3 times higher than that of total reported cases.

(5) The relapsing rate in 1982 epidemic year is 950 per 100,000 children with previous history of Kawasaki Disease. The rate is more than six times higher than the incidence rate at the same period, which is 151 per 100,000 children of age 0-4 years.

AGE AND SEX PATTERNS

Fig. 8 shows the age specific incidence rate sex in 1982. The incidence by age presents a unimodal curve with a peak at the age of 9-11 months. 50 % of all the cases is of age two or less. The sex ratio (M/F) is 1.4. The age of onset tends to be lower and the sex ratio tends to decrease during the year of epidemic.

CARDIAC SEQUELAE AND FATALITY

In the last nationwide survey the presence or absence of cardiac sequelae was asked to be reported. The cardiac sequelae were defined as the presence one month after onset of Kawasaki Disease of dilatation of the coronary artery (including aneurysm), stenosis (including occlusion), myocardial infarction or valvular lesion. The overall incidence of cardiac sequelae was 17.2 %. By age, the incidence was the highest in the 0 age group as shown in Fig. 9.

The average fatality rate of the cases reported in 1982 through 1984 was 0.3 %. The rate is higher in less than one year of age.

TREATMENT

Steroid was mainly used for the treatment of Kawasaki Disease in 1977 or before, as seen in Fig. 10, but recently doctors abstain from using it. Aspirin is most commonly used at the present time in Japan. Information

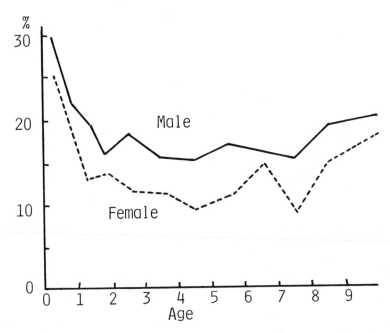

Figure 9. Proportion of cases with cardiac sequelae by sex and age.

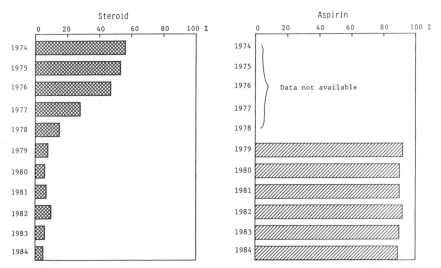

Figure 10. Proportion of cases treated with steroid and aspirin in Japan.

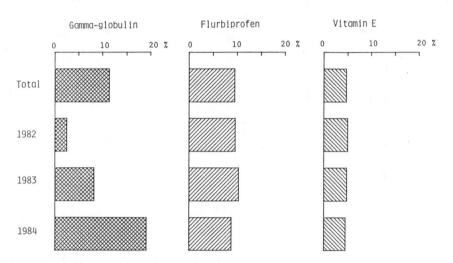

Figure 11. Proportion of cases treated with gamma-globulin, flurbiprofen and vitamin E.

on the use of other drugs was obtained in the 8th nationwide survey as illustrated in Fig. 11. Cases treated with gamma-globulin increased from 2.5 % in 1982 to 19.1 % in 1984.

CONCLUSION

The epidemiological studies so far have not produced sufficient evidence to settle the question on the causal agent of the disease. However, the author has the impression that only an infectious process can produce such conspicuous outbreaks as seen three times in Japan and two times in Korea.

REFERENCES

Fujita Y, Nagai M, Nakamura Y, Yanagawa H (1986). Measurement of familial aggregation of Kawasaki Disease. Jpn J Pub Hlth 33: 67-72. (In Japanese with English abstract)
Imada Y (1984). Clinical-epidemiological study on siblings with Kawasaki Disease. J Showa Med Association 44:605-

625. (In Japanese with English abstract)

Kawasaki T, Kosaki F, Shigematsu I, Okawa S, Yanagawa H (1974). A new infantile acute febrile mucocutaneous lymph node syndrome (MLNS). Pediatrics 54:271-276.

Lee DB (1985). Epidemiological survey of Kawasaki syndrome in Korea (1976-1984). J Catholic Med Coll 38:13-19.

Yanagawa H (1986). Nationwide surveys on Kawasaki Disease. In Shigematsu I, Kawasaki T, Yanagawa H (Eds): "Kawasaki Disease -Epidemiological Data Book-", Tokyo: Soft Science Pub Co, pp 196-200.

Yanagawa H, Nagai M, Kawasaki T (1985). Surveillance of Kawasaki Disease -Summary of the results in 1984-. SHONI-NAIKA 17(5):653-658. (In Japanese)

Yanagawa H, Nagai M, Ohgane H, Hashimoto T, Nakamura Y (1985). An epidemiological study on relapsed cases and household cases of Kawasaki Disease. Jpn J Pub Hlth 32:3-7. (In Japanese with English abstract)

Yanagawa H, Shigematsu I (1983). Epidemiological features of Kawasaki Disease in Japan. Acta Pediatrica Japonica 25:94-107.

Kawasaki Disease, pages 19–32
© 1987 Alan R. Liss, Inc.

TEMPORAL AND GEOGRAPHICAL CLUSTERING OF KAWASAKI DISEASE IN
JAPAN

Yosikazu Nakamura, Hiroshi Yanagawa
and Tomisaku Kawasaki

Department of Public Health, Jichi Medical School,
Minamikawachi, Tochigi, 329-04 Japan (Y. N. , H. Y.)
Japan Red Cross Medical Center, Shibuya, Tokyo,
150 Japan (T. K.)

INTRODUCTION

About twenty years have passed since Kawasaki Disease
(KD) was first reported by one of the authors. However, the
etiology of this disease is still unclear. Many epidemiological researches suggest that the cause of KD is related
to infection because of its epidemic curves (Yanagawa and
Shigematsu, 1973), geographical (Nakamura et al. , 1984) and
temporal (Yoshida, 1984; Nakamura et al. , 1984a) clustering,
movement of epidemics (Yosida, 1984; Nakamura et al. , 1984a)
and excess incidence among siblings (Tominaga et al., 1977;
Imada, 1984; Fujita et al. , 1986). Recent reports from
Japan (Furusho et al. , 1984) and the U. S. A. (Newburger et
al. , 1986) that gamma-globulin is effective to prevent
coronary lesions of the disease also support the infectious
theory.

The authors analyzed the temporal and geographical
patterns of KD and discussed the etiology of the disease.

METHODS

The Japan Kawasaki Disease Research Committee has
carried out 8 Nationwide Surveys of KD in Japan since 1970.
Information was collected about the patients treated in
pediatric departments in hospitals with more than 100 beds
in Japan from 1977 to 1984. It was estimated that more than
90 percent of KD patients throughout Japan had been included
in these Surveys (Kubota, 1978).

Analysis in Temporal Clustering

The weekly number of the patients was observed by prefecture, calculating the cluster index (H), which represents the level of temporal clustering, proposed by Yokoyama et al (Yokoyama et al., 1976). This index has the effect of Coulomb potential type for all the pairs of observation units with the occurrence of cases. The index is defined in the following formula:

$$ H = \frac{1}{2 N^2} \sum_{i=1}^{\ell} \sum_{j=1}^{\ell} \frac{f_i \, f_j}{d_{ij}} $$

where, N is the total number of cases in the study period (units, one-year period with 52 or 53 units in this study); f_i and f_j are the number of cases observed at i-th and j-th

observation unit, respectively; d_{ij} (d_{ij}= i-j (d_{ij}=0.5,

when i=j)) is the temporal distance between i-th and j-th observation units. If all patients cluster in one observation unit, H takes its highest value, 1.00. The level of the statistical test (5% and 1%) was estimated by 100,000 time-simulations for each total number N.

Yearly incidence rates (per 100,000 children aged 0-9) were calculated by using the data of the National Census in 1980.

Analysis of Geographical Clustering

Yearly incidence rate (per 100,000 children aged 0-9) was calculated in each smallest governmental unit (municipality : 3,278 municipalities in Japan). The frequency and geographical pattern of the distribution of municipalities with high incidence rate of KD (Annual incidence rate is twice as high as the average rate (33.4 x 2 = 66.8) in 8-year period (1977-1984) or more) were observed. Such municipalities were defined as "high incidence municipalities".

Correlation coefficients of the incidence rate in each municipality between two different years were calculated. The municipalities with small population size were excluded from the correlation analysis. The observation was done on 410 municipalities whose populations aged 0-9 were more than 8,704, where the probability that there is no KD patients in the municipalities in one year is less than 5% with an assumption that the children may be attacked in the Poisson distribution with expected yearly incidence rate 33.4 per 100,000 children aged 0-9 (average incidence rate in 8-year period, 1977 - 1984).

The difference of incidence rates between municipalities in urban and rural areas was compared. All municipalities were classified by population size of ages 0-9. In each group, yearly incidence rates (total number of KD patients / total number of children aged 0-9) were calculated. The same analysis was done by population density.

RESULTS

Temporal Clustering

The analysis was made on 51,061 patients of KD observed in an 8-year period. The average annual incidence rate was 33.4 per 100,000 children aged 0-9. The incidence rate and H value of each year were shown in Table 1. In 1979 and 1982 when large epidemics were observed, the incidence rates

TABLE 1. Number of Patients and Relationship between Incidence Rates and Clustering Indices (H)

Year	All Japan			By prefecture
	No. of patients	Incidence rate*	H value	Correlation coefficients between incidence rate and H value
1977	2,774	15.0	.0907**	-.483**
1978	3,425	18.5	.0869	-.543**
1979	6,825	36.8	.1000**	.337**
1980	3,897	21.0	.0881**	-.064
1981	6,352	34.2	.0895**	.379**
1982	15,428	83.2	.1225**	.674**
1983	5,904	31.8	.0870	-.166
1984	6,456	34.8	.0927**	.135

*:p<0.05   **:p<0.01   (d. f. =45)

*:per 100,000 children of age 0 - 9

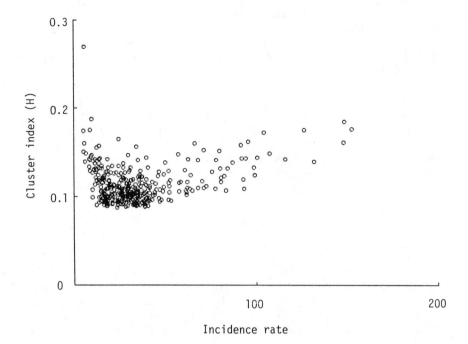

Number of dots is 376 (47 prefectures X 8 years)
Figure 1. The relationship between clustering index (H) and
incidence rate (per 100,000 children of age 0-9) by
prefecture in eight years (1977 - 1984).

and the H values were higher than any other non-epidemic
years. The H values were statistically significantly high
in all years except 1978 and 1983.

In the observation of the correlation coefficients
between the incidence rate and H value by prefecture, the
correlation coefficients were significantly positive in the
years with high incidence rates (1979, 1981 and 1982) (Table
1). In 1977 and 1978, when the yearly incidence rates were
rather low, the correlation coefficients were significantly
negative. Scatter diagram in which there is a relationship
between the incidence rate and H value for 8-years observed
by prefecture (n = 47 prefectures x 8 years = 376) is shown
in Fig. 1. It seemed that a high H value had a direct
relationship with a high incidence rate when incidence rate

TABLE 2. Clustering Indices (H) Based on Weekly Numbers of Cases by Prefecture and Year

Prefecture	H value							
	1977	1978	1979	1980	1981	1982	1983	1984
1 Hokkaido	.0951	.0979**	.1233**	.0938	.1017**	.1083**	.0937*	.0916
2 Aomori	.1502	.1419	.1207**	.1118*	.1054	.1136**	.1003	.1120*
3 Iwate	.1079	.1090	.1065**	.1090	.0961	.1168**	.0988	.1194**
4 Miyagi	.1264	.1085*	.1092**	.0976	.0953	.1063**	.0963	.1441**
5 Akita	.1570**	.1369	.1238**	.1152	.1077	.1512**	.0994	.1322**
6 Yamagata	.1208	.1209**	.1079*	.1050	.1487**	.0965	.1031	.1005
7 Fukushima	.1062	.0975	.1118**	.1134	.1030	.1317**	.1022	.1287**
8 Ibaraki	.1153**	.0947	.1219**	.1042	.0926	.1754**	.1004*	.1109**
9 Tochigi	.1417**	.1002	.1133**	.1202*	.1023*	.1719**	.1016	.1222**
10 Gumma	.1164	.1006	.1096**	.0996	.1032	.1381**	.0946	.1034**
11 Saitama	.0993**	.0896	.1141**	.0949	.0915	.1597**	.0933	.0968**
12 Chiba	.1000*	.0900	.1036**	.0928	.0917	.1329**	.0911	.0963**
13 Tokyo	.0907	.0891	.1111**	.0936**	.0889	.1441**	.0895	.0994**
14 Kanagawa	.0934	.0921	.0983**	.0914	.0913*	.1431**	.0901	.1058**
15 Niigata	.1299**	.1181*	.1019*	.0988	.0987	.1163**	.0892	.0939
16 Toyama	.1246	.0976	.1042	.1049	.0985	.1389**	.1018	.1053
17 Ishikawa	.1196	.1048	.1036	.0996	.1060	.1850**	.1013	.0982
18 Fukui	.1373**	.1180	.1088**	.1268*	.1141	.1427**	.1014	.1148
19 Yamanashi	.1879	.1464	.1468**	.1418	.1266	.1526**	.1087	.1043
20 Nagano	.1291	.1022	.1053**	.1005	.0943	.1614**	.0966*	.0958
21 Gifu	.1102	.0995	.1102**	.1413*	.1059**	.1021**	.0919	.1046**
22 Shizuoka	.1058*	.0926	.1060**	.0951	.0942*	.1763**	.0922	.0955**
23 Aichi	.0951	.0957	.0915	.0974*	.1104**	.1248**	.0878	.0937*
24 Mie	.1401**	.1207	.1007	.1049	.0989	.1228**	.0943	.1098**
25 Shiga	.1403	.1113	.1031	.1087	.1322**	.1158**	.1028	.1140*
26 Kyoto	.1161**	.0991	.1057**	.1019	.1053**	.1189**	.0909	.0977
27 Osaka	.0992*	.0908	.1011**	.0911	.0956**	.1167**	.0950**	.0928*
28 Hyogo	.0961	.0924	.1196**	.0936	.0918	.1215**	.0913	.0903
29 Nara	.1418*	.1154	.1196**	.1276*	.1478**	.1178**	.1101	.1087
30 Wakayama	.1211	.1278	.1087	.1109	.1011	.1415**	.0980	.1029
31 Tottori	.1320	.1345	.1288**	.1431	.1299	.1236**	.1101	.1378**
32 Shimane	.2693	.1376	.1222*	.1320*	.1130	.1407**	.1275	.1648**
33 Okayama	.1012	.1230**	.1149**	.1026	.0960	.1585**	.0970	.0968
34 Hiroshima	.0948	.0939	.1036**	.0948	.0949	.1614**	.0900	.0972
35 Yamaguchi	.1237	.0987	.1203**	.1100	.1129**	.1163**	.1019	.1018
36 Tokushima	.1311	.1266	.1099	.1184	.1043	.1312**	.1094	.1162*
37 Kagawa	.1325	.1236*	.1418**	.1210*	.1178**	.1089**	.1128	.1076
38 Ehime	.1447	.1137	.1414**	.1087	.1031	.1100**	.0937	.1133**
39 Kochi	.1257	.1150	.1074	.1257	.1215*	.1069*	.1046	.1074
40 Fukuoka	.0936	.0918	.1148**	.0912	.1067**	.1101**	.0903	.0924*
41 Saga	.1300	.1555	.1058	.1341	.1275**	.1274**	.1006	.1103
42 Nagasaki	.1124	.1179	.1053**	.1087*	.1016	.1238**	.0985	.1021
43 Kumamoto	.1596	.1750**	.1029	.1067	.1003	.1051**	.1129*	.1408**
44 Oita	.1333	.1179	.1276**	.1340**	.0986	.1117**	.0940	.0981
45 Miyazaki	.1200	.1188	.1076	.1186	.1173	.1053**	.1182**	.1019
46 Kagoshima	.1389	.1301	.1105	.1078	.1071	.1297**	.1085	.1063
47 Okinawa	.1487	.1742	.1314	.1557**	.1193**	.1310*	.1117**	.1157**

*:p<0.05 **:p<0.01

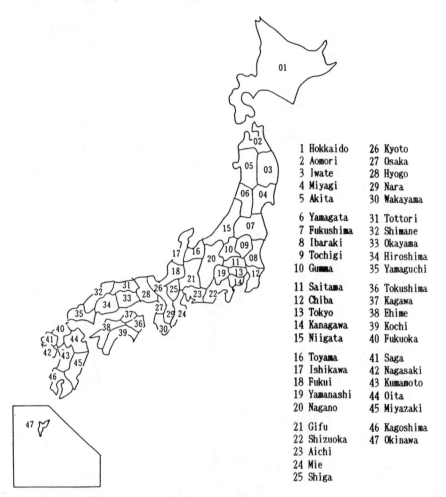

1 Hokkaido	26 Kyoto
2 Aomori	27 Osaka
3 Iwate	28 Hyogo
4 Miyagi	29 Nara
5 Akita	30 Wakayama
6 Yamagata	31 Tottori
7 Fukushima	32 Shimane
8 Ibaraki	33 Okayama
9 Tochigi	34 Hiroshima
10 Gumma	35 Yamaguchi
11 Saitama	36 Tokushima
12 Chiba	37 Kagawa
13 Tokyo	38 Ehime
14 Kanagawa	39 Kochi
15 Niigata	40 Fukuoka
16 Toyama	41 Saga
17 Ishikawa	42 Nagasaki
18 Fukui	43 Kumamoto
19 Yamanashi	44 Oita
20 Nagano	45 Miyazaki
21 Gifu	46 Kagoshima
22 Shizuoka	47 Okinawa
23 Aichi	
24 Mie	
25 Shiga	

Figure 2. Prefecture distribution in Japan.

was higher than 50.

Table 2 shows H values calculated by year and prefecture (Names of prefecture in Japan are shown in Fig. 2).
In 1982, when there was a nationwide epidemic, almost all
prefectures showed statistically significant H values.

Epidemic curves of all Japan and 4 selected prefectures
are shown in Fig. 3. Yamagata Prefecture was the only pre-

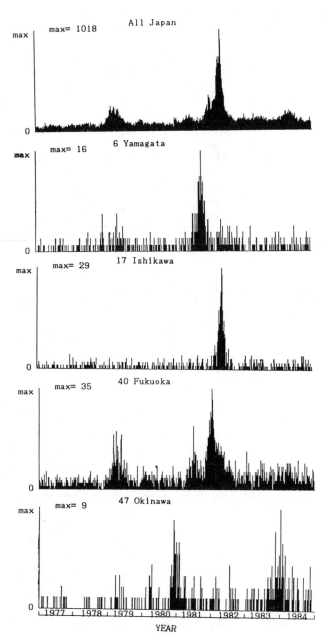

Figure 3. Weekly epidemic curves of Kawasaki Disease in all Japan and four selected prefectures.

fecture in which significant clustering was not seen in 1982. Ishikawa Prefecture showed the highest H value (0.1850) in 1982 and Fukuoka Prefecture showed an epidemic between 1981 and 1982. Okinawa Prefecture had epidemics in different periods than the rest of Japan.

Geographical Clustering

TABLE 3. Comparison of Incidence Rates and Proportion of High Incidence Municipalities* in Four Observation Years

	Average of 1981 - 1984	1981	1982	1983	1984
Incidence rate** (All Japan)	46.0	34.2	83.2	31.8	34.8
No. of high incidence municipalities (%)***		488 (14.9)	1,832 (42.2)	450 (13.7)	507 (15.5)

* : A municipality whose yearly incidence rate is over 66.8 per 100,000 children of ages 0-9.
** : Per 100,000 children of ages 0-9.
*** : There are 3,278 municipalities in Japan.

TABLE 4. Correlation Coefficients between Two Yearly Incidence Rates

	1981	1982	1983	1984
1981	—			
1982	.291**	—		
1983	.234**	.444**	—	
1984	.187**	.332**	.421**	—

Observation on 410 municipalities whose population of ages 0-9 were more than 8,704 (d.f. = 408).
* : $p < 0.05$ ** : $p < 0.01$

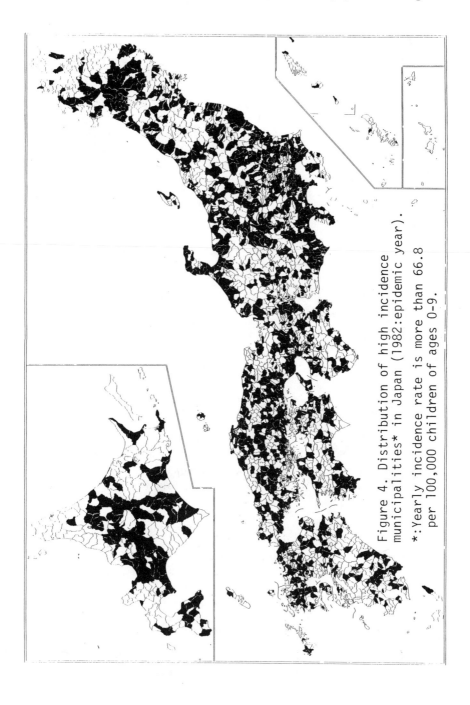

Figure 4. Distribution of high incidence municipalities* in Japan (1982:epidemic year).

*:Yearly incidence rate is more than 66.8 per 100,000 children of ages 0-9.

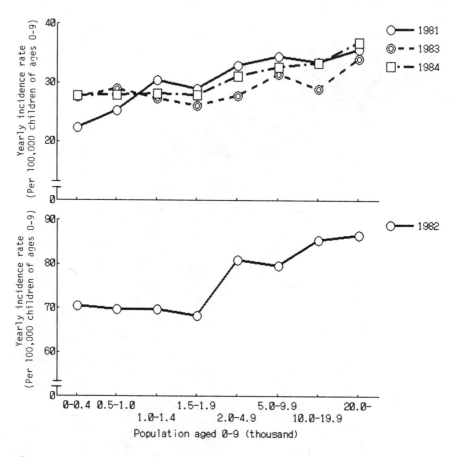

Figure 5. Yearly incidence rate in municipalities classified by the size of population of children aged 0-9.

Table 3 compares the yearly incidence rates of KD and numbers of high incidence municipalities in four observation years. Both the incidence rate and proportion of the high incidence municipalities in 1982, the second nationwide epidemic in Japan, were more than twice of those in other three years.

The geographical distribution of the municipalities with high incidence rate in 1982 (epidemic year) was shown in Fig. 4. Geographical clusterings were observes in many areas throughout Japan in 1982, for example, in Hokkaido

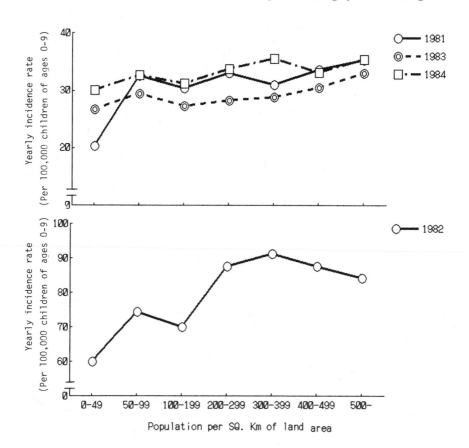

Figure 6. Yearly incidence rate in municipalities classified by population density of all residents.

(north island), in Tohoku district (north-east part of the main island), in Kanto district (around Tokyo), in Hokuriku district (north part of the center of the main island) and so on.

The numbers of high incidence municipalities in non-epidemic years were generally less than that in epidemic year. Nevertheless, there were still geographical clusterings in several areas.

Correlation coefficients between two yearly incidence

rates in municipalities whose population of ages 0-9 was
more than 8,704 were shown Table 4. The correlation coefficient was significantly positive in every combination of
the years. Correlation coefficients between adjacent two
years were higher than the others.

The results of observation of the difference between
incidence rates in urban areas and that in rural areas were
shown in Fig. 5 and Fig. 6. In both observations, by size
of population aged 0-9 and population density, incidence
rate is rather high in urban area (large population and high
population density), especially in epidemic year, 1982.

DISCUSSION

The level of temporal clustering of KD was evaluated by
cluster index H proposed by Yokoyama et al. (Yokoyama et
al., 1981) by year and prefecture in this study. It was
clarified that high H values were observed in many prefectures in 1979 and 1982 when nationwide epidemics of KD
were seen in Japan. When the yearly incidence rate was less
than 50 per 100,000 children aged 0-9, the H value did not
change or decrease in proportion to the incidence rate.
However, when incidence rate was more than 50, the H value
became higher as incidence rate went up. This fact
indicates that a high annual incidence rate is formed not by
many patients evenly disbursed throughout the year but by
clustering of cases in a short period, seeming less than six
months.

The outbreak of many patients in a limited time is
characteristic of infectious diseases. In fact, epidemic
curves of many infectious disease such as measles and
rubella in the surveillance of infectious diseases in Japan
were similar to that of KD (Nakamura et al., 1984a).
Geographical clustering of the incidence of KD were
observed in non-epidemic year as well as epidemic year in
this study. These results were reasonably explained by
the etiological agents widely spread and highly associated
with population density, such as infectious theory.

This theory is also supported by the higher incidence
rates in urban municipalities than in rural ones.

There may be more personal communications in cities

than in the country. So this result is also reasonable if some infectious agents are causally related to KD.

Positive correlation coefficients of incidence rate among different years may be caused by the environmental and social characteristics of the municipality, such as population size, population density, transportation system or others.

The epidemiological studies done so far in Japan have not produced sufficient evidence to settle the question on the causal agent of the disease. However, the result mentioned above strongly supports the hypothesis that the etiology of KD is related to some infectious agents widely spread in community.

SUMMARY

Statistical analysis of the data of Nationwide Surveys of Kawasaki Disease in Japan disclosed that (1) the incidence of the disease clustered temporally. The clustering levels were especially high in the years with high incidence rates. (2) Geographical clustering existed in both epidemic year (1982) and non-epidemic years. Incidence rate were lower in rural area than in urban area. These results support the hypothesis that the etiology of Kawasaki Disease is related to some infectious agents.

REFERENCES

Fujita Y, Nagai M, Nakamura Y, Yanagawa II (1986). Measurement of familial aggregation of Kawasaki Disease. Jpn J Public Health 33:67-72 (in Japanese with English abstract).

Furusho K, Kamiya T, Nakano II, Kiyosawa N, Shinomiya K, Hayashidera T, Tamura T, Hirose O, Manabe Y, Yokoyama T, Kawarano M, Baba K, Baba K, Mori C (1984). High-dose intravenous gammaglobulin for Kawasaki Disease. Lancet 2:1055-1058.

Imada Y (1984). Clinical-epidemiological study on siblings with Kawasaki Disease. J Showa Med Association 44:605-625 (in Japanese with English abstract).

Kubota S (1978). Epidemiological studies on so-called Kawasaki disease. J Nippon Med Sch 45:321-337 (in

Japanese with English Abstract).

Nakamura Y, Ohgane H, Yanagawa H (1984). Observation of the incidence of Kawasaki Disease in small geographic units in 1979 and 1982 epidemics in Japan. Jpn J Public Health 31:539-547 (in Japanese with English abstract).

Nakamura Y, Nagai M, Yanagawa H, Kusakawa S (1984a). An analysis on weekly incidence of Kawasaki Disease and selected infectious diseases. Acta Paediatr Jpn 26:108.

Newburger JW, Takahashi M, Burns JC, Beiser AS, Chung KJ, Duffy CE, Glode MP, Mason WH, Reddy V, Sanders SP, Shulman ST, Wiggins JW, Hicks RV, Fulton DR, Lewis AB, Leung DYM, Colton T, Rosen FS, Melish ME (1986). The treatment of Kawasaki Syndrome with intravenous gamma globulin. N Engl J Med 45:341-347.

Tominaga M, Ohshima K, Yanagawa H, Shigematsu I, Kawasaki T (1977). Epidemiological study of sibling cases of MCLS. Pediatrics of Japan 18:59-63 (in Japanese).

Yanagawa H, Shigematu I (1983). Epidemiological features of Kawasaki Disease in Japan. Acta Paediatr Jpn 25:94-107.

Yokoyama H, Hara N, Gotoh A, Hashimoto T, Yanagawa H (1981). A statistical index indicating the level of temporal cluster in the incidence of rare disease. Jpn J Public Health 28:3-12 (in Japanese with English abstract).

Yoshida I (1984). An epidemiologic study on an outbreak of Kawasaki Disease in Ehime Prefecture in 1978-1989. Jpn J Public Health 31:97-110 (in Japanese with English abstract).

Kawasaki Disease, pages 33–44
Published 1987 Alan R. Liss, Inc.

KAWASAKI SYNDROME: CRITICAL REVIEW OF U.S. EPIDEMIOLOGY

Alan M. Rauch, M.D. Division of Viral Diseases,
Center for Infectious Diseases, Centers for
Disease Control, Public Health Service, U.S.
Department of Health and, Human Services,
Atlanta, Georgia, U.S.A., 30333

The four main objectives of this presentation are to:

1. Describe the incidence of Kawasaki syndrome (KS) in
the United States from 1976 through 1985.

2. Identify who in the United States is at risk of
contracting KS.

3. Describe the clinical complications of KS.

4. Define environmental risk factors for contracting KS.

The information for the first three objectives come from
national surveillance of KS conducted by the Centers for
Disease Control (CDC). The information for the fourth
objective is from CDC investigations of KS outbreaks in
the United States.

CDC initiated a national surveillance system for KS in
July 1976. KS patients enrolled in the CDC surveillance
system include those reported to CDC by individual
physicians and health care professionals, those reported
to CDC by state and local health departments, and those
identified during outbreak investigations conducted by
CDC. KS is currently a reportable disease in
approximately 40 of the 50 United States. Nevertheless,
reporting of cases to CDC ultimately depends on
physicians recognizing KS and their interest in reporting
cases to public health officials. Clearly, as in any
large surveillance system, only a fraction of the total

cases in the United States is reported to CDC. Despite this limitation, the system allows us to obtain valuable information on KS in the United States.

The CDC epidemiologic case definition of KS used in surveillance is similar to that originally used in Japan:

Fever lasting 5 days or longer and at least four of the following five criteria:

1. Bilateral conjunctival injection
2. Oral mucosal changes
3. Extremity findings (swelling or redness of hands or feet or periungual desquamation which may occur later in the disease)
4. Rash
5. Cervical lymphadenopathy

An additional requirement is that there be no other more reasonable explanation for the observed clinical findings.

All information that follows is derived from patients who met the case definition.

First objective: describe the incidence of KS in the United States from 1976-1985.

Figure 1 shows KS cases by month of onset from January 1977 through December 1984.

Seasonal peaks occur in the spring (usually April-May) and winter (usually November, December, January), with a relative paucity of cases during the summer months. This incidence curve also shows that the number of KS cases reported to CDC has been increasing each year from 1981-1984.

Cases have been reported from all 50 states in the United States. Although outbreaks or clusters do occur, there is no evidence of person to person transmission. It is extremely rare to see cases occurring in members of the same family, school, or day care center.

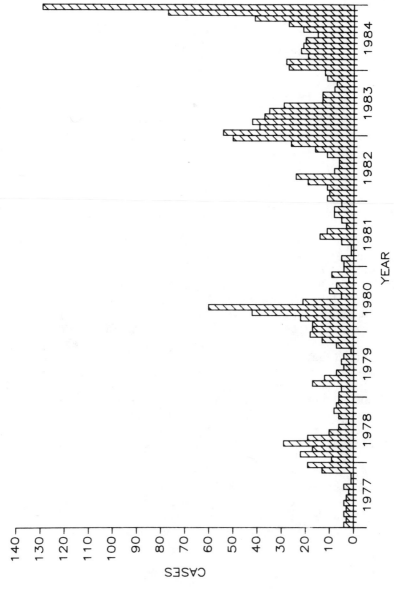

KAWASAKI SYNDROME CASES, BY MONTH OF ONSET, 1977–1984

Figure 1.

Table 1
Number of Cases of Kawasaki Syndrome by Year,
United States, 1976-1985

Year	Number of Cases
1976*	15
1977	61
1978	142
1979	99
1980	216
1981	71
1982	199
1983	300
1984	448
1985 (Preliminary)	547

*1976 only includes cases from July 1-December 31.

Table 1 shows the number of KS cases by year reported in our surveillance system. 1,551 confirmed Kawasaki syndrome cases having onset between July 1976 and December 1984 were reported to CDC. Preliminary analysis of 1985 data indicates a total of 547 reported cases. Including the preliminary 1985 data, more than 2,000 cases were reported between July 1976 and December 1985. From 1976 to 1984, 94.5% of reported KS patients were hospitalized.

Recurrences are rare. Only 0.6% of KS cases reported to CDC between 1976 and 1984 were recurrences.

Second objective: identify who in the United States is at risk of contracting Kawasaki syndrome.

Figure 2 shows the age distribution of KS patients in the United States. Peak incidence of KS in the United States occurs in children between 13 and 24 months old and 80% of cases occur in children under 5. Cases in persons > 14 years old are extremely rare.

KAWASAKI SYNDROME 1976–1984
Age at Onset

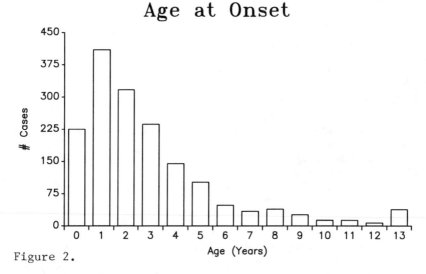

Figure 2.

Attack rates for KS in the United States vary markedly by race (Figure 3). For children under 5 years old the attack rate for Asians is over ,six times greater than for whites. Blacks have an attack rate approximately 1.5 times that in whites. Each of these differences in attack rate is statistically significant.

KAWASAKI SYNDROME 1976–1984
Incidence By Race
Age < 5

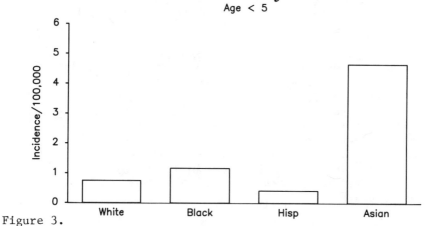

Figure 3.

Males get the disease 1.4 times more often than females.

Third objective: describe the clinical complications of Kawasaki syndrome.

Fifteen deaths from KS in the United States were reported to CDC from 1976-1984, resulting in a case-fatality rate of 1.0%.

Table 2 lists the frequency of reported cardiovascular complications of KS in national surveillance from 1976 through 1984. Coronary artery aneurysms and myocarditis were the most frequently reported complications.

Table 2

Frequency of Cardiovascular Complications, Kawasaki Syndrome, United States 1976-1984

Complication	% of Cases with Complication
Coronary artery aneurysm(s)	19.6%
other aneurysm(s)	0.2%
Myocarditis	10.1%
Pericarditis/Pericardial Effusion	5.1%
Myocardial Ischemia	3.6%
Arrhythmias	3.4%
Congestive heart failure	1.5%
Myocardial Infarction	0.9%

Clearly, the most important complication of Kawasaki syndrome is coronary artery aneurysm (Table 2). Echocardiograms were performed on 43.7% of patients reported in the surveillance system; coronary aneurysms were diagnosed in 19.6% of these . This percentage may be an underestimate because many case-reporting forms are completed early in the course of a patient's illness, sometimes preceding the time when aneurysms are detectable. Other complications of KS may also be underreported for the same reason or because they are not recognized.

One or more electrocardiograms were performed on 64.2% of reported KS patients; EKG abnormalities were reported in 19.8% of these.

We analyzed our data to attempt to define risk factors for developing coronary artery aneurysms. The results of our data analysis showed age less than 8 months and duration of fever were significantly correlated with formation of coronary artery aneurysms. Duration of fever was significantly linearly correlated with coronary aneurysm formation. Using a stepwise multivariate logistic regression analysis (a test which looks at the strength of association between variables and with an outcome in question), we found that elevation in erythrocyte sedimentation rate also significantly correlated with coronary aneurysm formation, even when elevated platelet count and white blood cell counts are considered. However, such clinical findings must be interpreted with caution because of the method by which surveillance data is obtained.

Table 3 lists the reported frequency of non-cardiovascular complications of KS reported in national surveillance from 1976 to 1984. Note that sterile pyuria and muscle symptoms were first included on the CDC surveillance form in 1981.

Table 3

Frequency of Noncardiovascular Complications, Kawasaki Syndrome, United States, 1976-1984

Complication	% of Patients Complication
Arthritis/Arthralgia	27.9%
*Meatitis/Sterile Pyuria	9.8%
Hepatitis	8.0%
Aseptic Meningitis	7.0%
*Myalgia/Myositis	3.6%
Hydrops of gallbladder	2.9%
Iritis/Uveitis	1.3%

*Data available only for 1981-1984.

Fourth objective: define environmental risk factors for contracting KS. CDC has conducted investigations of several outbreaks of Kawasaki syndrome in recent years that have suggested new potential risk factors for the disease.

In August 1984, I investigated a cluster of seven Kawasaki syndrome patients admitted during a 24-day period to a children's hospital in Houston, Texas. During this investigation I visited the homes of each of the seven KS patients. I found that six of the seven homes were located near water-containing drainage structures, bayous, or drainage ditches. As follow-up to this observation, a case-control study was conducted in which parents of KS patients and of matched controls were asked how far they lived from the nearest body of water, including bayous and drainage ditches.

Parents of KS patients reported living nearer bodies of water than did parents of matched controls (Table 4). The differences in distances reported by the two groups of parents are large and statistically significant. This finding suggested a potential new risk factor for KS. However, the sample size was small; further studies were required to test our hypothesis that living near a body of water is a risk factor for KS.

Kawasaki Syndrome Patients and Controls by Distance
of Residence from Bayou or Drainage Ditch,
Harris County, Texas, 1984

Distance in Yards	
Case	Control(s)
14	6160
	300
	200
30	8800
	7920
60	150
	100
70	2640
	1760
	880
	150
	100
100	2640
150	100
	50
	14
1760	2640

Table 4.

p < 0.05 by Wilcoxon stratified rank sum analysis

The month after this investigation, we had an opportunity to test our hypothesis when an outbreak of KS occurred in eastern North Carolina. Again we conducted a case-control study in which we asked how far homes of KS patients and controls were from the nearest body of water, and again KS patients lived significantly closer to bodies of water (creeks and drainage ditches) than did controls (Table 5).

Table 5
Kawasaki Syndrome Patients and Controls by Distance
of Residence from Nearest Body of Water,
Eastern North Carolina, 1984

Distance in Yards	
Case	Control(s)
5	700
10	2540
	>100
<25	5280
	100
50	17,600
	880
65	1760
	250
70	3520
	>1760
<100	200
	90

p < 0.05 by Wilcoxon stratified rank sum analysis

We have subsequently found that KS patients lived closer to bodies of water than did controls in two more KS outbreaks, one in 1984-1985 in Denver, Colorado (p < 0.07) and one in 1985 in Ohio (p < 0.05). In light of recent evidence suggesting a possible role of retroviruses in KS, it is interesting to speculate on what this association with living near water may mean; perhaps an animal reservoir or an arthropod vector is involved. Additional studies are required to clarify the nature of the association between KS occurrence and living near water.

Another environmental risk factor remains controversial, that is, the association between KS with rug or carpet cleaning. In 1982, Patriarca and others observed an association between rug or carpet cleaning in the home within 30 days and onset of KS in 11 of 23 KS patients (48%) compared with 10% and 11% of homes in two matched-control groups. These differences are statistically significant. Four subsequent CDC investigations as well as a study conducted by the Maryland State Health Department failed to reveal any such association with rug or carpet cleaning. However, the rug or carpet cleaning association was again suggested in our investigation of the small cluster of cases in Houston, Texas, the same cluster in which we first noted an association between occurrence of KS and living near a body of water.

In the winter of 1984-1985, another outbreak of Kawasaki syndrome occurred in Denver, Colorado. In this outbreak 16 of 26 (62%) KS patients were exposed to shampooed or spot-cleaned rugs or carpets within 30 days of onset of illness, compared with 12 of 49 (24%) of matched controls. This difference in exposure between KS patients and controls is statistically significant (p < 0.01)

Table 6.
Case-Control Study: Rug or Carpet Cleaning within 30 days of Onset of Kawasaki Syndrome, Denver, Colorado, October 1984 to January 1985

Cases	Controls	Number of Case-Control Sets
+	− −	9
+	−	2
+	+ −	3
+	+ +	2
−	+ +	1
−	+ −	3
−	− −	5
−	−	1
Total		26

Odds ratio = 7 (99% confidence interval=1.35 to 37.2)

The time interval between rug or carpet cleaning and onset of illness in three outbreaks of KS is shown in Table 7. As found in the 1982 Denver outbreak, timing of exposure during the 30 day period before onset of illness clustered during the period 13 to 30 days before onset of illness, with a notable absence of cases occurring during the 0- to 12-day period preceding illness. The likelihood of this distribution of timing between exposure to recently cleaned rugs or carpets and onset of KS illness occurring by chance alone is 5×10^{-6}. This interval between exposure and onset of illness suggests an incubation period or induction period for an infectious agent. Furthermore, being in the room where cleaning occurred, rather than actually being on the rug or carpet, was associated with illness. This finding suggests that inhalation is a likely way in which exposure through rug or carpet cleaning occurs. Again, during a KS outbreak in Los Angeles during February–March 1986, we found an association between occurrence of KS and rug or carpet cleaning. In that outbreak, rug or carpet cleaning occurred in 17 of 24 (71%) homes of KS patients compared with 17 of 44 (39%) homes of controls during the 60-day period preceding the KS onset date. This difference is statistically significant, $p = 0.01$. Furthermore, 12 of 13 exposed KS patients (92%) compared with 8 of 17 (47%) exposed controls were in the room where rug or carpet cleaning occurred within 1 hour of cleaning. This difference is also significant ($p = 0.02$) and is similar to previous findings in Denver, Colorado, in 1982 where KS patients were in rooms sooner after rug or carpet cleaning occurred than were controls. No arthropods were found in carpet samples from homes of KS patients and controls in Los Angeles. Why a significant association between rug or carpet cleaning and Kawasaki syndrome occurs in some outbreaks and not in others remains a mystery.

Table 7
Cases of Kawasaki Syndrome by Interval from Patient's
Exposure to Rug or Carpet Cleaning to Onset of Illness

Investigation	Interval in days 0-12 No.Cases	13-30 No.Cases	Rate Ratio* (13-30 days to earlier period
Denver and Eastern Colorado 1981-82	1	21	14
Harris County, Texas 1984	0	3	∞
Metropolitan Denver 1984-85	1	9	6
Total	2	33	11

*Rate Ratio equals $\dfrac{\text{cases/day in 13- to 30-day interval}}{\text{cases/day in 0- to 12-day interval}}$

To summarize, the incidence of Kawasaki syndrome in the United States has been increasing from 1981-1985.

Future epidemiologic studies are needed to further explore rug or carpet cleaning and living near water as potential risk factors for KS. Key questions remain: what is the reservoir for this disease? what is its mode of transmission? It will be exciting to see how the answers to these questions unfold and how they relate to the possible retroviral etiology suggested in recent laboratory studies.

Kawasaki Disease, pages 45–53
© 1987 Alan R. Liss, Inc.

THE DESCRIPTIVE EPIDEMIOLOGY OF KAWASAKI SYNDROME IN CANADA,
1979-1985

Vera Rose, Nancy E. Lightfoot, Anne Fournier, and
James E. Gibbons

Division of Cardiology, The Hospital for Sick
Children, Toronto, Ontario, Canada M5G 1X8.
(V.R., N.E.L.), Cardiology Service, Ste. Justine
Hospital, Montreal, Quebec (A.F.), and Cardiology
Service, Montreal Children's Hospital, Montreal,
Quebec, Canada (J.E.G.)

INTRODUCTION

The present information about Kawasaki syndrome in Canada
was acquired from two reviews. The first, was the
International Society and Federation of Cardiology (ISFC)
Canadian Survey which examined the period from 1979-1982,
retrospectively (in draft), and second a recent update using
the data (analyzed separately by centre) from two cities with
the largest pediatric centres in the country, the Hospital
for Sick Children (HSC) in Toronto and the Ste. Justine and
Children's Hospital in Montreal (from which 58% of the cases
in the first review were reported.)

The initial survey of 15 Canadian University Pediatric
Centres was conducted for the ISFC and identified 367
children who had been diagnosed as having Kawasaki syndrome
in the years 1979-1982 based on the criteria established by
the Japanese Mucocutaneous Lymph Node Syndrome Committee.
There were more males than females with a ratio of 1.7:1.
Many other features were consistent with the descriptions
received from other countries. Interestingly, 74% of
affected children were under four years-of-age and coronary
artery involvement was detected in 18% with marked
centre-to-centre variations. However, in view of non-uniform
assessments of coronary artery dimensions in different
centres this initial figure may have been excessively high.

The treatment at that time was fairly uniform across the
country and consisted of high dose aspirin, followed by low
dose with or without persantin. The overall mortality was
1.9%. There were seven patients who died, six of them
under 12 months of age (with a median age of six months).
The median interval from the onset of the disease to death
was 22 days in those patients. The data gathered in the
first survey also suggested that epidemics occurred in 1980
and 1982.

An examination of the 1981 Canadian census data showed
that the greatest number of children under age five were
recorded in the provinces of Ontario and Quebec; it was
therefore not surprising that 70% of the total number of
children in that early survey were recognized in these
provinces and more than half of the cases were reported from
the HSC in Toronto, and the Ste. Justine and Children's
Hospitals in Montreal. For this reason and in view of time
limitations, the updated information of the descriptive
epidemiology of Kawasaki syndrome was derived from the recent
experiences in these three large pediatric centres. Due to
the possibility of referral filter (Sackett, 1979) and
ascertainment bias (Schlesselman, 1982), particularly in more
recent times when fewer cases are referred to large centres
as a result of better recognition of the disease, as well as
an imprecisely defined population at risk, analysis using
rates was generally not undertaken. The update of the ISFC
worldwide study, which includes Canada, is presently underway.

EPIDEMIOLOGY

Case Distribution

An examination of the number of cases seen each year at
the HSC in Toronto and the Children's Hospital in Montreal
showed that apparent peaks in number of cases detected
occurred in 1980, 1982-83, 1984 and 1985 when the number of
cases seen was greater than in 1979 and 1981 (Fig. 1). The
total number of cases seen at HSC in Toronto was 278, and 72
and 149, respectively, for the Children's Hospital and Ste.
Justine Hospital in Montreal, during the period from
1979-1985 inclusive.

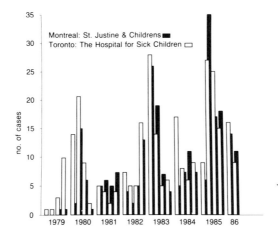

Figure 1. Distribution of cases with Kawasaki syndrome by trimester. January 1979-July 1986.

Seasonal Pattern

The seasonal trends for Kawasaki syndrome were not consistent (Fig. 2). Seasonal peaks were observed in the January to April interval in three of the seven years and in the September to December interval in two of those years. During 1980 and 1985, a May to August summer peak was noted.

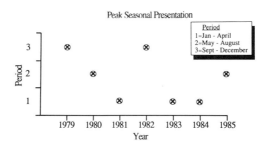

Figure 2. Seasonal pattern of Kawasaki syndrome (Toronto and Montreal experience).

Sex

A greater number of affected male children were observed
in all age categories; overall the sex ratio was 1.5 to 1.
The ratio was reduced in years when epidemics occurred. For
example, in 1985, which was an epidemic year, the male to
female sex ratio was 1.2 whereas it was as high as 1.8 in
non-epidemic years.

Age

Kawasaki syndrome occurred principally in young children
(Fig. 3). Using four age categories (less than 1, 1-4, 5-9
and 10 years or greater), the age of onset of Kawasaki
syndrome was commonest in children in the 1-4 year age
group. The age of onset pattern was similiar in both Toronto
and Montreal.

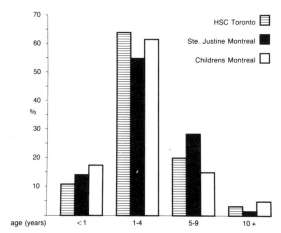

Figure 3. Age at onset of Kawasaki syndrome

Rates

Based on the 1981 census data for children 0-4 years
resident in the municipality of Metropolitan Toronto, the
rate per 100,000 children for the occurrence for the Kawasaki
syndrome varied from 7-8 per 100,000 in non-epidemic years to
21-46 per 100,000 in epidemic years (Fig. 4).

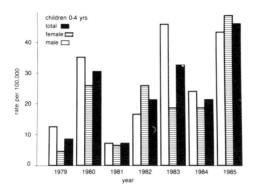

Figure 4. Rate per 100,000 children 0-4 years based on 1981 Canadian census data for the municipality of Metropolitan Toronto.

However, these rates must be interpreted with caution and are likely conservative estimates based on available and probably selective data. There are three possible explanations for the apparent rise in the attack rates over the seven year period: (1) better recognition of the syndrome, (2) errors in enumeration of base population, and (3) increasing numbers of cases.

Racial Origin

An ascertainment of racial origin is not required for patient records in Canada. Of 233 cases, however, of known race seen at the Hospital for Sick Children, 65% were white, 14% were black and 17% oriental, with 5% including East Indians and others (Table 1). When patients from the Metropolitan Toronto area only were considered, the proportion of non-white children with Kawasaki syndrome was greater and may reflect the "cosmopolitan" racial ethnic mix in Toronto (Table 1). The population of children with Kawasaki syndrome in Montreal was 89% French-Canadian. The remaining 11% included 20% of oriental and 10% of black origin. A precise estimate of the proportion of black and oriental children in Metro Toronto was not available, although a study in 1982 recorded 6% black and 5% oriental, a situation which may well have changed since.

Table 1. Racial Origin of Children with Kawasaki Syndrome
Seen at the Hospital for Sick Children, Toronto.

	% of patients seen at HSC (n=233)	% of patients from Metro Toronto (n=114)	% of Metro Population*
White	65	42	
Black	14	26	6
Oriental	17	25	5
Other	5	8	(* from 1982 study)
	100	~100	

Our data show an apparently increased proportion of children
of nonwhite origin affected with Kawasaki syndrome.

Coronary Artery Involvement

The coronary lesions which were included in this updated
review of Kawasaki syndrome were ectatic lesions over 4 mm in
dimension and definite aneurysms which were present at two
months after the onset of the disease. Dilatation lesions
less than 4 mm present in the acute and subacute phases were
not included. The total number of coronary aneurysms was 42
or 15.1%, of which 29 were males and 13 were females (or 17.6
and 11.5%, respectively) (Table 2). The proportion of
children with coronary artery aneurysms was 25.3% in males
and 7.5% in females, when children from the municipality of
Metro Toronto only were considered (X^2 test, p=0.01888).
Of interest was the low (7%) percentage of coronary aneurysms
in a review of 106 French-Canadian children with Kawasaki
syndrome seen during the period 1979-1983 from the Ste.
Justine Hospital in Montreal (Fournier et al, 1985). The
updated review from that hospital (176 cases) of Kawasaki
syndrome now reveals 12.5% with aneurysms, but transient mild
dilatation lesions may also have been included so this figure
may be elevated.

Table 2.   Coronary Artery Aneurysms in Children with
Kawasaki Syndrome (Hospital for Sick Children, Toronto)

	Total n	Aneurysm n	%
Males	165	29	17.6
Females	113	13	11.5
All	278	42	15.1

Coronary aneurysms occurred most frequently in children
under five years-of-age, (Fig. 5) and this held true for
cases from the Metro area and those referred from the rest of
the province of Ontario.

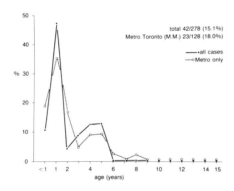

Figure 5.   Percentage of total number of coronary artery
aneurysms by age of onset of Kawasaki syndrome (Hospital for
Sick Children, Toronto)

Interestingly, in examining cases by age of onset category
85% of those with aneurysms were in the under 1 year and in

the 1-4 year age groups, and 19% were detected in the under 1 year of age category. Examination of those who did not develop coronary aneurysms revealed that the proportion of younger children was less. The age distribution of children with coronary aneurysms from the Ste. Justine Hospital in Montreal showed 77% under 5 years-of-age, of which 27% were under 1 year-of-age.

A review of the racial origin of children with and without coronary aneurysms (Fig. 6) reflected a 9% increase in non-white children in the aneurysm group in Toronto.

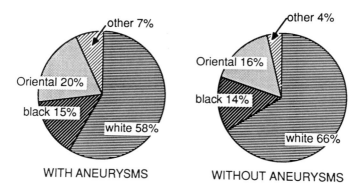

Figure 6. Kawasaki syndrome: racial origin of children with and without coronary aneurysms (Hospital for Sick Children, Toronto)

Mortality

The overall mortality in the updated review of the Toronto and Montreal experience over the seven year period 1979-1985 was 0.75%.

DISCUSSION

The question as to whether the Kawasaki syndrome is a new entity or disease previously prevalent but not well recognized remains unresolved. Although the etiology of Kawasaki syndrome remains unclear, many investigators have postulated either an infectious agent or immune response to an infectious agent or agents (Morens, 1981). Suggested etiologies have included: bacterial, viral, fungal, rickettsial, allergenic, and chemical agents (The Study Committee on Cause of Kawasaki Disease, Japan Heart Foundation, 1986). In the International Society and Federation of Cardiology Survey of Kawasaki Syndrome, 1979-1982, (in draft), the disease was not recorded in parts of the world where infectious diseases such as measles are still endemic. Clearly, it is possible that Kawasaki syndrome could have been previously existent, although unrecognized, and perhaps masked by various other febrile exanthems in the past, so that it may not be a new disease but merely better recognized. Further investigation is required in order to resolve this debate and to ascertain accurate temporal trends for Kawasaki syndrome.

REFERENCES

Fournier A, Van Doesburg NH, Guerin R, Lapointe N, Lacroix J, Fouron JC, and Davignon A (1985). La maladie de Kawasaki. Aspects epidemiologiques et manifestations cardio-vasculaires - A propos de 106 observations. Arch Mal Coeur 78: 693-698.

Japan MCLS Rsearch Committee (1978). Diagnostic Guideline of Infantile Acute Febrile Muco-Cutaneous Lymphnode Syndrome 3rd rev. ed. Tokyo: Dept. of Epidemiology, Institute of Public Health.

Morens DM (1981): Infectious diseases (unclassified), Kawasaki disease (muco-cutaneous lymph node syndrome). In Feigin RD and Cherry JD (eds): "Textbook of Pediatric Infectious Diseases. Volume II." Philadelphia, London, Toronto, and Sydney: W.B. Saunders Company, pp. 1637-1648.

Sackett DL (1979). Bias in analytic research. J Chron Dis 32:51-63.

Schlesselman JJ (1982). "Case-control studies." New York and Oxford: Oxford University Press, 354 pp. The Study Committee on Cause of Kawasaki Disease, Japan Heart Foundation (1986). "Kawasaki Disease - Epidemiological Data Book." Tokyo: Soft Science Publications, inc., pp. 194-195.

The authors would like to acknowledge the typing efforts of Beverley A. Foo, Division of Cardiology, Hospital for Sick Children, Toronto, Ontario, Canada.

Kawasaki Disease, pages 55–60
© 1987 Alan R. Liss, Inc.

EPIDEMIOLOGIC STUDY OF KAWASAKI DISEASE IN KOREA

Du Bong Lee

Department of Pediatrics, St. Mary's Hospital
Catholic Medical College
Seoul, Korea 150

INTRODUCTION

An epidemiologic survey of Kawasaki Disease in Korea
has been carried out each year since 1980. The questionnaires were mailed to 144 pediatricians in responsible
posts at general hospitals located all over the country.
They were asked to respond to questions concerned with K.D.
cases admitted to their hospital during the year.

The rate of reply to the questionnaire was 72.4% or
50/69 general hospitals.

The questionnaire included patient's name, address,
date of birth, sex, date of first visit, date of illness,
kinds of drugs used, accuracy of diagnosis, occurrence
among siblings, date of discharge, and outcome of illness.

Diagnosis of K.D. was based on the revised guidelines
of the Research Committee on MCLS in Japan.

RESULTS

The first K.D. cases in Korea were reported in 1972.
However, patient numbers increased obviously after 1978.
During the four years from 1972 to 1975, the patients were
few in number, totaling only 11 cases. Then 10 cases were
reported during the following two years, 1976 and 1977. In
1978, 29 cases were admitted which exceeded the total
number of patients in the previous six years.

The first Korean epidemic of K.D. occurred from November, 1979, to February, 1980, and 107 hospitalized patients were reported during this period. Since then, the number of patients remarkably increased by about fivefold compared with that of the previous years, with 132, 155, 149 and 136 cases in 1979, 1980, 1981 and 1982, respectively (Figure 1).

Figure 1

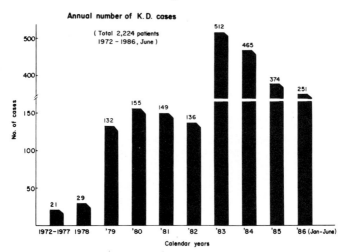

Three years and three months after the first epidemic, a second epidemic appeared from May to September 1983, with 394 cases identified during this period. The total of patients for the year 1983 was 512, higher by about 3.5 times than the previous years. It was the largest number of patients for a year since 1972.

In 1984, 1985 and the first six months of 1986, the totals of patients were 465, 374 and 251, respectively. These exceeded the number of patients identified in 1979 and 1980 despite the fact that a clear outbreak did not occur during this period (Figure 1).

The cumulative total for the past 15 years (1972-1986) in Korea was 2,224 cases; however, 72% (1,602 cases) had occurred during the most recent 3 1/2 years (1983-1986).

The yearly incidence of K.D. hospitalizations ranged from 1.2 to 4.1 per 100,000 population under 14 years of age with the mean incidence 2.3. The incidence during the most recent four years was significantly higher than that in 1979 and 1980 (P<0.005) (Table 1).

Table 1

Annual number of K. D. patients and Incidence
(1976 - 1986, June)

Yr Month	1972 1975	1976	1977	1978	1979	1980	1981	1982	1983	1984	1985	1986	Total
Jan	-	0	1	1	4	26	13	8	15	33	23	32	156
Feb	-	1	1	1	3	14	8	10	15	32	11	26	122
Mar	-	1	1	0	3	9	14	10	18	62	24	36	179
Apr	-	0	1	1	3	17	12	9	13	47	25	50	178
May	-	0	1	3	7	13	17	15	40	56	34	51	237
June	-	0	0	7	8	9	21	10	72	58	49	56	290
July	-	0	1	2	15	16	20	13	114	40	39	-	260
Aug	-	0	0	2	10	3	2	17	134	31	56	-	255
Sept	-	1	1	2	7	13	7	11	34	18	39	-	133
Oct	-	0	0	3	5	14	12	12	20	17	31	-	114
Nov	-	0	0	5	27	9	15	6	22	33	17	-	134
Dec	-	0	0	2	40	12	8	14	15	38	26	-	155
Total	(11)	3	7	29	132	155	149	136	512	465	374	251	2,213 (2,224)
Incidence (per 100,000)		-	-	-	1.2	1.3	1.3	1.2	4.1	3.6	3.0	2.0	2.3

This evidence suggests that K.D. is becoming a new endemic disease in Korea as in Japan. It is also noteworthy that the first and second epidemics in Korea occurred at intervals of about 7 months and 15 months after epidemics had occurred in 1979 and 1982 in Japan, respectively. These epidemiologic patterns of K.D. strongly suggest that this disease is caused by some biological agent which spreads easily in the community.

Regarding the seasonal occurrence of this disease, out of 2,213 patients, 594 (26.8%), 805 (36.4%), 381 (17.2%) and 433 (18.6%) were taken ill in spring, summer, autumn and winter, respectively. K.D. was most prevalent in the summer season, but the difference in number of patients between summer and other seasons was not statistically significant.

Figure 2.

Seasonal incidence of
patients during eight
years.

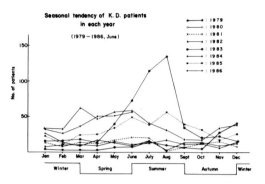

The regional distribution of the patients showed a
tendency to occur primarily in urban areas with high
density of population, such as Seoul, Taegu and Pusan
Cities areas (P<0.005). 1,454 cases of the total (65.7%)
occurred in Seoul City and its neighbor province. In
addition, 10.4% (230 cases) and 14.1% (313 cases) occurred
in Taegu and Pusan Cities and their neighbor provinces.

The regional incidences
of K.D. in 1985 and 1986
were 7.8 and 2.3 per 100,000
population under 14 years of
age in Seoul and Pusan areas
(Figure 3).

Figure 3

Regional distribution of 2,213 K.D. patients
(1976-1986, June)

: Number of patients

( ) : Incidence per 100000 population
under the 14 years of age

The number of patients in each age group were 553, 755,
244, and 96 for under one year, 1-2, 2-3 and 3-4 years of
age, respectively. The total of patients over 5 years of
age was 146 cases. Out of 2,213 patients, 553 (24.9%) and
755 (34.1%) cases were under one year and from 1-2 years of
age, respectively. The total number of patients under two
years of age was 1,308 cases (59.0%), which was over half
of all patients.

The yearly incidence in each age group were 7.1, 9.4, and 5.2 per 100,000 population for under one, 1-2 and 2-3 years of age, respectively, and the highest incidence occurred at 1-2 years of age (P<0.005) (Figure 4).

Figure 4

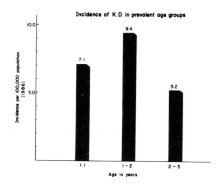

The totals of male and female patients were 1,440 and 773 cases each, and the male:female ratio was 1.8:1.0 (Figure 5).

Figure 5

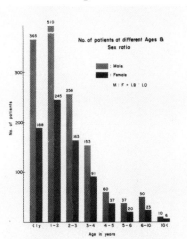

The mortality rate was 4.06 per thousand. Out of 2,213 patients, nine cases expired with coronary complications.

SUMMARY

The cumulative number of K.D. patients for the past 15 years in Korea was 2,224. There were two epidemics, in winter of 1979 and summer of 1983. The increase in patient numbers accelerated remarkably after each epidemic. This disease had a tendency to occur in urban areas with high density of population and was more likely to occur in male infants under two years of age than in females.

When it is taken into consideration that the first and second epidemics occurred in this country at intervals of seven months and 1 1/4 years, respectively, after epidemics in Japan, it is possible that the third epidemic in Korea may occur in the near future, in view of the large epidemic in Japan in the beginning of 1986.[2]

REFERENCES

1. Yanagawa H: Results of nationwide survey on Kawasaki Disease epidemiological data book, Tokyo, Soft Science Pub., 1986, p. 37-51.

2. Yanagawa H, Nakamura Y: Nationwide epidemic of Kawasaki Disease in Japan during winter of 1985-86, Lancet II:1138, 1986.

3. Lee DB: Epidemiologic survey of Kawasaki Disease in Korea (1976-1984), J Catholic Med Coll 38:13, 1985.

Kawasaki Disease, pages 61–65
© 1987 Alan R. Liss, Inc.

EPIDEMIOLOGY OF KAWASAKI SYNDROME IN GERMANY (FRG)

Hansjörg Cremer
Städt.Kinderklinik
7100 Heilbronn / Germany(FRG)
and
Christian Rieger
Universitätskinderklinik
3550 Marburg / Germany(FRG)

In the fall of 1978 we observed the first cases
of KAWASAKI Disease(KD) in Heilbronn Pediatric
Hospital. The following year in 1979 during the
German Pediatric Congress at Karlsruhe,a symposium
on the KD was held in the presence of Dr KAWASAKI.
We formed a workteam,the aim of this being to
obtain as complete a record as possible of all
cases of KD in West Germany.

Every one to two years we held meetings consisting of a selected group of immunologists,
cardiologists and haematologists. A bulletin is
sent regularly to all pediatric hospitals in West
Germany,giving the latest developments in therapy
and research.

At first we used detailed registration forms
(Fig.1) in which a large number of clinical data
were asked for. After we ascertained that the
symptoms of the disease we observed were identical
to those described in Japan,a simplified version
of the registration form was adopted at the beginning of 1986(Fig.2). In this new questionnaire
we only receive back part of the form which has
to be detached and returned to us with some basic
information,while the main part of the form containing therapy recommendations and addresses of
the pediatric cardiology centers in FRG is retained
by the hospital.

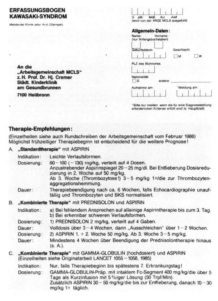

Figure 1. detailed registration form used until 1986

Figure 2. simplified version of the registration form used since 1986

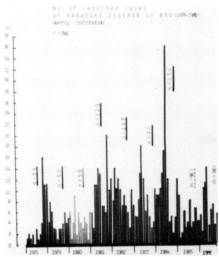

Figure 3. cases reported in West Germany till 1986

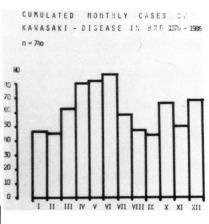

Figure 4. cumulated monthly distribution of cases reported 1978-1986

Altogether 740 cases of KAWASAKI Disease have been reported to us(Fig.3).Even though the number of cases registered is too small to make a definite statement,the information received by us,as in Japan,shows that a rise in the number of cases occurs every three years.The ratio male to female was 1.5 to 1.0. The cumulated monthly distribution does not show any clearcut preference (Fig.4).

The cases reported came from all over West Germany;however there was a higher number of cases reported in Baden-Württemberg-one of the states in the south of Germany.Heilbronn lies in Baden-Württemberg. I am sure that this does not mean that the disease is more prevalent in this part of Germany,I think this is probably due to more direct communication with us.

An analysis of the frequency with which KAWASAKI Disease occurs in the catchment area of Heilbronn Pediatric Hospital comprising approximately 450 000 inhabitants gives us the opportunity to make a fairly reliable estimate of the frequency of the disease occuring in 100 000 children under 5 years of age. (Fig.5)One can assume that in this area a large percent of the cases are diagnosed correctly and reported. Assuming that this is so,it can be estimated that about 8 cases occur annually in 100 000 children under the age of five.Thus in the entire Federal Republic of Germany one can assume that about 200 cases of KAWASAKI Disease occur annually. (Fig.6).We estimate that every 2nd case occuring in West Germany is reported to us.

KAWASAKI DISEASE in HEILBRONN

Nr. of inhabitants in this area	: 450 000
Nr. of children under 5 years in this area	:ca 22 500
Nr. of reported cases in this area between 1978-1985	: 14
average Nr per year in this area	: 1,75
calculated Nr of cases per 100 000 child.under 5 y	: 8 /year

KAWASAKI DISEASE in BRD

	1978	1979	1980	1981	1982	1983	1984	1985
Children under 5 years	2 360	2 340	2 360	2 390	2 390	2 390	2 380	2 380 (x 1 000)
Reported cases of M C L S	54	50	50	120	103	97	134	56
cases pro 100 000 child.under 5 year	2,3	2,1	2,1	5,1	4,3	4,1	5,6	2,4

Figure 5.calculated nr.of cases in Heilbronn area

Figure 6. calculated nr. of cases in West Germany

I was originally requested to give a survey of the situation of KAWASAKI Disease in other European countries as well as West Germany. Unfortunately this is extremely difficult to do, as West Germany is the only country in Europe so far where an attempt is being made to register all cases that occur. From 1979 to 1982 an international survey was made of which Prof. van der Hauwert from Belgium was one of the organisers. The results obtained were reported at the last international congress in New York.(Fig.7) The authors have based their conclusions on the frequency of KAWASAKI Disease in the countries concerned from the number of cases reported in publications and from the size of the population in the areas where the cases occurred. However I believe that the number of cases very often was too small to give any reliable information from which to draw conclusions. I am convinced that if a method similar to the one we use in West Germany were used in other European countries,the number of cases in these countries would probably be very similar to the frequency with which the disease occurs in the Federal Republic of Germany.

Results from International survey of KAWASAKI disease 1979-1982

Country	total reported cases	1979	1980	1981	1982	1983	(Luc van der HAUWERT) Children less than 5 y old	weighted average annual rate per 100 000 child 5 y	estimated annual no of KD cases
FINLAND	87-107	10	10	62	25		320 738	5,4-6,7	25
SWEDEN	15	3	2	3	7		487 482	1,0-3,5	15
SCOTLAND	22	3	1	12	6		320 738	1,3	5
ENGLAND	31	2	1	6	22		2 961 200	1,2	50
FRANCE	89	30	18	36	5		3 8000 322	10,8-30,7 (??)	1 000 (?)
BELGIUM	13	4	3	4	2		598 556	1,9-2,6	20
HOLLAND	10	1	2	4	3		882 115	4,0-6,-	45
BRD = West Germ.	403	50	50	120	102	81	2 931 200	3,9	120
DDR = East G	11	0	7	0	4		1 136 839	2,0	25
SWITZERLAND	27	2	4	9	12		353 300	18,0-15,5	60
AUSTRIA	29	11	2	5	11		433 261	6,0	30
ITALY	22	0	0	5	17		3 660 461	0,3-14,7	180 (?)

**=Population figures taken from U N Demographic Yearbook 1981

Figure 7.International survey of KAWASAKI Disease in Europe 1979-1982 (Luc van der Hauwert)

Now I should like to conclude with some remarks on
the therapy we use. In our latest bulletin to hospitals we have mentioned the high dosage Gamma Globulin therapy. So far,however,most mild cases are
treated with aspirin only,but more severe cases are
treated with a combination of Aspirin and Prednisolone.
In recommending this combination for severe cases
we differ from articles published in Japan,warning
against the use of cortisone. Comparing therapy
recommendations in Japan and Germany,I have noticed
that Japanese articles always compare cortisone
therapy alone to aspirin therapy. In West Germany
cortisone is never given alone but always together
with aspirin. So far I know of only one Japanese
study in which aspirin is compared to a combination
of prednisolone with aspirin (Fig.8). The observation
time of this study is a bit short but the combined
group of prednisolone and aspirin does not seem to
have fared badly. It is certainly possible that
impressed by the good results obained from using
gamma globulin therapy,our workteam will recommend
this therapy in future.

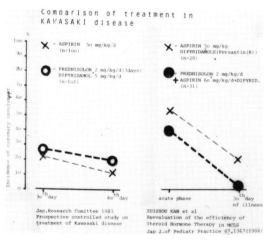

Figure 8. Comparison of treatment in KAWASAKI Disease-
Aspirin versus Prednisolone and Aspirin versus a
combination of Prednisolone and Aspirin.

Kawasaki Disease, pages 67–70
© 1987 Alan R. Liss, Inc.

EPIDEMIOLOGY OF KAWASAKI DISEASE IN NORTHERN EUROPE

Eeva Salo

Children's Hospital, University of Helsinki,
SF-00290 Helsinki, Finland

FINLAND

In Finland, the first cases of Kawasaki Disease were
diagnosed in 1977 (Hurme et al, 1978). After that,
scattered cases were recognized at several hospitals.

By the fall of 1981, a sharp increase in the incidence
was noted. In a period of 10 months, 83 new cases were
diagnosed (Figure) (Salo et al, 1986). The attack rate was
26 cases/100,000 children under 5 years of age, equivalent
to an annual attack rate of 31/100,000. During the three
most intense months of the outbreak, October to December
1981, the attack rate corresponded to an annual rate of
67/100,000.

The distribution of the patients roughly followed that
of the population. The first cases of the outbreak were
diagnosed on the south-western coast. In the north of
Finland, the first cases were seen four months later, thus
giving the impression of the outbreak expanding northward.
Patient-to-patient transmission was not noted. The mean
age of the patients was 2.6 years; 55% were under 2 years
of age and 92% under 5 years. The male:female ratio was
1.2:1.

After the outbreak the annual attack rate has been
about 5 cases/100,000 children under age 5 (Figure).
Altogether 200 children have been diagnosed, 180 of them
during and after the outbreak. There are two recurrences
and one sibling case.

Four children have died, all of them boys. A six-year-
old boy died of myocardial infarction four months after the
onset of the disease, and three infants in the third or
fourth weeks of the illness. The autopsies showed rupture
or thrombosis of coronary artery aneurysms.

On echocardiography, 10 of 76 children have been found
to have dilatation or aneurysm of the coronary arteries.
Since 1984, 26 patients have received intravenous gamma
globulin; a coronary aneurysm has been found in one.

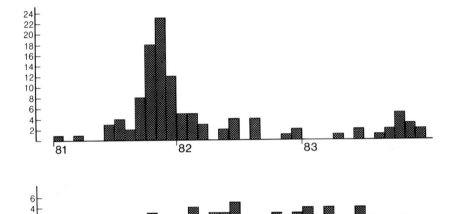

Figure.   Incidence of Kawasaki Disease in Finland in
          1981-86.

ICELAND

The first known case of KD occurred in 1979, an
American girl staying in Iceland. The child died soon
after admission to the hospital (K. Jönsdottir, personal
communication).

From August to October 1981, 8 patients with Kawasaki
Disease were diagnosed (Thorsson, 1981; Gudbrandsson et al,
1982; K. Jönsdottir). They recovered uneventfully. The
attack rate corresponds to 120 cases/100,000 children under
age 5. After this outbreak, only one suspected case could
be recalled (Prof. V. Arnorsson, Dr. A. Thorsson, personal
communication).

SWEDEN

In 1977, H. Ahlstrom et al. described four cases of infantile periarteritis nodosa/Kawasaki Disease over a period of ten years. Three of these children died (Ahlström et al, 1977). Since then, sporadic cases have been seen in Sweden (Hederos, 1981).

In 1984, Dr. Bodil Mykap made an informal survey, and altogether 120 cases from 1977 to 1984 came to light. The incidence in 1983-84 was calculated to be 6 to 11/100,000 children under age 5 (B.M., personal communication). One child has died, and one has undergone surgery because of aortic incompetence.

In the southern region of Sweden, 16 children had been examined by echocardiography during a period of 9 months in 1985 (Björkheim et al, 1985). Four of them had coronary aneurysms, which were confirmed by angiography. Some patients have received gamma globulin for KD, but it is not regularly used in Sweden (Johansen et al, 1984; Dr. K. Johansen, personal communication).

NORWAY

No nationwide investigations have been made. In Ulleval Hospital, Oslo, 4 cases have been seen in 1986 (Prof. Halvorsen, personal communication).

DENMARK

No surveys have been made. A rough estimate of 2 to 4 patients per year in Denmark was made by Dr. Nils-Henrik Rasmussen (personal communication). One child has died. Coronary aneurysms have not been found in other patients.

REFERENCES

Ahlström H, Lundström N-R, Mortensson W, Östberg G, Lantorp K (1977). Infantile periarteritis nodosa or mucocutaneous lymph node syndrome. Acta Paediatr Scand 66:193-198.

Björkheim G, Lundström N-R, Sandtröm S (1985). Koronärkärls-aneurysm vid Kawasakis sjukdom. Läkartidningen 82:3066-3068.

Gudbrandsson B, Jonsson B, Asgeirsson G, Benjaminsdottir S (1982). Letter to the editor. Acta Paediatr Scand 71: 141.

Hederos CA (1981). Kawasakis sjukdom - en översikt och fyra fallbeskrivningar. Läkartidningen 78:6394-6.

Hurme P, Terho P, Salmi TT (1978). Kawasakin tauti. Duodecim 94:1038-43.

Johansen K, Persson B, Elinder G, Marin L, Hammarström L, Smith E (1984). Gammaglobulin vid Kawasakis sjukdom - en my tänkbar terapimetod. Läkartidningen 81:3234-5.

Salo E, Pelkonen P, Pettay O (1986). Outbreak of Kawasaki Syndrome in Finland. Acta Paediatr Scand 75:75-80.

Thorsson A (1981). Kawasaki sjukdomur. Laeknabladid 67: 251-253.

Kawasaki Disease, pages 71-72
© 1987 Alan R. Liss, Inc.

DISCUSSION:

HISTORY AND EPIDEMIOLOGY OF KAWASAKI DISEASE

The potential role of rug shampoo or mite exposure was
discussed by several investigators. Drs. A. Rauch
(Atlanta) and M. Melish (Honolulu) pointed out that
Kawasaki Disease occurs in areas of the United States with
markedly different degrees of mite exposure as demonstrated
by the number of mites in vacuumed dust samples and by
serum levels of IgE and IgG antibodies to mite antigens.
Rauch pointed out that environmental sampling always occurs
some time after the putative exposure. Melish found mites
in dust samples from all case and control homes in Honolulu
as well as high levels of IgE and IgG in both cases and
controls with no difference. Dr. H. Yanagawa (Tochigi) in
a study of 300 Kawasaki cases and 300 controls in Japan
found no differences regarding the type of house or in rug
usage. He pointed out that the use of rug shampoo in Japan
is rare. Dr. M. Glode (Denver) pointed out that fewer than
10% of the cases and controls studied in Denver had any
mites identified in home dust samples and that very low
levels of mite antibody were present in cases and
controls. She suggested that, since rug cleaning materials
are 98%-99% water, water might function as a co-factor in
arid areas but not be important in other areas. Dr. Rauch
indicated that commercial rug cleaning in the U.S. occurs
year-around, with some increase in December. The association with Kawasaki Disease is intermittent, is with
commercial or non-commercial cleaning, and is unrelated to
the area of carpet cleaned or to the product used. All rug
shampoo products are characterized by high water content
and anionic and non-ionic detergents. In the outbreaks
with a rug shampoo association, the interval between

shampoo and onset of illness is more consistent with an
infectious rather than a toxic etiology.

Additional discussion focussed upon the relation of
Kawasaki Disease to humidity or proximity to bodies of
water. Dr. Melish noted that rainfall is high in Hawaii
but that there is essentially no correlation between areas
of high incidence of Kawasaki Disease and areas of highest
rainfall on Oahu. Dr. Rauch found no relationship between
U.S. outbreaks of Kawasaki Disease and rainfall or weather
patterns. However, he indicated that a CDC environmental
epidemiologic study in Ohio found that 9/10 Kawasaki cases
but only 1/10 controls had septic water within 440 yards of
their homes, with septic water defined as water that can
support arthropod vectors or that has high coliform counts.
Dr. Yanagawa noted that the 1985-1986 Japanese epidemic of
Kawasaki Disease corresponded with a period of low humidity
and that the two previous epidemics peaked at times of low
humidity.

Another topic of discussion related to whether cases of
Kawasaki Disease are seen in the Southern Hemisphere. Drs.
T. Kawasaki (Tokyo) and S. Naoe (Tokyo) indicated that
cases have indeed been seen in countries such as Brazil,
South Africa, and New Zealand.

Kawasaki Disease, pages 73–80
© 1987 Alan R. Liss, Inc.

CYTOPATHOGENIC PROTEIN (CPP) PRODUCED BY PROPIONIBACTERIUM
ACNES ISOLATED FROM   PATIENTS WITH KAWASAKI DISEASE

Shobun Tomita, Yuko Koga, Osamu Inoue,
Tamotsu Fujimoto and Hirohisa Kato

Department of Pediatrics and Child Health,
Kurume University, School of Medicine,
67 Asahi-machi Kurume City, Fukuoka 830, JAPAN.

INTRODUCTION

Kawasaki disease is an acute febrile illness with mucocutaneous involvement   affecting predominantly children under 4 years
old. (Kawasaki, et al, 1974)
The aetiology of this disease remains still unknown at the present time.
Many hypotheses on the aetiology have been proposed to date. However
none have been established. A recent epidemiological study suggests
the possibility of an infectious aetiological mechanism or a certain
immune response to infectious agents. (Yanagawa, et al, 1983)

We have postulated that a common microorganism may be a causative agent because this disease has been recognized widely in North
America and Europe as well as in Japan. Since 1983, we have reported that
Propionibacterium acnes (P. acnes) may have a causative role in Kawasaki
disease.

Evidence   supporting this hypothesis include (Kato, et al, 1983,
Kato, et al, 1985 Inoue, 1984);
    1 : We isolated P. acnes in higher incidence from Kawasaki dis-
ease patients' blood and lymph node specimens, than we did from controls. All strains isolated from patients were determined to be identical, and of serotype I.
    2 : In the agglutination tests against P. acnes, the patients
had significantly higher titers than had age-matched controls.
    3 : P. acnes isolated from patients was inoculated into guinea
pigs intraperitoneally. We observed weight loss, depilation of fur,
lymphadenopathy and hepatosplenomegaly in some of them.
Microscopically, lymphoid hyperplasia, focal necrosis of the liver
cells, myocarditis, and coronary arteritis were recognized.

4 : IgG circulating immune complex was detected in higher concentration by Raji cell assay in the patients. The cross-antigenecity to P. acnes was found in the circulating immune complex.

5 : In guinea pigs sensitized by BCG, the reaction on footpads by BCG was found to be increased by means of the subsequent inoculation of P. acnes intraperitoneally.

6 : After inoculation of the human embryo liver cells (HELi) with the culture filtrate of P. acnes isolated from the patient, cytoplasmic vacuola of various sizes appeared in the fetal liver cells. The culture filtrates of P. acnes isolated from the controls and also standard strain did not reveal any such abnormal findings. If the culture filtrates were either treated with the patients' convalescent sera or heated at 100 °C for 30 minutes, then cytoplasmic vacuoles did not appear.

From these results we postulate that the P. acnes isolated from the patients may produce an exotoxin or pathogenic protein. In this paper, we demonstrate the isolation of this cytopathogenic substance from the culture medium, and the detection of the IgG antibody against this substance in the sera of patients' and of the controls'.

MATERIALS AND METHODS

Microorganism

The method used for isolation and typing of P. acnes has been described previously by Kato et al. (Kato et al, 1983) The biochemical analysis of the culture filtrates were performed using the four strains of P. acnes isolated from the patients with Kawasaki disease, two strains from the controls, one strain from the house dust mite, and the standard strain (ATCC 11827). The same analysis was performed on the medium only as control.

Analysis of the culture filtrates

Each strain was cultured separately in GAM broth (1.0 g/dl peptone, 0.3 g/dl soy-peptone, 1.0 g/dl proteose peptone W, 1.35 g/dl peptide digest serum powder, 0.22 g/dl meat extract, 0.5 g/dl yeast extract, 0.12 g/dl liver extract, 0.3 g/dl glucose, 0.3 g/dl sodium chloride, 0.25 g/dl KH_2PO_4, 0.5 g/dl soluble starch, 0.03 g/dl L-cystine-HCl and 0.03 g/dl sodium thioglycollate in distilled water; pH 7.3±0.1) at 37°C for 4 to 10 days. The culture supernatant was passed through a filter with a pore size of 0.22 μm. The culture filtrate was precipitated by addition of ammonium sulfate to 80% saturation. The precipitate was harvested and dissolved in distilled water and dialyzed. The concentrated culture filtrate was fractionated on a Ultragel AcA 44 column. Each fraction was inoculated into HELi for observation of cytopathogenic effects and cytoplasmic vacuola. The active fractions were pooled, concentrated, and further purified by flat-bed isoelectrofocusing (Flat- Bed IEF). Each fraction was inoculated into HELi again. The fractions producing intraplasmic vacuola in HELi were analyzed by using sodium dodecylsulfate-polyacrylamide gel electrofocusing (SDS-PAGE).

Measurement of IgG antibody against the cytopathogenic substance

IgG antibody against the cytopathogenic substance, in the sera of patients with Kawasaki disease and in sera of controls, was measured by using the indirect Enzyme-Linked Immunosorbent Assay (ELISA).

Preparation of antigen

One strain from patients' lymph node and two strains from patients' blood were used for the preparation of antigen. The method of preparation is described as above.

Collection of serum samples

We collected serum samples from patients with Kawasaki dis - ease. 63 samples were collected on the 2 nd to 8th day of illness (mean, 5.2 days), 45 on the 14th to 33rd day of illness (mean, 23.6 days) and 42 in the 11th to 22nd month of illness (mean, 19 months) for this study.
We also used sera from three patients with recurrent case.

Control samples were collected during the same period. We divided controls into four groups by age; 102 samples from 0 to 4 years of age, 35 from 4 to 9 years of age, 15 from 9 to 14 years of age and 16 from adults. Each serum sample was diluted 1 : 4 in phosphate buffer saline (pH 7.2) with 0.05% Tween 20 and 2% fetal calf serum.

Tests

We detected the IgG antibody against the cytopathogenic sub-stance using indirect enzyme-linked immunosorbent assay (ELISA). The procedure of ELISA is as follows;

$100 \mu l$ of 0.05 M carbonate-bicarbonate buffer (pH 9.6) with 50 $\mu g/ml$ of cytopathgenic substance was placed into each well of the 96 well polystyrene flat bottomed microtitration plate, and stored overnight at 4°C. The plate was washed four times with phosphate buffer saline containing 0.05% Tween 20 (pH 7.2) (PBS-T) and added 100 μl of diluted sample sera to each well. The plate was incubated for two hours at 37°C, then washed four times with PBS-

T. A $100 \mu l$ volume per well of horse-radish peroxidase-conjugated anti-human IgG rabbit serum in a dilution of 1 : 2000 was added. After an additional two hours incubation at $37\,^{\circ}C$ and the washing procedure, a $100 \mu l$ volume of substrate solution, consisting of 0.4 mg of orthophenylene diamine per ml in 0.1 M citrate-Na_2HPO_4 buffer (pH 5.0) and $40 \mu l$ of 30% H_2O_2 per 100ml of same solution, was added to each well. The reaction was stopped by adding a $50 \mu l$ volume per well of 2.5M H_2SO_4 after the incubation for 30 minutes at room temperature in the dark. The OD at 486nm is read by an ELISA ANALYSER (ETY-96, TOYO).

RESULTS

Analysis of the culture filtrates

From the results of gel filtration, molecular weight peaks of approximately 200,000 and 20,000-30,000 dalton were identified in the culture filtrates of all strains and control medium. There were no changes in HELi of these fractions. However, in the culture filtrates from the strains of Kawasaki disease patients, a small peak of approximately 100,000 dalton in molecular weight was identified, which caused cytoplasmic vacuola in HELi.

The results of Flat-Bed IEF are shown in Fig 1. A specific fractionation band in the isoelectric range of approximately 7.0 was recognized in the culture filtrates of all strains from the patients with Kawasaki disease, and these fractionations formed cytoplasmic vacuola in HELi (Fig. 2). However there was no such band from the controls. These fractionations were evaluated with SDS-PAGE. The molecular weight was determined to be approximately 100,000 dalton.

We tentatively named this protein as the Cyto-

Fig. 1

Preparative Flat-Bed electrofocusing of culture filtrates

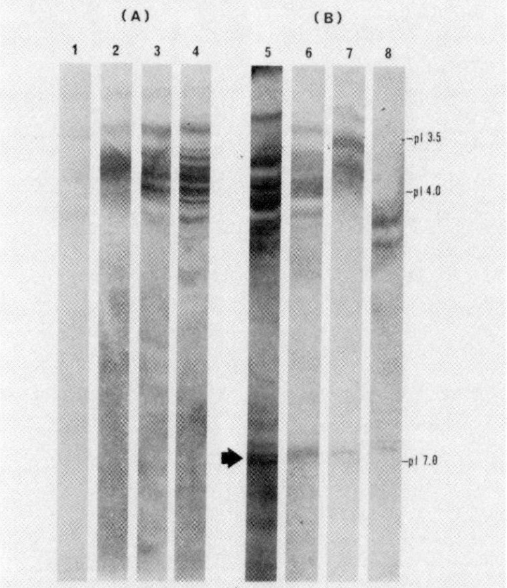

(A)   (B)

1 2 3 4   5 6 7 8

—pl 3.5

—pl 4.0

—pl 7.0

(A) culture filtrates of Controls
  1 pure GAM broth
  2 P.acnes isolated from house-dust mite
  3 P.acnes isolated from patient with Leukemia
  4 P.acnes standard strain (ATCC 11827)
(B) culture filtrates of P.acnes isolated from Kawasaki disease

Fig. 2   Human embryonic liver cells inoculated CPP

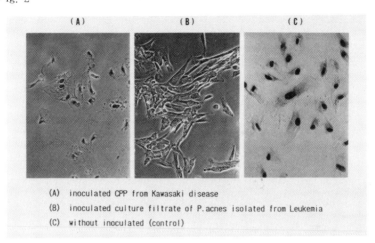

(A)   inoculated CPP from Kawasaki disease
(B)   inoculated culture filtrate of P.acnes isolated from Leukemia
(C)   without inoculated (control)

Fig. 3

IgG antibody against CPP (ELISA)
A   strain

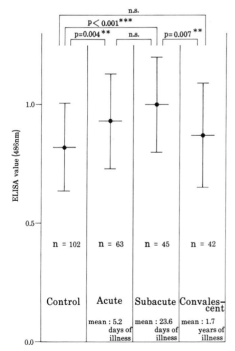

pathogenic Protein (CPP).

Measurement of IgG antibody against the CPP

The mean (plus minus standard deviation) of ELISA absorbance value at 486 nm of the CPP antigen produced by P. acnes isolated from patient's lymph node is shown in Fig. 3. The patients' sera from 2nd to 8th day of illness and from 14th to 33rd of illness showed significantly higher ELISA absorbance values than did age-matched controls' sera. On the other hand the patients' sera from 11th to 22nd month of illness showed similar ELISA absorbance values as did controls' sera. When the acute phase was compared with subacute phase, the subacute phase showed slightly higher ELISA absorbance values than did the

Fig. 4

**IgG antibody against CPP
of patient with recurrent MCLS**

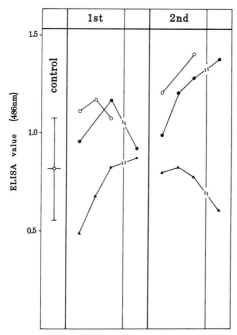

acute phase. However the difference between them was not significant.

The results of the three recurrent cases are shown in Fig. 4. Two cases showed an increased ELISA absorbance value in the first episode with subsequent decreased value in the convalescence phase. In the second episode, the ELISA absorbance value was again increased and was higher than in the first episode.

Meanwhile the results of the control groups are shown in Fig. 5. The controls' sera from the group 0 to 4 years of age had lowest ELISA absorbance values and the sera from adults had the highest. In the controls, ELISA absorbance values increased gradually by age.

We observed similar results with a further two strains of P. acnes isolated from patients' blood.

DISCUSSION

P. acnes is one of the principal indigenous flora of the skin and is found as a contaminant from adult skin in blood culture. Generally, P. acnes is not pathogenic in children. However, previous studies have suggested that P. acnes isolated from patients with Kawasaki disease may have a certain pathogenicity. (Kato et al, 1983, Kato et al, 1985, Inoue, 1984)

Here we have tried to isolate the cytopathogenic substance from the culture filtrates of P. acnes. Specific fractionations were successfully extracted only from the culture filtrates of P. acnes

Lambert et al., 1985), Ehrlichia canis (Edlinger et al., 1980), rickettsia-like (Hamashima et al., 1973a,b; Carter et al., 1976). Tasaka and Hamashima (1978 and Shishido (1979) were unable to confirm the rickettsia isolations originally reported by Hamashima et al. (1973b) and we have not been able to confirm the etiological association of these or any other bacteria with the syndrome (Table 1).

Table 1. Antibody to bacterial pathogens in KS patients in Hawaii

Organism	N	KS %+	Conv.*	Controls N	%+	Test
Propionibacterium acnes	72	65	6	85	64	IFA**
Ehrlichia canis	76	11	5	55	24	IFA
E. sennetsu	54	15	3	55	20	CF
Coxiella burnetii	44	2	1			IFA
Chlamydia trachomatis	58	5	0			CF
C. psittaci	31	0	0			MIF
Rickettsia typhi	26	0	0			Agg.
R. rickettsii	26	0	0			Agg.
Proteus OX-2	31	0	0			Agg.
Proteus OX-K	29	0	0			CF
Proteus OX-19	31	0	0			CF
Legionella pneumophila	18	0	0			CF
Mycoplasma genitalum	19	0	0			ASO
Spiroplasma mirum	18	0	0			IFA
Streptococcus	96	8	0			IFA
Anaplasma marginale	40	0	0			RIA
Toxoplasma gondii	55	0	0			
Staphylococcus	22	5	0			

* Number of patients with a four fold or greater rise in antibody titer from acute phase of illness to convalescence.

**IFA=Indirect immunofluorescence; CF=Complement fixation;
MIF=Microimmunofluorescence; Agg.=Agglutination;
ASO=Anti-streptolysin O; RIA=Radioimmunoassay.

Although leptospirosis can resemble KS clinically (Humphrey et al., 1977), there has been no report of

serological or bacteriological evidence for leptospiral
infection in any confirmed case of KS tested (Humphrey et
al, 1977; Ohtaki et al., 1978; Dean et al., 1982).
Recently we have investigated the possible relationship to
KS of another spirochaete, Borrelia burgdorferi, the
etiological agent of Lyme disease in North America and
erythema chronicum migrans in Europe (Steere et al., 1983;
Burgdorfer et al., 1983; Johnson et al., 1984). It is a
natural symbiote of hard-bodied (ixodid) ticks (Barbour et
al., 1983), which are solely responsible for its
transmission to man as far as is known. A recent report,
however, claims the isolation of B. burgdorferi from deer
flies, horse flies, and mosquitoes (Magnarelli et al.,
1986), all potential vectors of the agent to man from
their natural wild mammal (Lohen et al., 1985) and bird
(Anderson et al., 1986) hosts.

In Hawaii, 18 per cent of KS patients had antibody to
B. burgdorferi at titers of 1:160 or greater compared to
only 5 percent of controls by indirect immunofluorescence
assay (IFA) (Table 2). Serum from Wisconsin supplied by
Dr. Bruce Klein and from Japan provided by Dr. Hirohisa
Kato gave quite different results. There was essentially
no difference in prevalence of antibody between Wisconsin
KS patients and controls; none of the Japanese had
antibody.

Table 2. Antibody to Borrelia burgdorferi at a
titer of ≥160 by indirect immunofluorescence assay

Location	KS N	KS %+	Controls N	Controls %+
Hawaii	68	18	87	5
Wisconsin	13	15	20	20
Japan	20	0	20	0

One Hawaii patient, a two year old boy, had an antibody
response to B. burgdorferi typical of an acute infection,
and the antibody persisted for more than two years (Table
3). Western blot analysis of sera from this and other KS

Table 3. B. burgdorferi antibody
in a 2 year old KS patient

DOD	IFAT titer
9	<80
19	160
46	1280
350	160
850	160

patients and controls with or without detectable antibody
by IFA suggests infection of some children with the Lyme
disease or related spirochaete. Not everyone had antibody
to all the major B. burgdorferi proteins to which all or
most Lyme disease patients react (Table 4). Some

Table 4. Reactivity of sera from KS patients with
B. burgdorferi proteins by Western Blot analysis

Protein Band(MW)	Lyme Disease Patients(U.S.)	Hawaii	
		KS Patients	Controls
41K	100*	18	43
60K	97	0	0
66K	91	6	29
83K	88	24	14
61K	79	18	14
75K	74	35	29
29K	65	0	0
17K	59	41	14
25K	44	0	0
31K	38	0	0
34K	18	0	0

*Percent reacting

individuals had antibody to the 41 KDa protein which
appears to be unique to Borrelia species (Barbour et al.,
1986), but none had antibody to the 60KDa protein to which
97 per cent of Lyme disease patients react (Barbour et
al., 1983). The significance of these data is not known
since Lyme disease is rarely seen in infants, and few have
been tested serologically.

The antibody may be due to a nonspecific polyclonal antibody response, but it is also possible that children are being exposed to an agent which shares some antigens with B. burgdorferi. The relatively poor tick fauna in Hawaii makes it   unlikely that there is transmission of any tick-borne borreliae to which the organism is related (e.g. the relapsing fever spirochaete), and there is no evidence of infection with Treponema pallidum. There are, however, numerous spirochaetes in the normal flora of the mouth, and practically all these children are in the tooth eruption or replacement phase of their lives. Consequently, the data might be explained by transient, localized gum infection with oral treponemes or borreliae, which share antigens with B. burgdorferi, and stimulation of an antibody response.

A preparation of Treponema denticola kindly supplied by Dr. William Faukler at the University of Maryland Dental School, was used in Western blot analyses with serum from KS patients and controls. Polyacrylamide gel electrophoresis and Coomassie blue staining identified 17 major protein bands ranging in molecular weight from approximately 200 KDa to 14KDa. Some sera contained antibodies that detected an additional broad band, possibly lipopolysaccharide, not stained by the protein stain. Not surprisingly, all individuals had antibodies to many of these antigens; all had antibody to either major band 9 or the adjacent minor band e or both (Table 5). There were some differences between adults and children (bands b, 6, d), but no consistent differences between KS patients and age-matched controls.

Both IgM and IgG antibodies reacted with T. denticola proteins. In some cases, IgM antibodies to specific proteins in early serum samples were not present in samples collected weeks to months later; and IgG antibodies not present in early samples appeared in later samples; but the reverse was also true. This might be related to recurrent teething activity, but appropriate data are not available.

Table 5. Reactivity of sera from KS patients with
proteins of <u>Treponema denticola</u> by Western Blot analysis

Band No.*	Normal Adults N=10	Control Children N=11	KS N=11
1	80**	36	45
2	60	64	54
3	90	91	91
a	60	73	64
4	100	64	54
b	0	82	45
c	50	54	54
5	70	73	54
6	10	64	82
7	50	45	54
8	60	64	64
d	20	45	27
e	10	45	45
9	90	54	100
10	50	18	18
f	0	9	0
11	30	27	45
#	0	36	9
g	80	36	54
h	0	9	0
i	0	0	0
j	70	9	0
k	0	0	0

* Numbers refer to deeply staining bands,
  letters to weakly staining bands.
  # = non-protein band.

**Percent reacting.

There was no apparent correlation with reactivity to
any of the <u>T</u>. <u>denticola</u> proteins and antibody to <u>B</u>.
<u>burgdorferi</u> (Table 6).

Only one of the five or more <u>Treponema</u> species known
to be part of the normal oral flora (Tall and Nauman,

Table 6. Reactivity to T. denticola proteins of sera from KS patients with or without B. burgdorferi antibody

	Borrelia ≥160 N=10	Borrelia ≤80 N=12
1	50	33
2	70	50
3	90	91
a	60	75
4	60	58
b	58	67
c	60	42
5	60	58
6	80	58
7	50	50
8	60	50
d	30	42
e	40	50
9	70	83
10	10	25
f	0	8
11	30	42
*	20	25
g	50	42
h	10	0
i	0	0
j	0	8
k	0	0

*Percent reactivity

1986) was tested, but the data illustrate the complexity of the antibody response to these organisms in infants and young children. It appears that oral treponemes actually cause localized infection or invasion of the tissues during tooth eruption or loss and stimulate production of antibody, some of which may cross-react with related organisms. The antigenic similarity of these organisms to other spirochaetes is not known. The major T. denticola proteins are physically unlike any of the B. burgdorferi proteins, and there are distinct differences in protein patterns by polyacrylimide gel electrophoresis within the Treponema genus, but there may be antigenic similarities.

Infection with oral treponemes may also stimulate a nonspecific polyclonal antibody response, and this may explain the presence of B. burgdorferi antibody in children not at risk of being infected with it.

These data do not support the hypothesis that the spirochaetes tested are etiologically associated with KS. Neither do they rule out the possibility that some spirochaete or other fastidious microorganism is the cause of KS or is significantly involved in the pathogenesis of the disease.

REFERENCES

Anderson JF, Johnson RC, Magnarelli LA, Hyde FW (1986). Involvement of birds in the epidemiology of the Lyme disease agent, Borrelia burgdorferi. Infect Immun 51:394-396.

Arita K, Ikuta K, Nishy Y, Kato S, Yamauchi E, Maki S, Naiki M (1982). Heterophile Hanganutziu-Deicher antibodies in sera of patients with Kawasaki disease. Biken J 25:157-162.

Arneborn P, Biberfeld G (1983). T-lymphocyte subpopulations in relation to immunosuppression in measles and varicella. Infect Immun 39:29-37.

Bach MA, Bach JF (1981). Imbalance of T-cell subsets in human diseases. Int J Immunopharmacol 3:269-274.

Baranda L, Moncarda B, Gonzalez-Amaro R (1984). Decrease of helper T-cells in children with recurrent respiratory tract infection. J Infect Dis 149:123.

Barbour AG, Hayes SF, Heiland RA, Schrumpf ME, Tessier SL (1986). A Borrelia-specific monoclonal antibody binds to a flagellar epitope. Infect Immun 52:549-554.

Barbour AG, Burgdorfer W, Grunwaldt E, Steere AC (1983). Antibodies of patients with Lyme disease to components of the Ixodes dammini spirochete. J Clin Invest 72:504-515.

Barbour AG, Urueger GG, Feurino PM and Smith CB (1979). Kawasaki-like disease in a young adult associated with Epstein-Barr virus infection. JAMA 241:397-398.

Barnaba V, Zaccari C, Levrero M, Ruocco, G, Balsano F (1983). Immunoregulatory T-cells in hepatitis B virus-induced chronic liver disease as defined by monoclonal antibodies. Clin Immunol Immunopathol 26:83-90.

Barnaba V, Musca A, Cordova C, Levrero M, Ruocco G, Albertini-Pertroni V, Balsano F (1983). Relationship between T-cell subsets and suppressor cell activity in chronic hepatitis B virus (HBV) infection. Clin Exp Immunol 53:281-288.

Baum L, James K, Glaviano R, Gewurz H (1983). Possible role for C-reactive protein in the human natural killer cell response. J Exp Med 157:301-311.

Bertotto A, Gentili F, Caccaro R (1982). Immunoregulatory cells in varicella. Lancet II:1271-1272.

Bowen DL, Lane C, Fauci AS (1984). Immune function in the acquired immunodeficiency syndrome. In: MS Gottleib and JE Groopman (Eds.). Acquired immune deficiency syndrome. Alan R Liss, Inc: NY pp 211-221.

Brettle RP, Gray JA, Sangster J, Murdoch JM, DIck HM (1982). The mucocutaneous syndromes-erythema multiforme, Stevens-Johnson and ectodermosis erosiva pluriorificialis. J Infect 4:149-160.

Burgdorfer W, Barbour AG, Hayes SF, Peter O, Aeschlimann A (1983). Erythema chronicum migrans-a tickborne spirochetosis. Acta Trop 40:79-83.

Carney WP, Iacoviello V, Hirsch MS (1981). Analysis of T lymphocyte subsets in cytomegalovirus mononucleosis. J Immunol 126:2114-2116.

Carter RF, Haynes ME, Morton J (1976). Rickettsia-like bodies and splenitis in Kawasaki disease. Lancet II:1254-1255.

Dean AG, Melish ME, Hicks R, Palumbo NE (1982). An epidemic of Kawasaki syndrome in Hawaii. J Pediat 100:552-557.

Edlinger EA, Benichou JJ, Labrune B (1980). Positive Ehrlichia canis serology in Kawasaki disease. Lancet I:1146-1147.

Fisher-Hoch S, Swaby D, Stern H, Lambert H (1980). Kawasaki disease and Q fever in Tooting. Comm Dis Rep Weekly Ed 18 July.

Fishman JA, Martell KM, Rubin RH (1983). Infection and T-lymphocyte subpopulations: changes associated with bacteremia and the acquired immune deficiency syndrome. Diagnostic Immunol 1:261-265.

Fujiwara H, Kao T, Shimizu J, Fujiwara T, Oo MM, Hamashima Y, (1983). Microorganisms in the heart in Kawasaki disease. Lancet II:620-621.

Furukawa F, Ohishio G, Hamashima Y (1986). Possible polyclonal B cell activation in mucocutaneous lymph node syndrome. Euro J Pediat 145:104-108.

Gewurz H, Mold C, Siegel J, Fiedel B (1982). C-reactive protein and the acute phase responses. Adv Intern Med 27:345-372.

Goldstein G, Lifter J, Mittler R (1982). Immunoregulatory changes in human disease detected by monoclonal antibodies to T-lymphocytes. In: A McMichael and W Fabre (Eds.) Monoclonal antibodies in clinical medicine. Academic Press, London. pp 39-70.

Griffin DE, Hirsch RL, Johnson RT, de Soriano IL, Roedenbeck S, Vaisberg A (1983). Changes in serum C-feactive protein during complicated and uncomplicated measles virus infections. Inf Immun 41:861-864.

Griffin DE, Moench TR, Johnson RT, de Soriano IL, Vaisberg A, (1986). Peripheral blood mononuclear cells during natural measle virus infection: cell surface phenoypte and evidence for activation. Clin Immunol Immunopathol 40:305-312.

Hamashima Y, Kishi K, Tasaka K (1973). Rickettsia-like bodies in infantile acute febrile mucocutaneous lymph-node syndrome. Lancet II:42.

Hamashima Y, Kishi K, Tasaka K (1973). Discovery and isolation of rickettsia-like bodies from mucocutaneous lymph node syndrome patients. Igaku-no-Ayumi 87:189-193 (in Japanese).

Humphrey T, Sanders S, Stadius M (1977). Leptospirosis mimicking mucocutaneous lymph node syndrome. J Pediat 91:853.

Iwanaga M, Takada K, Osato T, Saeki Y, Noro S, Sakurada N (1981). Kawasaki disease and Epstein-Barr virus. Lancet 1:938-939.

Joffe MI, Sukha NR, Rabson AR (1983). Lymphocyte subsets in measles. J Clin Invest 72:971-980.

Johnson RC, Schmid GP, Hyde FW, Steigerwaldt AG, Brenner DJ (1984). Borrelia burgdorferi sp. nov.: etiologic agent of Lyme disease. Int J Syst Bact 34:496-497.

Kao T, Shimizu J, Furukawa F, Saito Y, Iwamoto H, Fujiwara H, Hamashima Y (1984). Reevaluation of microorganisms in skin lesions in mucocutaneous lymph node syndrome. Report of 18 cases. Acta Dermatol (Kyoto) 79:293-298.

Kato H, Inoue O, Koga Y, Shingu M, Fujimoto T, Kondo M, Yamamoto S, Tominaga K, Sasaguri Y (1983). Variant strain of Propionibacterium acnes: a clue to the aetiology of Kawasaki syndrome. Lancet II:1383-1387.

Keren G, Cohn BE, Barzilagi Z, Hiss J, Imolman M (1979).
Kawasaki disease and infantile periarteritis nodosa: is
Pseudomonas infection responsible? Report of a case.
Israel J Med Sci 15:592-600.
Kikuta H, Mizuno F, Osato T, Konno M, Ishikawa N, Noro SI,
Sakurada N (1984). Kawasaki disease and an unusual
primary infection wtih Epstein-Barr virus. Pediatrics
73:413-414.
Kuta AE, Baum LL (1986). C-reactive protein is produced
by a small number of normal human peripheral blood
lymphocytes. J Exp Med 164:321-326.
Lambert HP, Fisher-Hock SP, Grover SR (1985). Kawasaki
disease and Coxiella burneti. Lancet II:844.
Leung DY, Siesel RL, Grady S, Krensky A, Meade R,
Reinherz EL, Geha RS (1982). Immunoregulatory
abnormalities in mucocutaneous lymph node syndrome.
Clin Immunol Immunopathol 23:100-112.
Leung DYM, Chu ET, Wood N, Grady S, Meade R, Geha RS
(1983). Immunoregulatory T-cell abnormalities in
mucocutaneous lymph node syndrome. J Immunol
130:2002-2004.
Levandowski RA, Ou DW, Jackson GG (1986). Acute-phase
decrease in T-lymphocyte subsets in rhinovirus
infection. J Infect Dis 153:743-748.
Lohen KI, Wu CC, Johnson RC, Bey RF (1985). Isolation of
the Lyme disease spirochaete from mammals in Minnesota.
Proc Soc Exp Biol Med 179:300-302.
Ludlam GB, Bridges JB, Benn EC (1964). Association of
Stevens-Johnson syndrome with antibody for Mycoplasma
pneumoniae infections. Lancet 1:958-959.
McCarthy PL, Frank AL, Ablow RC, Masters SJ, Dolan PF
(1978). Value of the C-reactive protein test in the
differentiation of bacterial and viral pneumonia. J
Pediatr 92:454-456.
Magnarelli LA, Anderson JJ, Barbour AG (1986). The
etiologic agent of Lyme disease in deer flies, house
flies, and mosquitoes. J Infect Dis 154:355-358.
Matsumi F, Ueno T (1979). Streptococci as a causative
agent for Kawasaki disease (MCLS). Jap J Med Sci Biol
32:247-249.
Melekian B (1982). Kawasaki-like infectious
mononucleosis. Acta Paediatr Scand 71:843.
Ohtaki C, Tomiyama T, Suzuki M, Hayakawa H, Kaga M (1978).
Leptospiral antibodies and mucocutaneous lymph node
syndrome. J Pediat 93:896.

Reinherz EL, O'Brien C, Rosenthal P, Schlossman SF (1980). The cellular basis for viral-induced immunodeficiency: analysis by monoclonal antibodies. J Immunol 125:1269-1274.

Ruuskanen O, Putto A, Sarkkinen H, Meurman O, Irjala K (1985). C-reactive protein in respiratory virus infections. J Pediat 107:97-100.

Salonen EM, Vaheri A (1981). C-reactive protein in acute viral infections. J Med Virol 8:161-167.

Shannon K, Fink CW, Buchanan GR, Punaro M, Stastny P (1983). Lymphocyte subpopulations in Kawasaki disease. Clin Exp Rheumatol 1:59-62.

Shishido A (1979). Failure to confirm the rickettsial etiology of mucocutaneous lymph node syndrome (Kawasaki disease). Jap J Med Sci Biol 32:250-251.

Steere AC, Grodzicki RL, Kornblatt AN, Craft JE (1983). The spirochetal etiology of Lyme disease. New Engl J Med 308:733-740.

Strohm J (1^69). Herpes simplex virus as a cause of allergic mucocutaneous reactions (ectodermosis erosiva pluriorificialis, Stevens-Johnson syndrome, etc.) and generalized infection. Scand J Infect Dis 1:3-10.

Tall BD, Nauman RK (1986). Microscopic agglutination and polyacrylamide gel electrophoresis analyses of oral anaerobic spirochetes. J Clin Microbiol 24:282-287.

Tasaka K, Hamashima Y (1978). Studies on rickettsia-like body in Kawasaki disease. Attempts at the isolation and characterization. Acta Pathol Jap 28:235-245.

Vetter MA, Gewurz H, Hansen B, Baum LL (1983). Effects of C-reactive proteins on human lymphocyte responsiveness. J Immunol 130:2121-2126.

Weir WRC, Bouchet VA, Mitford E, Taylor RFH, Smith H (1985). Kawasaki disease in European adult associated with serological response to Coxiella burneti. Lancet II:504.

Kawasaki Disease, pages 101-111
© 1987 Alan R. Liss, Inc.

EVALUATION OF EVIDENCE RELATED TO STREPTOCOCCI IN THE
ETIOLOGY OF KAWASAKI DISEASE

Shozo Kotani

Department of Microbiology and Oral Microbiology,
Osaka University Dental School, Yamadaoka, Suita,
Osaka 565; Director, Osaka College of Medical
Technology, Higashitenma, Kita-ku, Osaka 530, JAPAN

INTRODUCTION

Epidemiological evidence strongly suggests that some
infectious agent is responsible for the occurrence of Kawasaki disease (MCLS), either directly or indirectly, for
instance by triggering immunopathological responses. Thus,
a variety of microbes, bacterial, viral and fungal, have so
far been proposed as a candidate for the etiological agent
of MCLS (Study Committee on Cause of Kawasaki Disease, Japan
Heart Association, 1986).

Regarding bacterial candidates, Streptococcus pyogenes,
viridans group of streptococci, particularly Streptococcus
sanguis, a variant strain of Propionibacterium acnes (Kato
et al., 1983), rickettsia-like bodies (Hamashima et al, 1973;
Carter et al., 1976), Pseudomonas (Keren and Wolman, 1984),
Yersinia pseudotuberculosis (Ouchi et al., 1985) and others
have been proposed as possible agents associated with MCLS.
This minireview will be centered on the streptococci that
have been the most extensively studied among these bacteria.

HYPOTHESIS ON S. PYOGENES AS A POSSIBLE MCLS AGENT

Ueno and Matsumi suggested that S. pyogenes is related
to the etiology of MCLS (Ueno and Matsumi, 1983). The draw-
back of their hypothesis, primarily based on the close
similarity in symptomatology between MCLS and streptococcal
infections such as scarlet fever (Yamamoto, 1983), is the
fact that S. pyogenes is only rarely isolated from infants
and children of the age group susceptible to MCLS (Katsukawa

and Harada, 1984) as well as from MCLS patients (Harada et al., 1986). To deal with this problem, they devised a "specific fibrin precipitation test" to detect a "derivative" of streptococcal pyrogenic exotoxin (SPE) instead of S. pyogenes in the blood plasma of MCLS patients by reaction with antiserum of the rabbits immunized with extracellular products of S. pyogenes. They reported significantly higher positive rates with the plasma of MCLS patients than the plasma of age-matched control subjects. Unfortunately, this test does not yield reproducible and objective results, and the findings reported by Ueno and Matsumi have not yet been confirmed by other investigators. Also, their observation that many L form-like structures, possibly originating from streptococci, were found in the blood of patients with MCLS could not be verified.

Akiyama's group is pursuing the possible role of S. pyogenes in MCLS along another line of approach. In their studies, comparison was made among patients with MCLS, streptococcal pharyngitis and illnesses not related to streptococcal infections, by the guinea pig macrophage migration inhibition test for the reactivity of peripheral blood mononuclear cells with S. pyogenes cells, SPE, the water-extracts of the transformed human B cell line, human needle-size arteries and guinea pig heart muscle. By analysis of changes in the reactivity during the course of diseases, Akiyama proposed a hypothesis that an "intracellular strain" of S. pyogenes might be the pathogen of MCLS (Akiyama et al., 1985, 1986). This unique hypothesis, however, has not yet been supported by actual demonstration of an "intracellular strain" of S. pyogenes.

NEW SEROTYPE STRAINS OF S. SANGUIS PROPOSED BY THE KITASATO INSTITUTE GROUP TO BE RELATED TO MCLS

A few years ago, a research group at the Kitasato Institute, Tokyo, isolated S. sanguis-like organisms at significantly higher rates from the dental plaque materials of MCLS patients and their mothers (Nakagawa et al., 1985; Takeuchi et al., 1986). These streptococci, which were tentatively named "MCLS" strains of S. sanguis, have biochemical properties similar to reference biotype B strains, although there are some subtle differences in fermentation of raffinose and melibiose ("MCLS" strains fermented both sugars, while the reference biotype B strains did not). The "MCLS" strains are more readily discriminated from the conventional strains of

S. sanguis by demonstration of the antigens that are not shared by reference strains of serotype I, II, III and IV (Hamada et al., 1980) by immunodiffusion analysis using Rantz-Randall extracts and adsorbed anti-S. sanguis rabbit sera (serotyping sera). Table 1 shows that "MCLS" strains of S. sanguis can be grouped into two new serotypes, MCLS-1 and MCLS-2, both of which are clearly distinguishable from the so-far established four serotypes. The Rantz-Randall extracts of "MCLS" strains as well as the reference strains did not react with serotyping sera against Streptococcus mitis reference strains (see the footnote in TABLE 1).

TABLE 1. Serological characteristics of the "MCLS" strains of S. sanguis

Rantz-Randall extracts from strain	serotype	Serotyping serum against					
		ATCC 10556	ATCC 10557	ATCC 10558	ST-7	MCLS 1	MCLS 2
ATCC10556	I	+	−	−	−	−	−
ATCC10557	II	−	+	−	−	−	−
ATCC10558	III	−	−	+	−	−	−
ST-7	IV	−	−	−	+	−	−
SSH-83	MCLS-1	−	−	−	−	+	−
KIH-T	MCLS-2	−	−	−	−	−	+

All the Rantz-Randall extracts from the above reference and "MCLS" strains did not react with serotyping sera against Streptococcus mitis reference strains (ATCC 9811, 9895, 15910, 15911, and 15912).
[Cited with modification from Nakagawa et al., 1985)]

TABLE 2 summarizes the survey of the Kitasato Institute group on prevalence of "MCLS" strains in MCLS patients and the age-matched control infants and children. Although no information is available of the number of MCLS cases examined, the "MCLS" strains were isolated from two thirds of the MCLS cases from whom S. sanguis were isolated, namely at a rate of 36% with MCLS-1 strain and at 30% with MCLS-2, while these new serotype strains were rarely isolated from the control group.

TABLE 2. Detection rates of the "MCLS" strains of S. sanguis in MCLS and control groups

Subjects	No. of subjects	No. of subjects from whom S. sanguis were isolated (A)	"MCLS" strain-postive subjects (B) (percent, B/A)		
			MCLS-1	MCLS-2	Total
MCLS group					
KIH		40	15(37.5)	11(27.5)	26(65.0)
KWH		130	44(33.8)	42(32.3)	86(66.2)
TIH		11	5(45.5)	0	5(45.4)
SSH		12	6(50.0)	4(33.3)	10(83.3)
Total		193	70(36.3)	57(29.5)	127(65.8)
Healthy control group					
Pediatric outpatients (0 to 8-year-old)	30	18	0	0	0
4-month-old infants	90	3	0	0	0
One and half-year-old infants	94	57	0	0	0
3-year-old children	92	66	1(1.5)	0	1(1.5)

[Modified from Nakagawa et al., 1985]

EVALUATION OF THE RESULTS OF KITASATO INSTITUTE GROUP BY NIH, TOKYO GROUP

The study committee on Cause of Kawasaki Disease, Japan Heart Foundation, requested Shigeyuki Hamada, the head of Oral Biology Division, NIH, Tokyo to evaluate the results reported by the Kitasato Institute group as an impartial investigator.

The evaluation study was performed in the following way. Cotton swab specimens of the labial surface of incisor teeth of each jaw, were collected at the Japan Red Cross Medical Center by Tomisaku Kawasaki and Yoshio Yanase. Sonicated dental plaque materials were cultivated on Mitis-Salivarius medium (Difco) plates. After 48-h incubation at 37°C, the colonies showing S. sanguis-like colonial morphology (50 col- onies randomly selected, if it is possible) were inoculated in brain-heart-infusion broth. Pure cultures thus obtained were subjected to biochemical test and serotyping. The latter was done by two dimensional immunodiffusion in agarose gel be- tween the Rantz-Randall extracts and adsorbed serotyping sera against serotypes I, II, III, IV, MCLS-1 and MCLS-2 as re- ported by Nakagawa et al. (1985). The serotyping results were collated with the origin of test specimens after comple- tion of serotyping of S. sanguis-like organisms isolated from each test material having only the code number, in the pres- ence of both laboratory workers and medical doctors in the clinic; in other words, the study was carried out on a strict- ly blind basis.

Since the study is still in progress, only the results so far obtained can be reported here (Akada et al., 1986). From 10 out of 14 MCLS cases, all of whom have teeth, the habitat of S. sanguis, MCLS-2 strains were isolated as the predominant S. sanguis-like organisms (detection rate was 71%). The remarkable finding was that MCLS-2 strains were isolated as almost a homogeneous culture from 5 MCLS cases. The percentage of MCLS cases showing the predominance of the MCLS-1 strain and reference serotype I to IV strains were 29% and 7%, respectively. With the age-matched 13 healthy children (all were after tooth eruption), the number of sub- jects showing the predominance of MCLS-2 was 3, namely the detection rate was 23%, and only one case gave the MCLS-2 strain as a homogeneous culture. Serotype I to IV strains were most prevalent in this group (the detection rate was about 46%). The MCLS-1 strain was recovered at a rate of about 15%. The third group, although small in number, con-

sisted of children (after tooth eruption) suffering from
acute febrile diseases. Three out of 4 cases showed the predominance of MCLS-2 strain among S. sanguis-like isolates.
These three cases having the predominant MCLS-2 strain were
associated with MCLS; each one of the patients with acute
febrile disease after MCLS recovery, possibly abortive form
of MCLS and measles 8 months after MCLS.

Table 3 summarized the results of the NIH, Tokyo, research group. The difference in the detection rate of the
MCLS-2 serotype strain between the MCLS patient group and
the age-matched healthy group is highly significant. Thus,
the finding of the Kitasato Institute group was confirmed
with MCLS-2 serotype strains. However, no significant difference was found in the detection rate of MCLS-1 serotype
strain between MCLS and healthy control groups. This finding is not consistent with that of the Kitasato Institute
group, and the reason for this discrepancy is still unknown.

TABLE 3. Summary of detection rates of S. sanguis, serotype
MCLS-1 and MCLS-2, in MCLS and control groups

Children suffering from	No. of subjects	No.(%) of subjects harboring predominantly S. sanguis, serotype	
		MCLS-1	MCLS-2
MCLS	14	4(28.6)	10(71.4)*
None	13	2(15.4)	3(23.1)
Acute febrile diseases	4	1(25.0)	3(75.0)[a]

[a] Acute febrile disease after recovery form MCLS; abortive form of MCLS; and measles (MCLS 8 months earlier).
    * Significantly different from the none control value
(P < 0.02).

STUDIES ON PECULIARITIES OF "MCLS" STRAINS NOT SHARED BY THE
CONVENTIONAL S. SANGUIS STRAINS

The findings described in the preceding section indicate
that the high detection rate of the "MCLS" strains, at least
MCLS-2 serotype strain in MCLS and MCLS-associated patient
groups and the low detection rate of the particular serotype
strain(s) in the age-matched, healthy control group seem to

conform, although not quite satisfactorily, to criter
II of the Koch's postulates.

Nevertheless, it is difficult to understand the role of
"MCLS" strain(s) of S. sanguis in the manifestation of clinical symptoms, pathological changes and epidemiological features of MCLS on the basis of hitherto known bacteriological
or pathogenic properties of the conventional S. sanguis
organisms (Hardie, 1986). If the "MCLS" strain(s) of S. sanguis were the etiological agent of MCLS, the "MCLS" strain(s)
should have some particular, pathogenic traits, namely
traits not shared by the conventional S. sanguis strains.

Recently, the Kitasato Institute group reported the presence of a toxic substance in the culture supernatant fluid
of the "MCLS" strains, but not in that of the reference S.
sanguis strains (Nakamura et al., 1986; Takeuchi et al.,
1986). Test S. sanguis strains were grown in a dialysate medium prepared from TTY medium. From the culture supernatant
of the "MCLS" strains, a protein fraction with a molecular
weight of 140 K was concentrated and purified by successive
precipitation with ammonium sulfate, gel filtration and ion-
exchange chromatography, as outlined in Fig. 1. The purified protein thus obtained caused marked swelling of ingui-
nal lymph nodes by intra-footpad injection into mice at doses
of one to 5 ug. Keizo Kageyama, a pathologist who examined
the section of the swollen lymph nodes noted that the pathological findings had some similarity to those of cervical
lymph nodes of MCLS patients (personal communication). The
toxic substance was recovered from MCLS-1 as well as MCLS-2
stains at a yield of around 10 mg per 20 liters of the culture supernatant fluid, but was not obtained at a comparable
yield from the culture fluid of the reference serotype I to
IV serotype strains. The toxic substance was reported to be
immunogenic and detoxified by formalin treatment. Serum specimens of the rabbits immunized with the toxic fractions of
MCLS-1 and MCLS-2 strains gave one major and one minor precipitation line in immunodiffusion with the immunogens.
The major bands produced by the toxic substance of both
strains fused and showed the reaction of identity. The interesting findings described above are waiting confirmation
by impartial investigators.

In this connection, Miyamoto isolated viridans group
streptococci from the blood of 5 out of 16 MCLS patients. In
a subsequent study, he showed that some S. sanguis strains,

which grew abundantly like a homogeneous culture on the isolation plates inoculated with throat swabs from MCLS patients,
caused systematic perivasculitis and/or vasculitis by repeated intravenous injection of a concentated cell suspension into mice (Miyamoto et al., 1985). However, no comparative
study on reference S. sanguis strains has been reported.
Further, there is no information on the relationship between
the strain used in Miyamoto's study and the "MCLS" strains
isolated by the Kitasato Institute or the NIH, Tokyo groups.

Test S. sanguis strain

    Cultured in dialysate medium prepared from
    TTY medium at 37°C for 24-h.

Culture supernatants

    Salted out with ammonium sulfate (80%),
    and dialysed against 0.05 M Tris-HCl buf-
    fer (pH 7.6).

Crude fraction

    Fractionated with Sephacryl S-300

Pooled active fraction

    Concentrated by salting out with ammonium
    sulfate (50 to 80% sat) and dialysed against
    the buffer.

Concentrates

    Fractionated with Q-Sepharose by linear
    sodium chloride concentration gradient
    (0 to 1 M) in the buffer.

Active fraction

    Lyophilized, dissolved in water, and dialy-
    sed against the buffer. Fractionated with
    Superose-6 by elution with the buffer added
    with 0.15 M sodium chloride.

Purified toxic substance (140K)

Figure 1. Purification method of a toxic substance
of "MCLS" strains of S. sanguis.
[Constructed from the description of Nakamura et al.
(1986)]

    Finally, Ohtsu et al. (1985) suggested the role of a
protein with calcium-inhibitable phosphatidylinositol phos-

pholipase C activity in the etiology of MCLS, on the basis
of findings that the in vitro production of this enzyme protein was greater in S. sanguis isolates from 20 MCLS
patients than from those of eleven 3-month-old and ten 3-
year-old control children, and that MCLS patients developed
antibody responses to the enzyme protein. These findings,
however, need to be confirmed.

CONCLUSION

The newly described serotype strain(s) of S. sanguis
may be worth further studying with respect to the etiology
of MCLS. Nevertheless, it is premature to draw a conclusion
on the pathogenic significance of "MCLS" strains of S. sanguis, because the information available is still limited,
and in view of recent studies that retroviruses may be the
agents associated with the occurrence of MCLS.

REFERENCES

Akada H, Asakawa H, Fujiwara T., Koga T, Yamamoto T, Okaha-
    shi N, Hamada S (1986). Classification and possible asso-
    ciation with Kawasaki disease of Streptococcus sanguis-like
    organisms isolated from oral cavity of Kawasaki patients.
    Jpn J Oral Biol 28(suppl): 243. [in Japanese]
Akiyama T, Osawa N, Yashiro K, Hiraishi S (1985). Possible
    role of Streptococcus pyogenes in mucocutaneous lymph node
    syndrome. Acta Paediatr Jpn 27: 205-213.
Akiyama T, Osawa N, Yashiro K, Hiraishi S (1986). Possible
    role of Streptococcus pyogenes in mucocutaneous lymph node
    syndrome. II. Hightened cellular reactivity to stimulation
    by mammalian myocardial and arterial antigens in MCLS pa-
    tients. Acta Paediatr Jpn 28: 788-796.
Carter RF, Haynes ME, Morton J (1976). Rickettsia-like
    bodies and splenitis in Kawasaki disease. Lancet ii: 1254-
    1255.
Hamada S, Torii M, Tsuchitani Y, Kotani S (1980). Isolation
    and immunobiological classification of Streptococcus sanguis
    from human tooth surfaces. J. Clin. Microbiol. 12: 243-249.
Hamashima Y, Kishi K, Tasaka K (1973). Rickettsia-like bodies
    in infantile acute febrile mucocutaneous lymph-node syn-
    drome. Lancet ii: 42.
Harada K, Katsukawa T, Kotani S, Kanoh S, Takemasa N, Iida
    Y, Usami H, Yanase Y, Kawasaki T (1986). Bacteriological
    study on the etiology of Kawasaki disease (MCLS) - Search
    for non-β-hemolytic bacteria which are capable of producing

streptococcal pyrogenic exotoxin. Pediatr Jpn 27:921-928. [in Japanese]

Hardie JM (1986). Genus Streptococcus: Oral streptococci. In Sneath PHA, Mair NS, Sharpe ME, Holt JG (eds):"Bergey's Manual of Systematic Bacteriology," Baltimore, Williams & Wilkins, pp 1054-1063.

Kato H, Fujimoto T, Inoue O, Kondo M, Koga Y, Yamamoto S, Shingu M, Tominaga K (1983). Variant strain of Propionibacterium acnes: A clue to the etiology of Kawasaki disease. Lancet ii: 1383-1387.

Katsukawa T, Harada K (1984). An epidemiological study of group A streptococci. Proc Osaka Prefectural Institute. No. 22: 29-34. [in Japanese]

Keren G, Wolman M (1984). Can Pseudomonas infection in experimental animals mimic Kawasaki's disease. J. Infect. 9: 22-29.

Miyamoto Y, Yamai S, Shimoda Y, Nikkawa T, Obara Y, Kazuno Y, Takeda Y, Sasaki H, Kawamoto H, Takemura T (1985). Mouse model and human studies on Kawasaki's disease(mucocutaneous lymph node syndrome) with special reference to Streptococcus sanguis. In Kimura Y, Kotani,S Shiokawa Y (eds): "Recent Advances in Streptococci and Streptococcal Diseases," Bracknell, Berkshire, pp 357-358.

Nakagawa N, Sato T, Tsurumizu T, Hashimoto T, Sato M, Nakamura R, Ozaki F, Ohara S, Kawaguchi Y, Okada S (1985). A study of Streptococcus sanguis isolated from dental plaque of MCLS patients and their mothers. I. Classification and characterization. J Dental Health 35: 435-443. [in Japanese with English summary]

Nakamura N, Nakagawa N, Tsurumizu T, Hashimoto T, Sato M (1986). Characteristics of Streptococcus sanguis isolated from MCLS patients and their family. J Dental Health 39: 496-497. [in Japanese]

Ohtsu E, Yamai S, Kuroki T, Obara Y, Hachimura K, Ohnuki Y, Takamiya H, Takayama K, Ohsawa N, Suzuki S, Shirai S, Yashro K (1985). Possible role of streptococcal exotoxins in the etiology of Kawasaki disease. In Doyle EF, Engle MA, Gersony WM, Rashkind WJ, Talner NS (eds): "Pediatric cardiology; Proc 2nd World Congress," New York, Spring-Verlag, pp 1077-1082.

Ouchi K, Sato K, Takahashi R, Taki M, Tateishi K (1985). Importance of differentiation of Yersinia pseudotuberculosis infections from Kawasaki disease. J Jpn Soc Pediatr 89: 449-454.

Study Committee on Cause of Kawasaki Disease, Japan Heart Association (1986). Kawasaki disease - Epidemiological

Data Book -. Tokyo, Soft Science Publications, pp 1-318. [in Japanese with English abstract]

Takeuchi Y, Tsurumizu T, Hashimoto T (1986). Is Streptococcus sanguis like organisms the etiological agent of mucocutaneous lymph node syndrome ? Abstracts of Scientific Presentations; XVIII International Congress of Pediatrics (Honolulu - Hawaii). No. 299.

Ueno T, Matsumi F (1983). Kawasaki syndrome and streptococcal infection. Acta Paediatr Jpn 25: 130-146.

Yamamoto T (1983). Etiology of the mucocutaneous lymph node syndrome, and the streptococcus hypothesis. Acta Paediatr Jpn 25: 118-126.

Kawasaki Disease, pages 113-116
© 1987 Alan R. Liss, Inc.

KAWASAKI DISEASE AND EPSTEIN-BARR VIRUS INFECTION

Toyoro Osato, Hideaki Kikuta, Motohiko Okano, Fumio Mizuno, Mutsuko Konno, Nobuyoshi Ishikawa, Kanji Hirai and Shuzo Matsumoto

Department of Virology, Cancer Institute (T.O., H.K., M.O., F.M), and Department of Pediatrics (H.K., M.O., S.M), Hokkaido University School of Medicine, Sapporo 060, Japan; Kitami Red Cross Hospital (M.K., N.I), Kitami 090; Department of Molecular Biology, Tokai University School of Medicine (K.H), Isehara 259-11

INTRODUCTION

The number of children with Kawasaki disease (mucocutaneous lymph node syndrome) has been increasing both in Japan and other countries. We have some probable reasons to study Epstein-Barr virus (EBV) (Epstein and Achong, 1979; Osato et al., 1986) in Kawasaki disease. First, EBV infects humans in early life, especially in Japan, and Kawasaki disease is an infant illness. Second, EBV is lymphotropic as seen in infectious mononucleosis, and lymph nodes are also involved in Kawasaki disease. Third, EBV potentially affects immune system through persistence in B cells, and Kawasaki disease has some immunologic changes.

EBV SEROLOGIC RESPONSE IN KAWASAKI DISEASE

Our initial studies (Iwanaga et al., 1981) in the 1979 nationwide outbreak of Kawasaki disease in Japan with 69 patients showed that only 2 (2.9%) of 69 were EBV-seropositive, in sharp contrast with 58 positives (84.1%) in 69 healthy children. Although only one serum sample was collected during the acute phase, an abnormal immune response to EBV was strongly suggested.

The second nationwide outbreak came in 1982, and 45 new Japanese patients (27 boys and 18 girls; mean age of 2.3 years) were then investigated (Kikuta et al., 1984).

The control subjects were 153 age-matched and sex-matched children with common acute febrile respiratory infections. EBV-specific serology was mainly carried out with 3 different antibody categories: IgG antibodies to viral capsid antigen (VCA-IgG), IgM antibodies to VCA (VCA-IgM), and IgG antibodies to nuclear antigen (EBNA-IgG). VCA-IgG and VCA-IgM were examined by indirect immunofluorescence and EBNA-IgG by anticomplement immunofluorescence. This time, serum samples were frequently collected from each individual patient weekly, following the onset of Kawasaki disease. As a result, the first month after diagnosis, 18 (40.0%) of the 45 Kawasaki patients were EBV-seropositive, lower than 72.5% (111 of the 153 children) positive in common acute febrile illnesses. However, all of the 18 seropositive Kawasaki patients had characteristics of a primary EBV infection, VCA-IgM-positive or VCA-IgG-positive with EBNA antibody negative, as compared with 25.2% in the control children. It was particularly noted that a high frequency of 72.2% of EBV-seropositive Kawasaki patients was VCA-IgM-positive, in sharp contrast to 6.3% in the controls. Most of the control children were VCA-IgG-positive, EBNA-IgG-positive, thus representing a past EBV infection. Quite unusually, this particular EBV seropositive status in the acute phase of Kawasaki disease seemed transient for 1 to 2 week periods after the first detection of EBV antibodies. Another EBV antibody response was evident in a small number of Kawasaki patients. Five (11.1%) of the 45 children turned first EBV-seropositive considerably later, 3 months after the onset of the disease. This antibody response was not transient but consistent, as normally seen in EBV infection.

These results suggested that half of Kawasaki disease patients were closely associated with a primary infection with EBV, and the EBV events seemed suppressed and unusual. To look for a small amount of EBV antibodies in seronegative patients, not feasible with conventional tests, we reassessed the previously examined 45 Kawasaki serum specimens together with the 153 control sera, following development of a more sensitive assay (Kikuta et al., 1984). Since all Kawasaki patients' sera were negative for EBNA antibodies as mentioned above, anticomplement immunofluorescence became available for the assessment of VCA antibodies. Specificity was quite evident with a 4-fold or more sensitive VCA antibody detection, in comparison to the conventional indirect method. Using this sensitive assay, the first month after diagnosis, 40 (88.9%) of the 45 Kawasaki patients were VCA-seropositive, in contrast to 40.0% positivity in the previous indirect immunofluorescence . All of the 40 VCA-seropositive patients were totally negative for EBNA antibodies, thereby indicating a primary EBV infection. In controls, the seropositivity was increased from 72.5% to 77.1% and 29.7% showed anti-EBNA-negative, as compared with 25.2% in the previous indirect test.

DETECTION AND CHARACTERIZATION OF EBV IN KAWASAKI DISEASE

Through spontaneous establishment of EBNA-positive peripheral lymphocyte lines and immortalization of cord blood lymphocytes exposed to throat swabs, EBV was seen shortly after diagnosis from a small number of the patients converting late, consistently seropositive after 3 months (Kikuta et al., 1983). EBV, however, was not totally detectable in the early, transiently seropositive patients. Preliminary data indicate that the EBV isolated from Kawasaki disease seem to have much lower B-cell immortalizing ability than the standard EBV strain, B95-8 virus. Restriction enzyme analysis showed that the BamHI-H fragment of the Kawasaki virus was partially deleted (Kikuta et al., 1985). This particular EBV DNA fragment is closely associated with EBV immortalization of B lymphocytes.

EBV INDUCIBILITY OF B CELLS IN KAWASAKI DISEASE

Finally, Kawasaki patients' B lymphocytes seem to be different from those of control children, in terms of inducibility of latent EBV genomes. Although the number of EBV genomes in spontaneously immortalized Kawasaki patients' B lymphocytes was the same as that in control children's immortalized B cells, EBV induction in Kawasaki lymphocytes was significantly lower than control lymphocytes, when exposed to phorbol ester TPA (12-0-tetra-decanoylphorbol-13-acetate) and when superinfected with P3HR-1 strain EBV (Okano et al., 1985).

Taken all together, our findings seem to indicate that the patients with Kawasaki disease have an associated unusual primary infection and this might be due to a defective mutant EBV and also impaired patients' B cell responsiveness to EBV. There was, however, no significant difference between Kawasaki patients and control children in antibody response to other viruses, such as cytomegalovirus, herpes simplex virus, poliovirus type 1, measles virus, and influenza viruses. Also, no significant difference was there between patients' family members and control children's families in EBV serology.

REFERENCES

Epstein, MA, Achong, BG (1979). Discovery and general biology of the virus. In: The Epstein-Barr Virus (Epstein MA, Achong BG, eds), Berlin, Springer-Verlag, pp 1-22.

Iwanaga M, Takada K, Osato T, Saeki Y, Noro S, Sakurada N (1981). Kawasaki disease and Epstein-Barr virus. Lancet 1: 938-939.

Kikuta H, Mizuno F, Osato T, Konno M, Ishikawa N, Noro S, Sakurada N (1984). Kawasaki disease and an unusual primary infection with Epstein-Barr virus. Pediatrics 73: 413-414.

Kikuta H, Mizuno F, Osato T, Konno M, Ishikawa N, Nanbu H, Anakura M, Oka Y, Matsumoto S, Noro S, Sakurada N (1983). Occurrence of Kawasaki disease and a primary Epstein-Barr virus infection. Jpn Clin J 41: 2069-2074 (in Japanese).

Kikuta H, Koizumi S, Tachibana K, Mizuno F, Osato T, Hirai K, Sakiyama Y, Matsumoto S (1985). Establishment of a marmoset line producing Kawasaki patient-born EB virus and its virus characteristics. Abstracts of Papers, 33rd Japanese Virologists Meeting, p 165 (in Japanese).

Okano M, Sakiyama Y, Matsumoto S, Osato T (1985). Epstein-Barr virus susceptibility and inducibility of Kawasaki disease patients' lymphocytes. Abstracts of Papers, 33rd Japanese Virologists Meeting, p 166 (in Japanese).

Osato T, Mizuno F, Fujiwara S, Koizumi S (1986). Human Epstein-Barr virus and Cancer. In: The Human Oncogenic Viruses (Luderer AA, Weetall HH, eds), Clifton, The Humana Press, Inc, pp 185-211.

Kawasaki Disease, pages 117-124
© 1987 Alan R. Liss, Inc.

THE ETIOLOGY OF KAWASAKI DISEASE: RETROVIRUS?

S.T. Shulman*, A.H. Rowley*, R. Fresco**, D.C. Morrison*.

*Division of Infectious Diseases, The Children's Memorial
Hospital, Department of Pediatrics, Northwestern University
Medical School, **Department of Pathology, Loyola
University Stritch Medical School.

A childhood illness that is characterized by fever,
rash, inflammatory changes of hands, feet, lips, oral
mucosa, bulbar conjunctivae, and enlarged cervical lymph
nodes would seem to be a prime candidate for having an
infectious etiology. Likewise, an illness that manifests
time and space clusters occurring at two- to three-year
intervals, superimposed upon an endemic occurrence in many
geographic areas, and demonstrating wave-like spread (Yanagawa, 1983) would appear to behave like a disorder caused
by an infectious agent. Thus, in January, 1984, at the
Makaha Kawasaki Symposium on Oahu, it was not surprising
that virtually all in attendance agreed that Kawasaki
Disease has an infectious etiology.

Reports by Leung et al (Leung et al, 1982) that striking immunoregulatory lymphocyte abnormalities are present
during the acute stage of Kawasaki Disease prompted us in
1984 to begin to give serious consideration to the possibility that a human lymphotropic viral agent such as a retrovirus might be etiologically related to this disorder. We
studied this possibility by co-culturing peripheral blood
mononuclear cells (PBMC's) from acute stage Kawasaki
Disease patients with established human lymphoblastoid cell
lines.

We have now studied 33 children admitted to The Children's Memorial Hospital in Chicago with acute Kawasaki
Disease. This represents an update of the data that were
first submitted in abstract form for presentation to The

American Federation of Clinical Research in December,
1985,(Rowley and Shulman, 1985) and reported in The Lancet
in September, 1986(Shulman and Rowley, 1986). All patients
fulfilled classic diagnostic criteria and were within 14
days of onset of illness except for two patients studied at
21 and 23 days and one at six weeks. After informed consent was obtained, 3-6 ml of heparinized blood was obtained
from patients and from healthy laboratory or febrile childhood controls. PBMC's were isolated by Ficoll-Hypaque sedimentation. We co-cultured 1×10^6 PBMC's with 1×10^6
of one of the human T lymphoblastoid cell lines MOLT-3,
MOLT-4, HUT-78, and NC-37 in the presence of 10% inter-
leukin-2 and 2.5 mcg/ml phytohemagglutinin in RPMI 1640
medium containing 10-20% fetal calf serum, L-glutamine,
penicillin and streptomycin at 37°C in humidified 5% CO_2.

Aliquots of co-culture supernates were removed from
each flask at weekly intervals for four to five weeks and
assayed for Mg^{++}-dependent reverse transcriptase, an RNA-
dependent DNA polymerase that is characteristic of retroviruses and promotes synthesis of DNA from viral RNA. Aliquots were centrifuged at 75,000g for 60 minutes, and the
pellet resuspended in a reaction mixture comprised of
TRIS-HCl with KCl, dithiothreitol, $MgCl_2$, Triton X-100,
poly (rA) oligo (dT) as a template, and tritiated thymidine
triphosphate. After incubation for 15 minutes at 0°C and
one hour at 37°C, transfer RNA was added and duplicate aliquots were spotted onto Whatman glass fiber filters, washed
immediately with trichloroacetic acid containing sodium
pyrophosphate and HCl, dried and counted. Duplicate counts
were averaged. Values were disregarded when the coefficient
of variation exceeded 20% between duplicate specimens with
a mean of at least 5,000 cpm/ml. Specimens were considered
positive for reverse transcriptase when they yielded
≥10,000 cpm/ml culture supernatant. Positive controls
included avian myeloblastosis virus reverse transcriptase,
the L1210 mouse leukemia cell line, and a fibroblast cell
line infected with murine Moloney virus. We compared the
frequency of reverse transcriptase activity in co-culture
supernatants from patients and controls by Chi square
analysis with the Yates correction for small numbers and by
Fisher's exact test. The results obtained are shown in
Table I.

TABLE I: Co-Culture Supernate Aliquots Containing
          Reverse Transcriptase Activity

	Kawasaki Disease	Controls
NC-37	1/40	0/11
HUT-78	1/86	0/74
MOLT-3	4/91	0/68
MOLT-4	10/124	2/125
Total	16/341	2/278

$$\chi^2 = 7.21, \; p < 0.01$$

Not all cell lines were used for each patient or control
accounting for the different numbers of assays in the
patient and control groups. Fourteen of the 16 positive
Kawasaki Disease supernate specimens were obtained after
co-cultivation of patient PBMC's with either the MOLT-3 or
MOLT-4 lymphoblastoid lines. Co-cultivation with HUT-78
yielded only one positive aliquot. At least one co-cultivation supernatant aliquot from 10/33 acute stage Kawasaki
Disease patients but from only 2/37 adult or childhood
controls demonstrated reverse transcriptase activity
($p < 0.02$ by Chi square analysis).

Reverse transcriptase activity was most commonly detected 7 to 14 days after initial establishment of co-
cultures, was present in one or two aliquots, and then declined. In limited experiments, this co-culture supernatant reverse transcriptase activity was not inhibited by
actinomycin D, which blocks the activity of DNA-dependent
DNA polymerases.

Several technical modifications to increase the frequency of reverse transcriptase activity in co-culture
supernates and to sustain this activity beyond one or two
determinations have been attempted. Feeder PHA-stimulated
normal adult lymphocytes, feeder PHA-stimulated human cord
blood lymphocytes, as well as the CEM and H9 cell lines
have been utilized for co-cultivation. These efforts have
not appeared to yield a higher rate of transcriptase positivity of specimens. Likewise, the addition of 1 mcg/ml Polybrene as well as anti-alpha interferon to co-cultured cells
has not been associated with more frequent supernatent
transcriptase activity. Twice-weekly or even daily supernatent assays have not yielded more frequent enzyme detection.

Attempts to passage transcriptase activity by cell-free material have met with only limited success to date. Clearly other technical modifications will be required to increase the proportion of Kawasaki Disease patients whose co-cultured lymphocytes produce reverse transcriptase and to sustain this activity in tissue culture.

We also have examined whether reverse transcriptase activity was present in sera of Kawasaki Disease patients, as had been reported in patients with non-A, non-B hepatitis.[5] We studied 19 acute sera from Kawasaki patients and 16 sera from control children for Mg^{++}-dependent reverse transcriptase activity, as well as 16 Kawasaki sera and 16 control sera for Mn^{++}-dependent enzyme activity. No significant differences in serum RT activity were detected between Kawasaki and control subjects.

Electron microscopic studies of patient PBMC's cultured alone and PBMC's co-cultured as described above have failed to date to demonstrate convincing viral particles. However, we have seen suspicious viral-like structures (160 nm in diameter) (Figure 1), but we do not believe that the structures shown in Figure 1 nor those recently published by Burns et al (Burns et al, 1986) are convincing.

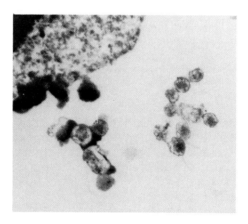

Figure 1: Co-cultured Kawasaki Disease patient PBMC's and MOLT-4 cell line. Viral-like structures (160 nm in diameter) can be seen near the cell surface, in right half of micrograph.

By electron microscopy we have also observed cytoplasmic tubuloreticular structures, which are typically induced by interferon, in a number of cultured Kawasaki Disease lymphocyte specimens (Figure 2). These structures are consistent with but are not diagnostic of viral infection.

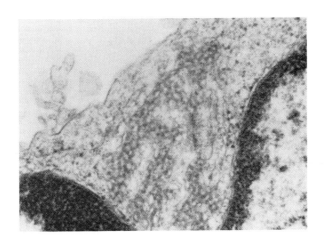

Figure 2: Co-cultured Kawasaki Disease patient PBMC demonstrating intra-cytoplasmic tubulorecticular structures consistent with viral infection (15,000X)

Prior to initiating the co-culture experiments described above, we had sought serologic evidence of human retroviral infection in Kawasaki Disease. Twenty-five acute or convalescent sera from Kawasaki Disease patients and an equal number of matched childhood controls were studied by Western blot analysis for antibody to HTLV-I and HTLV-II by Dr. Jorg Schupbach, then at the National Cancer Institute. Faint bands were initially thought to be present in six acute and one convalescent Kawasaki sera, but this was not reproducible, and it was finally concluded that no definite bands were present. In addition, a large number of Kawasaki Disease sera have been negative by both ELISA and Western blot for anti-HIV/anti-HTLV-III. By a highly sensitive immunodot method, antibody to gp120 (an HIV outer membrane envelope protein) and to gp41 (a transmembrane envelope protein of HIV and HTLV-I) was not detected in Kawasaki and matched control sera. The latter studies were performed in collaboration with Dr. John Sullivan at the University of Massachusetts. We have studied 8 convalescent Kawasaki and control sera with ELISA's that utilize whole disrupted HTLV-I and HTLV-II in collaboration with Dr. Bernard Poiesz at State University of New York, Syracuse. All sera were negative for IgG anti-HTLV-II and for IgG and IgM anti-HTLV-I.

Thus, these serologic data are essentially negative, indicating that, if a retroviral agent is involved in the etiology of Kawasaki Disease, it is apparently not closely related antigenically to currently identified human retroviruses.

However, several additional observations lend support to the possibility that Kawasaki Disease has a retroviral etiology. In collaboration with Dr. Olivia Preble of the Uniformed Services Medical School, we have measured serum interferon levels in Kawasaki patients and childhood controls. The preliminary results indicate that 17/20 Kawasaki sera but only 2/7 control sera had elevated levels of interferon (p <0.005), with alpha and/or gamma interferon found in the Kawasaki sera. Further interferon studies are in progress.

Additional support for the retroviral hypothesis of Kawasaki Disease comes from a recent report by Drs. Vijay Joshi and Ed Connor of the New Jersey Medical School in Newark (Joshi, Connor et al, 1986). They recently reported on the cardiac findings at autopsy of 15 children who died of pediatric AIDS. Seven of the 15 autopsied children demonstrated cardiovascular involvement, including three with a cardiomyopathy similar to that recently reported in adult AIDS patients. Of more interest was the finding that four of the seven children manifested an arteriopathy that involved various medium-sized arteries, including cerebral, splenic, renal, and brachial arteries. In one patient, dramatic abnormalities of the right coronary artery were present, including gross aneurysmal enlargement of the vessel (Figure 3), striking medial fibrosis and calcification, impressive intimal proliferation, and occlusion by a thrombus with resultant fatal myocardial infarction. No active inflammatory changes were apparent. Such changes appear identical to the sequelae that may be observed in "burnt-out" Kawasaki Disease. These findings

were observed in a three year old black female with AIDS
who was the daughter of an IV drug abuser. She was relatively well clinically except for severe progressive
encephalopathy. Dr. Connor served as her primary physician
for all but the first few months of her life. No acute
illness suggesting Kawasaki Disease was present at anytime.

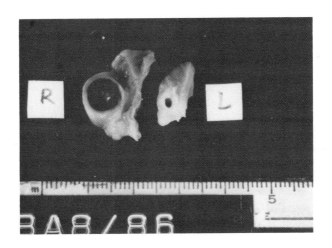

Figure 3: Cross-section of aneurysmally dilated right
coronary artery and normal sized left main coronary
artery from fatal case of pediatric AIDS (Dr. Vijay
Joshi).

We believe that the very striking similarity between
the coronary artery findings in this pediatric AIDS patient
and those observed in late or "burnt-out" Kawasaki Disease
provides additional support (albeit circumstantial) to the
thesis that Kawasaki Disease, like AIDS, may have a retroviral etiology.

Finally, if the retroviral hypothesis proves correct,
careful consideration of the epidemiologic features of
Kawasaki Disease, including its age distribution and the
apparent lack of person-person transmission, will prompt
reassessment of certain concepts of infection by human
retroviruses. This will include expansion of the spectrum
of human retroviral disorders from solely lymphoreticular
malignancies and immunodeficiency to include the broader
variety of retroviral diseases observed in animals.

REFERENCES

1. Yanagawa H, Shigematsu I (1983). Epidemiological Features of Kawasaki Disease in Japan. Acta Pediatrica Japonica. 25:94-107.
2. Leung DYM, Siegel RL, Grady S, et al (1982). Immunoregulatory abnormalities in mucocutaneous lymph node syndrome. Clin Immunol Immunopath 23:100-112.
3. Rowley AH, Pachman LM, Shulman ST (1986). Does Kawasaki Syndrome Have A Retroviral Etiology? American Federation for Clinical Research. (Abstract)
4. Shulman ST, Rowley AH (1986). Does Kawasaki Disease Have A Retroviral Etiology? Lancet II, 545-546.
5. Burns JC, Geha RS, Schneeberger EE, et al (1986). Polymerase activity in lymphocyte culture supernatents from patients with Kawasaki disease. Nature 323:814-16.
6. Joshi VV, Connor E, Oleske JM, et al (1986). Abstract #448 of the Interscience Conference on Antimicrobial Agents and Chemotherapy, New Orleans, LA.

Kawasaki Disease, pages 125-130
© 1987 Alan R. Liss, Inc.

POLYMERASE ACTIVITY IN LYMPHOCYTE CULTURE SUPERNATANTS
FROM PATIENTS WITH KAWASAKI DISEASE

Jane C.Burns *, Raif S. Geha, Jane W.
Newburger, Alice S Huang, Donald Y.M.
Leung +
Children's Hospital, Boston

INTRODUCTION

The etiology of Kawasaki disease has eluded
investigators for the last two decades since the first
report of 50 patients published by Dr. Kawasaki in
1967.

During these 20 years, epidemiologic observations
coupled with the clinical features of the illness
supported the concept that KD is an infectious disease.
At the same time, however, a substantial body of
negative data was accumulating in the search for the
etiologic agent. Candidate agents that were pursued and
then dismissed included a wide range of microbes from
rickettsiae to spirochetes, from toxin-producing
bacteria to viruses. Body secretions of every type were
subjected to various laboratory culture systems
including tissue culture and animal inoculation in an
attempt to find the elusive agent. Clues from the
remarkable immunologic abnormalities seen during acute
KD and described by Leung et al. (1982, 1983) lead us
to postulate that a lymphotropic virus with affinity for
endothelial and lymphoid cells might explain the
observed vasculitis and immunologic abnormalities in KD.
We, therefore, undertook the culture of peripheral blood
mononuclear cells (PBMC) from patients with KD in search
of a viral agent. We focused first on the retroviruses,
a family of viruses known to have tropism for lymphoid
and endothelial cells and to be difficult to cultivate
directly from patient specimens. We began by assaying

the supernatants of KD and control PBMC for
particle-associated reverse transcriptase (RT) activity.
As described in our published results (Burns et al.
1986) we found polymerase activity in the supernatants
from KD but not control PBMC cultures. This RT activity
could be transmitted to an established T cell line
(HUT-78) and thus may be due to an exogenous agent
infecting KD lymphocytes.

METHODS

Peripheral blood mononuclear cells (PBMC) were
obtained following informed consent from patients with
KD after diagnosis by one of the authors (JB or JN)
according to standard clinical criteria (Kawasaki 1967;
Melish et al. 1976). The mean age of the 14 KD
patients studied was 35.7 months (range 19 - 61 months).
A total of 27 control patients were studied. Twelve of
the controls were hospitalized patients age 9 days-19
mos. with fever and with known bacterial (6), viral (2),
or suspected viral (4) illnesses; 6 afebrile controls
were patients aged 14 mos. 30 yrs. with non-infectious
gastrointestinal, hepatobiliary, or allergic conditions;
and 9 patients with circulating DR+-T cells (Marker for
T cell activation) included 3 adults with systemic lupus
erythematosus, 5 patients with atopic dermatitis age 6
mos. - 9 yrs., and one patient (age 5 years) with acute
onset of systemic juvenile rheumatoid arthritis.

KD and control PBMC were separated from heparinized
venous blood by Ficoll-Hypaque density gradient
centrifugation and cultured as previously reported.(5)
Co-cultivation experiments were performed by subjecting
cultured PBMC from KD patients and controls to 10,000
rads on culture day 8-15, and incubating the irradiated
PBMC (density 5 x 10^8 cells/ml) with polybrene-treated,
PHA-stimulated HUT-78 cells (density: 1-2 x 10^6
cells/ml). The cultures were then maintained and
harvested in the same manner as the PBMC cultures.
Supernatants from all cultures were harvested at
3-4 day intervals and the cells split and re-fed to
maintain a density of 0.5 - 2.0 x 10^6 cells/ml.

Culture supernatants were prepared for assay by low
speed centrifugation (9,000 x g for 30 min.) to remove

cellular debris. The supernatants were then subjected to centrifugation at 100,000 x g for 90 min. and the resultant pellet resuspended in 15 μl of buffer (Buffer A) containing 50 mM Tris HCl pH 7.5, 20% (V/V) glycerol, 1 mM dithiothreitol (DTT), and 250 mM KCl. Reverse Transcriptase Assay: Specimens (15 μl) were thawed and incubated x 2 hr at 37°C with 40 μl of the following reaction mixture: 1.25 uCi ^{32}P-dTTP (NEN, Boston, MA, specific activity 600-800 Ci/mmol), 62.5 mM Tris HCl, pH 8.0, 6.25 mM DTT, 0.625% Triton X-100, 90 μM dTTP (some assays performed with all 4 dNTP's: dATP, dCTP, dGTP, and dTTP) (Boehringer Mannheim, Indianapolis, IN), 2.9 μg of poly (rA): oligo (dT) (Sigma, St. Louis, MO), and 7.5 mM MgCl . The reaction was stopped by addition of 10 mM disodium$_2$pyrophosphate and yeast RNA (1 mg/ml). Incorporation of ^{32}P-dTMP was measured by TCA precipitation and collection of the acid insoluble fraction on 0.45 micron nitrocellulose filters (Millipore). Filters were placed in liquid scintillant (Biofluor, NEN, Boston, MA) and counted in a Beckman model LS-1801 scintillation counter.

Disintegrations per minute were converted to picomoles of dTMP incorporated (specific activity: 400-850 cpm/pmole). The non-specific background (Buffer A alone) for each assay was subtracted from all values. Duplicate assays on a single specimen were averaged and this value used for statistical comparisons. The dTMP incorporation (mean picomoles + S.E.) for the particulate fraction of the HTLV I cell supernatants used as positive controls for each assay was 17.7 + 1.8 picomoles (MJ), 12.5 + 3.7 picomoles (HUT-102), and 12.3 + 1.3 picomoles (MT-2).

Culture supernatants for sucrose density gradient analysis were pooled and concentrated by centrifugation (Beckman SW27 rotor; 25,000 rpm x 90 min at 4°C). The pellet was resuspended in 100 ul of a mixture containing 10 mM Tris-HCl, pH 7.6, 100 mM NaCl, and 1 mM EDTA, pH 7.8 (TNE), layered onto a 20-60% sucrose gradient in TNE and centrifuged (Beckman SW50.1 rotor; 35,000 rpm x 16 hrs at 4°C). Fractions (500 μl) were collected from the bottom, diluted in TNE, centrifuged (Beckman SW50.1 rotor; 35,000 rpm x 90 min at 4°C), the pellet resuspended in Buffer A and assayed for reverse transcriptase activity as described. Density of sucrose was determined by refractive index measurement.

RESULTS

Over a 9 month period (3/85 - 1/86) 17 cultures were established from the PBMC of 14 KD patients. Culture supernatants from PBMC of KD patients exhibited a peak in polymerase activity between day 10 and 17 of culture. In contrast, culture supernatants of PBMC from controls contained no such activity.

Maximal polymerase activity measured at any point in the lifetime of the culture was significantly higher for KD patients than for controls (mean dTMP incorporated + S.E. was 15.3 + 5.7 picomoles for KD vs. 3.2 + 0.5 picomoles for controls; $P < .05$ by two-tailed unpaired T test). Culture supernatants of PBMC from patients with other diseases characterized by circulating activated T cells bearing HLA-Dr+ antigens (systemic lupus erythematosus, severe atopic dermatitis, and juvenile rheumatoid arthritis) showed no increase in polymerase activity compared to controls ($p > 0.1$).

Experiments to characterize the nature of this polymerase activity were performed. Heat treatment (80°C for 10 min) of the pellet, omission of template plus primer (poly rA:oligo dT) from the reaction mix, and omission of exogenous divalent cation plus addition of EDTA to the reaction mixture all greatly reduced the polymerase activity of the positive HTLV I control (MT-2) and the KD lymphocyte culture supernatants. Substitution of Mn^{++} (0.5 mM) for Mg^{++} reduced the polymerase activity by 60% (data not shown). The capacity of PBMC from KD patients to transmit this polymerase activity to the HUT-78 T cell line was also investigated. Three of the 5 co-cultures with KD PBMC showed a significant polymerase activity ($>$ mean + 2 S.D. of activity in culture supernatants from control patients) 7-12 days following the co-cultivation. Co-culture supernatants from a KD patient were pooled and the density of the particulate fraction associated with the polymerase activity was determined by sucrose density gradient. A single peak in activity was found at a buoyant density between 1.18 and 1.22 grams/ml of sucrose.

As previously reported (Burns et al. 1986) we have detected a polymerase activity which appears during the second week in culture in the supernatants of PBMC cultures from patients with KD. No such activity was associated with similar cultures from febrile patients or patients with other illnesses characterized by in vivo T cell activation. Characteristics of the polymerase from KD cultures are consistent with a Mg^{++}-dependent reverse transcriptase and suggest the possibility of a retrovirus as the causative agent of KD. The profile of polymerase activity in the PBMC cultures over time is similar to that seen with HTLV I and HIV (Yoshida et al. 1982; Levy et al. 1984). The loss of polymerase activity may be explained by: 1) culture conditions that fail to support continued growth of the agent; 2) depletion of a suitable host cell population through lytic infection; or 3) development of non-productive infection (latency) with no further production of new infectious particles and the associated polymerase.

While the current assays were performed using conditions of pH, divalent cation concentration, and template/primer specificity designed for an RNA-dependent DNA polymerase, it is possible that a polymerase with a different in vivo template preference (i.e., DNA-dependent DNA polymerase) could utilize dTTP under these experimental conditions. Insufficient data exist to permit conclusions regarding the optimal template/primer conditions.

In collaboration with Dr. Eveline E. Schneeberger, we have examined PBMC from 3 patients with acute KD by transmission electron microscopy. Rare PBMC from all 3 of these patients contained virus-like particles within intracellular vacuoles. The particles were 105-118 nm in diameter, contained an electron dense core and an outer membrane, and some appeared to bud from the vacuole membrane. Similar viral particles have not been observed in cultured PBMC from 5 control subjects. These preliminary observations support the possibility that the polymerase activity found in PBMC cultures of KD patients is associated with a virus.

While previously described human retroviral illnesses caused by HTLV I, II and HIV are usually thought of as chronic syndromes, acute infection with HIV has been reported to be associated with a self-limited illness characterized by fever, rash, lymphadenopathy, and mucositis (Cooper et al. 1985) In contrast to most patients with HTLV infection, KD patients return to their normal immunologic baseline following resolution of their acute illness. Further studies are needed to elucidate the potential role of lymphocytotropic viruses in the pathogenesis of Kawasaki Disease.

REFERENCES

Leung DYM, Siegel RL, Grady S, Krensky A, Meade R, Reinherz EL, Geha RS (1982). Immunoloregulatory abnormalities in MCLNS. Clin Immunol and Immunopathol 23:100-112.

Leung DYM, Chu ET, Wood N, Grady S, Meade R, Geha RS (1983). Immunoregulatory T-cell abnormalities in MCLNS. J Immunol 130:2002.

Kawasaki T (1967). Acute febrile MCLNS: Clinical observations of 50 cases. Japan J Allerg 16:178-222.

Melish ME, Hicks RM, Larson EJ (1976). MCLNS in the United States. Am J Dis Child 130:599.

Burns JC, Geha RS, Schneeberger EE, Newburger JN, Rosen FS, Glezen LS, Huang AS, Natale J, Leung DYM (1986). Polymerase activity in lymphocyte culture supernatants from patients with Kawasaki disease. Nature 323:814-816.

Yoshida M, Miyoshi I, Hinuma Y (1982). Isolation and characterization of retrovirus from cell lines of of human adult T-cell leukemia and its implications in the disease. Proc Natl Acad Science 79:2031-2035.

Levy JA, Hoffman AD, Kramer SM, Landis JA, Shimbabukano JM (1984). Isolation of lymphocytopathic retro-retroviruses from San Francisco patients with AIDS. Science 225:840-842.

Cooper DA, Gold J, Maclean P, Donovan B, Finlayson R, Barnes TG, Michelmore HM, Brooke P. Penny R (1985). Acute AIDS retrovirus infection. Lancet 1:537-539.

Kawasaki Disease, pages 131–139
© 1987 Alan R. Liss, Inc.

SEARCH FOR RETROVIRUS ETIOLOGY OF KAWASAKI SYNDROME.

Nyven J. Marchette*, David Ho**, Susan Kihara*,
Faith Caplan*, Marian E. Melish*

Departments of Pediatrics, Tropical Medicine and
Medical Microbiology, University of Hawaii* and
Department of Medicine, Harvard Medical School,
Massachusetts General Hospital**.

INTRODUCTION

The clinical course of Kawasaki Syndrome with its
acute febrile onset, exanthem and enanthem, basically
self-limited character, and virtual restriction to young
children has convinced nearly all workers in the field that
the disease is caused by or triggered by a microbial
agent. Conventional techniques used to search for
bacterial agents, rickettsial agents, spirochetal agents,
have not definitively demonstrated an etiologic agent
although champions of various viral, bacterial and
rickettsial agents can be found.

Conventional viral techniques have demonstrated a wide
variety of viral agents which infect children with Kawasaki
Syndrome. Using techniques of viral isolation and
serologic confirmation we have demonstrated a recent or
concomitant viral infection in over 50 percent of children
with Kawasaki Syndrome. The wide variety of agents
encountered and failure to demonstrate any unique serologic
relationships indicates that these viruses are likely to be
either incidental or to play a "helper" role in the
pathogenesis of Kawasaki Syndrome. Review of the
epidemiology of this disease suggest that the agent we are
searching for is likely to be a highly human associated
agent rather than a zoonosis. The past health history of
children with Kawasaki Syndrome does not differ from
healthy age, race and sex matched controls and demonstrates
no common parenteral exposures. The marked age restriction
of this disease to young children suggest that infection

and/or immunity occurs early in life. This etiologic agent is likely to be efficiently transmitted as suggested by the regular appearance of community-wide epidemics.

As new microbiological approaches are developed, it is logical that they should be applied to etiologic searches into disease of unknown cause. We attempted to look for evidence of reverse transcriptase activity as a possible marker or footprint for the presence of retroviruses in children with Kawasaki Syndrome. Our initial experimental approach was to attempt to precipitate virus particles with polyethylene glycol and then attempt to detect reverse transcriptase. In the first 12 patients studied by this approach, we did obtain some samples which we felt had evidence of DNA polymerase activity. However, we became aware that we were dealing with polymerase activity of a relatively low magnitude and that polyethylene glycol was inhibiting its detection. Therefore we abandoned that approach. In this communication we discuss 11 patients with acute Kawasaki Syndrome who were evaluated using techniques for reverse transcriptase detection modified from several protocols of established retrovirus investigators.

MATERIALS AND METHODS

Patients - Eleven consecutively encountered patients with Kawasaki Syndrome were studied at least once during the course of their illness. All patients met strict diagnostic criteria for Kawasaki Syndrome and all had initial studies in the first 10 days of illness.

Peripheral blood mononuclear samples are collected by Ficoll-Hypaque sedimentation and set up in culture at a density of 1×10^6 cells/ml in tissue culture medium RPMI with 10 ugm/ml of phytohemagglutinin. Cultures are incubated for 2 days at 37° in 5% CO_2. At 2 days the media is replaced with fresh medium containing 0.5 ugm/ml of interleukin-II, .1% anti-alpha interferon and 1 ugm/ml polybrene. This is incubated for a further 2 days after which the supernatant fluid is again harvested and replaced with HUT 78 cells or MOLT-4 cells in fresh media. Cell number is maintained at a density of 0.5 to 1×10^6/ml. Supernatant fluids are harvested at 2-3 day intervals for the remainder of the culture.

The DNA polymerase assay is performed by clarifying
the supernatant fluid by slow centrifugation to precipitate
cells and debris. The supernatant fluid is pelleted at
25,000 rpm in a swinging bucket rotor in an
ultracentrifuge. The pellet is resuspended in 10 uM Tris,
100 uM NaCl, 1 uM EDTA, freeze thawed twice and allowed to
react with Tris-HCl buffer, Dithiothreitol, bovine serum
albumin, freshly prepared glutathion EDTA and the
synthetic homopolymer template primer Poly rA:Oligo dT.
After addition of labelled tritiated thymidine triphosphate
the mixture is incubated at 37° for 60 minutes. The
reaction is then stopped with transfer RNA and sodium
pyrophosphate. The product is precipitated with cold 10%
TCA and collected on a TCA soaked glass fiber filter,
rinsed with sodium phyrophosphate and counted. For each
assay, a negative control of supernatant fluid from 3 day
cultures of MOLT-4 and HUT 78 cells were run. All results
are given with values for this negative control subtracted
from the experimental findings. In addition, positive
controls of supernatants from tissue culture cells infected
with HTLV-I virus, HTLV-III virus and human syncytia
forming virus were run in every assay.

RESULTS

9 of 11 patients had
elevated values of reverse
transcriptase-like
activity compared with
none from 10 child
controls with other
febrile exanthematous
illnesses. It can be seen
that, with one exception,
the peak values for
picomoles of labelled
thymidine monophosphate
incorporated were
generally low; in the same
range but slightly lower
than that encountered with
HTLV-I infected cells and
considerably lower than
that seen in cells
infected with HTLV-III.
(Figure 1)

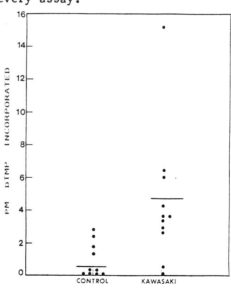

Fig. 1. Peak reverse
transcriptase activity for
11 K.S. pts. and 10 controls.

The general pattern was for peak polymerase values to occur on days 8 to 13 in culture. (Figure 2)

FIGURE 2

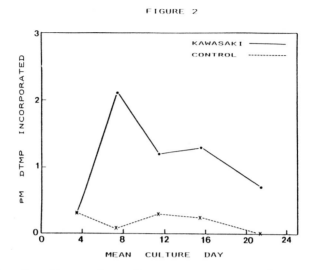

Fig. 2. Mean values for reverse transcriptase activity expressed as pM dDTMP incorporated by day in culture of 11 K.S. patients and 10 controls.

Individual patterns can be seen in Figures 3-5. Patient 1, studied on day 5 of disease, had a sharp peak in

FIGURE 3

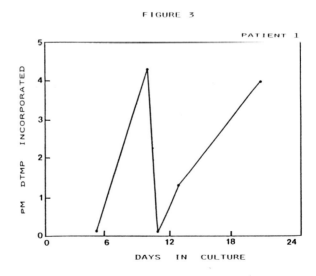

polymerase activity when tested on day 9 in culture. By
day 11 no activity could be detected, however on day 13 the
value of almost 2 times baseline was obtained and on day 21
another peak of activity was seen. After this
determination the culture was no longer viable.

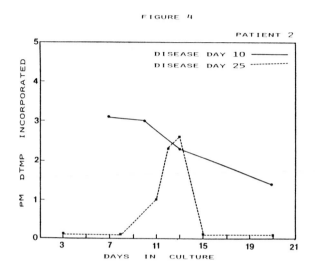

FIGURE 4

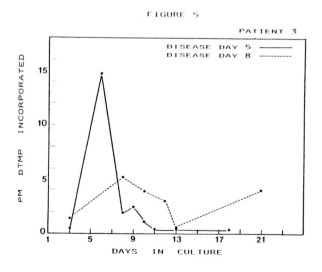

FIGURE 5

Patient 2 (Fig. 4) had modestly elevated values on culture days 7, 9, 12, and 21 when tested on disease day 10. Later in the illness he was retested and found to have elevated values on days 12 and 13 in culture.

Patient 3 (Fig. 5) showed a sharp peak of activity to higher than usual levels in our experience when tested on day 5 at 7 days in culture. When tested on day 8 of disease, a more modest elevation was seen and when tested on days 14 and day 80 after onset, no RT activity could be detected.

DNA polymerase activity was characterized by comparing results with different template primer combinations. Using our usual template combination Poly rA:Oligo dT we have demonstrated elevated values in 9 of 11 patients tested. Several patients had multiple elevations noted. Using the template primer combination Poly rC:Oligo dG, we found essentially no activity in 5 of 5 samples tested which had been positive with the Poly rA:Oligo dT template. The template Poly dA:Oligo dT is usually utilized as a marker for cellular polymerases. Nearly equivalent quantities of polymerase were detected using this template. (Table I)

TABLE I

Template:Primer	Culture	Comment
Poly rA:Oligo dT	9/11	Usual Template
Poly rC:Oligo dG	0/5	Usual Retrovirus Preference
Poly dA:Oligo dT	5/5	Usual Cellular Polymerase

Serologic study of the 11 Kawasaki Syndrome patients showed that all were negative to HTLV-I and HIV at less than 10 days of illness and week 8 of illness.

During the course of these investigations, we saw evidence of syncytia-forming activity in peripheral blood mononuclear cell cultures from 2 patients. Electronmicrographs showed the presence of myxovirus-like virus particles within cultured lymphocytes. Further investigation demonstrated that both of these children had recently been immunized with measles vaccine and both seroconverted to measles concomitant with their Kawasaki Syndrome.

DISCUSSION

Our investigations have demonstrated elevated levels of DNA polymerase in the particulate fraction of PBMC culture supernatants. We detected this activity in 9 of 11 Kawasaki patients compared with 0 of 10 febrile child controls. We demonstrated that peak polymerase activity is present in a strictly time limited fashion in cultures from 6 to 22 days. The peak polymerase activity detected was present at relatively low concentrations, generally equal to or below that seen with HTLV-I infected cells and considerably lower than seen with HIV infected cells. These characteristics were also noted by Shulman, et al[1] and Burns, et al[2] in their reports of reverse transcriptase-like activity in K.S. patients' PBMC cultures. Preliminary studies with template preference indicate that artifactual detection of reverse transcriptase due to the presence of cellular polymerases is a distinct possibility in our system. We have tested all of our patients for evidence of antibody to human retroviruses HTLV-I and HIV and have found all to be negative, thus proving that infection with these retroviruses is not the reason for their elevated DNA polymerase activity. Finally we noted that measles vaccine virus was isolated from 2 PBMC cultures and seen in cultured cells studied by electron microscopy, thus demonstrating non-specificity of visualization of virus particles.

The fact that recurrent disease occurs occasionally in Kawasaki Syndrome suggests that a highly cell associated agent may be the cause of Kawasaki Syndrome. A cell associated virus such as a herpes virus or a retrovirus would be able to establish persistent infection of cells, establish latency and occasionally emerge to again cause typical illness. From 1971 to 1986 we encountered 9 (2.3%) of 390 patients who had documented recurrent disease. More undocumented recurrences have been suggested by clinical history but could not be confirmed by physician examination and/or laboratory testing. 8 patients had 2 episodes of Kawasaki Syndrome and 1 patient had 3 episodes. Recurrence interval was a mean of 1.6 years but ranged from 2 months to 8 years. 4 patients had recurrence within 6 months of their original attack. In each case, return of sedimentation rate and all clinical parameters to normal was documented prior to recurrent disease.

Figure 6 shows a most interesting patient who had lymphocyte subset studies done during his first and second recurrences of Kawasaki Syndrome. The first attack of Kawasaki Syndrome had occurred 6 months previously; we have no data of lymphocyte subsets during that attack. A low level of T suppressor cells resulting in an elevated T_4/T_8 ratio, persisted despite clinical resolution and return of sedimentation rate, C-reactive protein and alpha-1 antitrypsin measures of acute inflammation to normal. This patient was treated with aspirin in his first recurrence and gamma globulin in his second recurrence. Coincident with the administration of gamma globulin, the T_8 level returned to the normal range for the first time in our observation of this child. This case particularly suggests persistent infection.

FIGURE 6

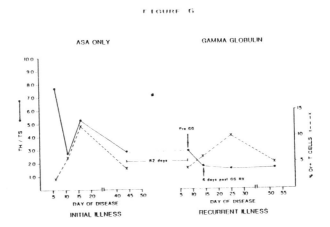

In conclusion, elevated DNA polymerase activity in cultured PBMC from K.S. patients has been reported by 2 other groups using different methodologies, Drs. Stanford Shulman and Anne Rowley and their group at Northwestern University and Dr. Jane Burns and her group at Harvard University. These exciting discoveries have opened new avenues for research. Because of clinical features of acute illness with fever, rash and mucositis such as has been reported with acute HIV infections and the phenomenon of recurrent disease in Kawasaki Syndrome, a highly cell associated retrovirus is a particularly attractive candidate etiologic agent. We are hopeful that reverse transcriptase-like activity may be a footprint of the presence of a novel human virus or retrovirus as the etiologic agent in Kawasaki Syndrome. However, preliminary data on template preference indicates in our system at least "reverse transcriptase" detection may be an artifact.

Our experience also demonstrates the need for caution in interpreting virus particles seen in electronmicrographs. Other agents which are incidental or concomitant infections during the course of Kawasaki Syndrome such as vaccine viruses and other common viruses may be "fellow travellers" rather than the etiologic agent of K.S. Isolation, characterization and demonstration of a unique serologic relationship will still be required to establish that any potential candidate etiologic agent is the cause of Kawasaki Syndrome.

REFERENCES

1. Shulman, Stanford T., Rowley, Ann H.: Does Kawasaki disease have a retroviral aetiology? Lancet, September 6, 1986:545-546.

2. Burns, J.S., Geha, R.S., Schneeberger, E.E., Newburger, J.W., Rosen, F.S., et al.: Polymerase activity in lymphocyte culture supernatants from patients with Kawasaki disease. October 30, 1986, Nature, 323:814-16.

Kawasaki Disease, pages 141-144
© 1987 Alan R. Liss, Inc.

DISCUSSION OF ETIOLOGY

Alfred S. Evans

Department of Epidemiology
and Public Health
Yale University School of Medicine
60 College St. Box 3333
New Haven, CT, 06510

While much work has been presented in this
symposium on the possible etiology of Kawasaki
Disease, it is still not clear if it is a single
disease or a syndrome, whether the cause is, in
fact, an infectious agent, and if so, if there
are one or more causative agents. Certainly,
other risk factors are involved. The limitations
to the age group around two suggests three pos-
sibilities: the agent is common but the disease
is unique, the agent is unique but usually clinically expressed, or the immunological response
is unique to several agents. I favor the first
possibility on the basis of general analogies in
the field of viral infections but I have no
proof. We have been presented with evidence in
support of several possible etiological agents
including spirochetes, bacteria and viruses.
Perhaps it would be wise to review the historical
evolution of the criteria for proving causation,
a subject I have reviewed in the past (1) and
where the references to which I allude can be
found.

The gold standard of the postulates of causation are the Henle-Koch postulates. Henle
proposed some guidelines in 1840, 42 years before
Koch described the isolation of the tubercule
bacillus in 1882 and proposed the postulates that
bear his name; they were further elaborated in
his paper of 1890. I should also acknowledge the

work of Edwin Klebs with which I recently became familiar who isolated the tubercule bacillus before Koch and in 1877 proposed a similar set of postulates for causation.

The Henle-Koch postulates are shown below:
1. The parasite occurs in every case of the disease in question and under circumstances which can account for the pathological changes and clinical course of the disease.
2. It occurs in no other disease as a fortuitous and nonpathogenic parasite.
3. After being fully isolated from the body and repeatedly grown in pure culture, it can induce the disease anew.

Note that the organism must be <u>consistently</u> isolated from the lesion and its's effect must make biological sense in terms of the pathological and clinical picture. The limitations of the postulates must also be recognized, some of which Koch discussed himself. For example, cholera, typhoid fever, diphtheria and leprosy did not fulfill his criteria, the first three as the disease could not be reproduced in experimental animals and leprosy because it also could not be grown in pure culture, an achievement which we have not yet made. So Koch thought it necessary to fulfill only two of the postulates. Later the asymptomatic and long term healthy carrier state was recognized so his postulate two was in invalid - the parasite could exist at a nonpathogen under certain circumstances. We later learned that such carrier organisms can exist in the experimental animal or tissue culture system we are using and be mistaken for the real causative agent.

After viruses were discovered, Tom Rivers re-stated the postulates in 1937 and introduced the concept of the need to show an immune response. Twenty years later Bob Huebner added epidemiological criteria and the critical requirement that a vaccine prepared from the putative causative agent should protect against the disease. In 1976 I emphasized that any

single syndrome could be produced by several
different causes depending on the age, geographic
location, season and other factors and that the
same agent could also produce other clinical
syndromes. I emphasized that we are ignorant of
many of the causative agents involved in our
syndromes of common illnesses of the respiratory,
gastrointestinal, and central nervous systems.
I also suggested a set of "Unified Guidelines"
(1) that might be useful for both infectious and
non-infectious diseases. On a simplified basis
for Kawasaki syndrome, it is important to show
that cause preceded the effect -ie that any
putative agent and it's antibody be shown to be
absent prior to the disease and to be
demonstrable during the course of illness. The
presence of latent agents in our tissues that
might be reactivated during the acute infection
makes this very important. One should also
realize that the later manifestations of the
infection might not be due to the agent directly
but to immunological consequences induced by it.

Finally, the importance of other risk factors
that provoke the infection into clinical
expression must be recognized. In order to
proceed in a systematic fashion I recommend that
a bank be established with sera and secretions
not only from patients but also from siblings and
other close contacts. A collection from healthy
children between six and 24 months in an area of
high incidence bled prior to the disease may also
be of great value in establishing causation, the
occurrence of other clinical and subclinical
forms of the disease and in the temporal relation
of the agent to the disease. Even now, such
collections would be useful in evaluating the
current candidate agents. At present, I would
look for reverse transcriptase, alterations in
platelet count and in the sedimentation rate in
close contacts of cases in the hopes of
elucidating the epidemiology of the disease. In
these endeavors, one must forget the clinical
criteria once provided with an index case.

As one who struggled for over 20 years seeking the epidemiology and etiology of infectious mononucleosis, I can speak with authority on the many false leads along the way, the need for innovative techniques, and the importance of prospective serological proof of causation. Good luck.

1. Evans, A.S. Causation and Disease: The Henle-Koch postulates revisited. Yale J. Biol. and Med. 1976: 49:149-195.

Kawasaki Disease, pages 145–147
© 1987 Alan R. Liss, Inc.

DISCUSSION:

ETIOLOGY OF KAWASAKI DISEASE

Dr. M. Takahashi (Osaka) reported preliminary findings
of reverse transcriptase activity in cell culture
supernatents from two Kawasaki patients and one sibling.
Dr. H. Kato (Kurume) found 1 of 4 Kawasaki patients whose
lymphocytes were co-cultured with H9 cells to manifest
reverse transcriptase activity, but at levels below that
seen with HIV. In response to Dr. L. Schonberger's
(Atlanta) question, Dr. J. Burns (Boston) indicated that
reverse transcriptase activity was detected in lymphocyte
cultures established as long as 9 years after Kawasaki
Disease. Dr. D. Leung (Boston) suggested that assay for
reverse transcriptase activity 3 times weekly enabled much
better detection than twice weekly sampling, suggesting
that positives could be missed with lower frequency
sampling. Drs. S. Shulman (Chicago), J. Burns and M.
Melish (Honolulu) agreed that no relationship between
reverse transcriptase positivity and aneurysm formation or
racial background had been demonstrated, and Dr. Melish
pointed out that the etiologic agent would be expected to
be recovered from patients with all degrees of illness.
Dr. W. Parks (Miami) noted that reverse transcriptase is a
difficult assay to standardize and suggested that sudden
changes in transcriptase activity could represent death of
a susceptible cell population which might be associated
with release of cellular DNA polymerases. He suggested
that the latter needs to be excluded very carefully by
extensive kinetic and template studies as well as sizing
and banding experiments, and pointed out that template
specificity is less important than some believe.

Retroviral serologic data were discussed. Dr. Kato reported negative HTLV-I, -II, and -III antibody levels in sera of 40 Kawasaki patients and controls. Dr. A. Rauch (Atlanta) reported negative HTLV-I, -II, and -III serology on 41 Kawasaki patients by ELISA and Western blot, in addition to negative antibody to STLV-III which cross-reacts with HTLV-IV. Dr. Shulman agreed that to date all serologic data in Kawasaki Disease are negative re known human retroviruses and suggested that this would be consistent with either that Kawasaki Disease is unrelated to a retrovirus, or that a retrovirus quite different antigenically from known human retroviruses is involved.

Dr. Ikawa (Tokyo) asked whether the electron micrograph shown by Dr. Burns had the morphology of the Spumavirinae. Dr. Parks indicated that Spumavirinae possess a small electron dense core that is completely formed before the particle buds externally or internally and have electron-dense glycoprotein surface projections. The published electron micrograph showed budding particles lacking both a completely formed nucleoid and cell surface projections.

Dr. A. Rowley (Chicago) asked whether any cellular changes were observed by light microscopy in lymphocyte cultures in Boston, and Dr. Leung indicated that some decreased cell viability, very rare giant cells and occasional intracellular vacuoles had been seen.

Dr. G. Koren (Toronto) asked whether there was any evidence of an increased susceptibility to infection in patients with Kawasaki Disease. Dr. Melish indicated that her case-control study failed to show an increase in infectious or allergic disorders before the development of Kawasaki Disease, and that patients appeared healthy in follow-up. Dr. Leung reported that a blinded study of the frequency of atopic dermatitis during Kawasaki Disease follow-up found a higher frequency of atopic dermatitis compared to a control group of cardiac patients. He speculated that this might be related to suppressor T cell changes.

Dr. A. Brown (New York) inquired about a potential interplay between vaccination and Kawasaki Disease, and Dr. Ikawa asked about the percentage of Kawasaki Disease patients that have not been vaccinated. Dr. Melish responded that most but not all Kawasaki Disease children have been exposed to polio vaccine but more than 30% have not received measles vaccine. Dr. Rauch noted that a small number of U.S. patients had never been immunized against polio and that, when the age of measles vaccination in the U.S was increased from 12 to 15 months, there was a decrease in the mean age of Kawasaki Disease with a higher percentage of cases occurring in children less than 15 months. Dr. H. Yanagawa (Tochigi) pointed out that the increase in cases of Kawasaki Disease in Japan antedated routine measles vaccination, that the mean age of measles vaccination in Japan is greater than the peak age for Kawasaki Disease, and that a detailed case-control study indicated no difference re measles vaccination rates. Drs. W. Mason and M. Takahashi (Los Angeles) reported on two very young children (2 weeks and 2 months old) who had never been vaccinated but who developed Kawasaki Disease with giant coronary aneurysms.

Dr. N. Kobayashi (Tokyo) noted that some years ago Dr. Ben Landing had suggested the possibility that Kawasaki Disease could represent a virus-induced vasculitis, and the recent retrovirus data would support this. However, questions re the route of spread and how to account for the epidemiologic characteristics of Kawasaki Disease remain unanswered.

Kawasaki Disease, pages 149-157
© 1987 Alan R. Liss, Inc.

ANIMAL MODELS OF KAWASAKI   DISEASE

THOMAS J. A. LEHMAN MD,FAAP,FARA,

Assistant Professor of Pediatrics, University
of Southern California School of Medicine,
and Director, Rheumatology Research
Laboratory, Division of Rheumatology,
Childrens Hospital of Los Angeles, 4650
Sunset Blvd, Los Angeles, CA 90027.

The etiology and pathogenesis of Kawasaki
disease remain uncertain. Etiologies as diverse
as chemical toxins, allergic reactions, and
bacterial or retroviral infection have been
proposed, but none has been conclusively established. In the absence of a recognized etiologic agent the role of immune responses in the
pathogenesis of Kawasaki's disease remains uncertain. In animal model studies, asymmetric
inflammatory coronary arteritis has been elicited
in mice by the injection of Candida albicans
[Murata, 1979] Streptococcus pyogenes [Cromartie
and Craddock, 1966], and Lactobacillus casei
[Lehman et al, 1985]. Pseudomonas aeruginosa has
also been utilized to induce coronary arteritis
in mice, but is effective only if the mice are
pretreated with alkylating agents which impair
the normal immunologic response [Keren and
Wolman, 1984]. A periarteritis-like picture has
also been induced in rats by the injection of
live Erysipelothrix rhusiopathiae [Shinomiya and
Nakato, 1985].

In my laboratory we have concentrated on the arteritis which follows a single intraperitoneal injection of nonviable Lactobacillus casei cell wall fragments in aqueous suspension [Lehman et al, 1985]. Knowledge of the precise time of disease initiation and the initiating 'antigen' has allowed us to study the natural history of the coronary arteritis and the accompanying immune response as they evolve from the earliest phases into the static, chronic phase of the disease. This model appears to be unique in demonstrating not only acute myocarditis with aneurysm formation, but also chronic scarring of the coronary arteries with the formation of stenotic segments, luminal obstruction, and evidence of coronary artery thrombosis. These findings closely parallel those descibed in children who have undergone either coronary artery biopsy or late followup coronary artery angiography [Sasaguri and Kato, 1982], [Suzuki et al, 1986].

The group B L. casei cell wall fragments utilized in this study were derived from ATCC strain 11578. As previously described in detail [Lehman et al, 1983], the bacteria were harvested from log phase growth in Lactobacillus MRS broth (Difco), washed, and subjected to detergent lysis by suspension in 4 % SDS overnight at room temperature. Following detergent lysis the bacterial fragments were washed extensively to remove all residual SDS then further purified by sequential incubation with DNAse, RNAse, and trypsin to remove noncell-wall materials. These cell wall fragments were then sonicated for two hours using a Heat Systems Ultrasonic W 375 sonicator (Ithaca, NY) while being maintained in a dry ice ethanol bath. The resultant small fragments remaining in the supernatant following centrifugation for 1 hour at 20,000 g were quantitated using a phenol:sulphuric acid extraction method. Within three days following the intraperitoneal injection of 500 micrograms of L. casei cell wall fragments, mononuclear cells can be seen accumulating in the fibrous tissues adjacent to the

coronary arteries and aortic root. This lesion
progresses over the following days, and by day 14
an asymmetric inflammatory lesion invading all
layers of the vessel wall is evident, with disruption of the arterial intima, media, and
adventitia (Figures 1 and 2). This destruction
of the vessel wall is often accompanied by true
aneurysm formation. Also found during the early
stage of the illness are varying degrees of
myocarditis and involvement of the aortic valve.
Following a large dose of cell wall materials
some mice develop severe arteritis which may be
accompanied by inflammatory invasion of the
aortic root. The lesions consist primarily of
large mononuclear cells including lymphocytes,
fibroblasts, plasma cells, and macrophages.
Polymorphonuclear cells are relatively few in
number, but 'nuclear dust' which may represent
polymorphonuclear cells is frequently seen in
early active lesions. Electron micrographic
studies performed on mice sacrificed 14 days
following injection have confirmed that the
majority of cells in the lesion are 'activated'
fibroblasts surrounding large numbers of
macrophages and histiocytes within the lesion.
Plasma cells and mast cells are also present in
increased numbers. Scanning electron microscopic
evaluation of the lesions has demonstrated the
adherence of lymphocytes and macrophages to the
endothelial surface of both the aortic root and
the coronary arteries, and on transmission
electron microscopy apparent fusion of macrophage
and endothelial cell cytoplasm can be seen.

Sequential sacrifice of mice following the
induction of disease has indicated that there is
progressive adventitial fibrosis surrounding the
coronary arteries. In mice sacrificed 180 days
after injection of L. casei cell walls evidence
of thrombosis and recanalization is seen in some,
while in others there is complete obliteration of
the coronary artery orifice. Marked smooth
muscle hyperplasia producing thickened stenotic
coronary artery segments occurs frequently
(Figures 3 and 4). These stenotic coronary

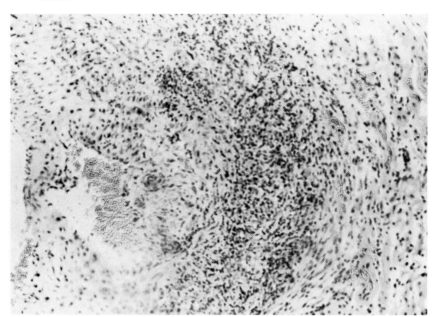

Fig. 1

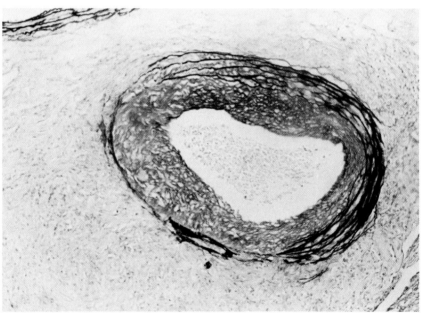

Fig. 2

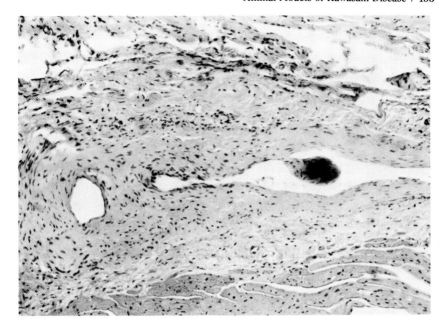

Fig. 3

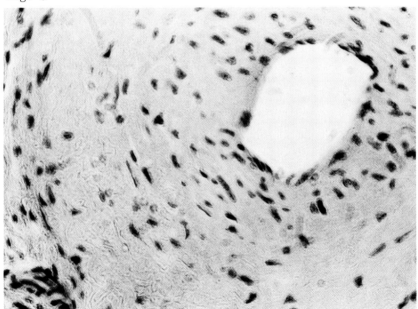

Fig. 4

artery segments would not be expected to increase
in caliber as the animal grows and may therefore
be expected to predispose the mouse to myocardial
infarction long after the acute phase of the
illness has resolved. Lesions such as this are
of particular concern because similar fibrosis
has been described in the coronary arteries of
children 'recovered' from Kawasaki's disease.

In order to improve our understanding of
the role of various components of the immune
system in this disease process we have evaluated
the induction of coronary arteritis in a variety
of inbred mouse strains with well-characterized
defects of their immune responses. Immunologically intact C57BL/6, BALB/C, and C3H/HebFej mice
all developed obvious coronary arteritis following the intraperitoneal injection of L. casei
cell wall fragments. A/J mice which lack C5
developed typical appearing coronary arteritis,
and also Aschoff-like lesions previously thought
to be pathognomonic of rheumatic fever-like
illnesses. CBA/N mice with defective antibody
production because they lack Lyb5$^+$ B cells, nude
A/J and nude C57BL/6 mice which lack normal T
cell function, C57BL/6-G 'beige mice which lack
natural killer cell function, and WBB6 mice which
lack normal mast cell function all developed
coronary arteritis of varying intensity following
the injection of L. casei cell wall fragments,
but in each case the disease in these mice lacked
the full intensity seen in immunologically intact
mice. Only the C3H/Hej mouse with its LPS
response defective macrophages completely failed
to develop evidence of coronary arteritis among
all the inbred strains tested. These studies
appear to confirm the important role of the
macrophage in the initiation of coronary arteritis in this model system and suggest that it may
play a significant role in the initiation of
Kawasaki's disease. However, full expression of
the inflammatory lesion appears to require intact
humoral and cell-mediated immunity as well.

An important advantage of this model is the
opportunity to study the effect of a variety of
potential therapeutic regimens for both their
short term effect on the preservation of coronary
artery architecture as evidenced by the histologic appearance of the coronary arteries following treatment and their effect on survival in
longer term studies. Hydroxychloroquine therapy
was associated with superior preservation of the
coronary artery architecture and lumen in short
term animal studies [Katz et al, 1986].
Unpublished anecdotal reports also suggest that
hydroxychloroquine may be an effective therapy in
children with Kawasaki's disease. However, long
term studies which may demonstrate its super-
iority in mice are not yet completed, and its
safety and efficacy for use in children with
Kawasaki's disease remain to be established.

The goals of an animal model are to allow
the study of the natural history of a disease
throughout its time course, to allow the evaluation of potential drug therapies, and to
provide insight into the etiology and pathogenesis of the disease being modeled. Studies of
the Lactobacillus casei cell wall-induced model
of coronary arteritis have demonstrated it to be
a useful model for the study of the natural
history of the cardiac and coronary artery
lesions which accompany Kawasaki's disease.
Whether this model also provides insight into the
etiology of Kawasaki's Disease in children
remains to be determined.

Studies of the pathogenesis of atherosclerosis have led to the hypothesis that a
number of agents can injure the endothelial or
subendothelial surface, all leading to subsequent
damage which appears similar [Ross et al, 1984].
The Lactobacilli are a unique genus of gram
positive bacteria which are widespread in the
environment including standing bodies of water,
and commonly found in the normal mammalian
enteric flora [London, 1976]. In additon they

are commonly found in fermenting food stuffs
where they are able to survive far greater levels
of acidity than other genera [Jay, 1986].
Fermenting vegetable products which have not been
pasturized are consumed in increased amounts by
oriental peoples with peak consumption during the
winter. These findings are suggestive. However,
whether the Lactobacilli play a role in the
initiation of Kawasaki's disease in children is
unknown. I do not personally believe that a
single etiologic agent for Kawasaki's disease
will be discovered. In addition to L. casei, L.
acidophillus has also been shown to be capable of
initiating coronary arteritis in my laboratory.
It is likely that a variety of agents will prove
capable of initiating an inflammatory response
leading to Kawasaki's disease just as a variety
of bacteria have been shown to initiate some but
not all cases of Reiter's syndrome [Calin, 1985].
Only by understanding the subsequent immune
response will we be able to better understand
Kawasaki's disease and decrease its morbidity and
mortality.

REFERENCES

Calin A (1985). Reiter's syndrome, in Textbook of
  Rheumatology, Kelley WN, Harris ED, Ruddy S,
  Sledge CB edits, WB Saunders, Philadelphia.

Cromartie WJ, Craddock JG (1966). Rheumatic-like
  cardiac lesion in mice. Science 154:283-284.

Jay JM edit (1986). Modern Food Microbiology.
3rd edition. Reinhold, New York City.

Katz AR, Mahnovski V, Lehman TJA (1986). The
  influence on healing of various treatment
  regimens in an animal model of the coronary
  arteritis associated with Kawasaki disease.
  Arthritis Rheum 29:S25 (abstract).

Keren G, Wolman M (1984). Can Pseudomonas
  infection in experimental animals mimic
  Kawasaki's disease. J Infect 9:22-29.

Lehman TJA, Allen JB, Plotz PH, Wilder RL (1983). Polyarthritis in rats following the systemic injection of Lactobacillus casei cell walls in aqueous suspension. Arthritis Rheum 26:1259-1265.

Lehman TJA, Walker SM, Mahnovski V, McCurdy D (1985). Coronary arteritis in mice following the systemic injection of group B Lactobacillus casei cell walls in aqueous suspension. Arthritis Rheum 28:652-659.

London JC (1976). The ecology and taxonomic status of the Lactobacilli. Annu Rev Microbiol 30:279-301.

Murata H (1970). Experimental Candida-induced arteritis in mice: Relation to arteritis in the mucocutaneous lymph node syndrome. Microbiol Immunol 23:825-831.

Ross R, Faggiotto A, Bowen-Pope D, Raines E (1984). The role of endothelial injury and platelet macrophage interaction in athero-sclerosis. Circulation 70(sup III):77-82.

Sasaguri Y, Kato H (1982). Regression of aneurysms in Kawasaki disease: A pathological study. J Pediatr 100:255-231.

Shinomiya K, Nakato H (1985). An experimental model of arteritis: Periarteritis induced by Erysipelothrix Rhusiopathiae in young rats. Int J Tiss Reac 7:267-271.

Suzuki A, Kamiya T, Kuwahara N, Ono Y, Kohata T, Takahashi O, Kimura K, Takamiya M (1986). Coronary arterial lesions of Kawasaki disease: Cardiac catheterization findings of 1100 cases. Pediatr Cardiol 7:3-7.

Kawasaki Disease, pages 159-165
© 1987 Alan R. Liss, Inc.

IMMUNOLOGIC ABNORMALITIES IN KAWASAKI SYNDROME

Donald Y. M. Leung

Department of Pediatrics, Harvard Medical School;
Division of Allergy, The Children's Hospital,
Boston, Massachusetts 02115

Kawasaki Syndrome (KS) is an acute illness of unknown
etiology which occurs primarily during infancy and early
childhood. Its clinical course is characterized by prolonged
fever, diffuse mucosal inflammation, indurative edema of the
hands and feet, skin rash, and lymphadenopathy (Kawasaki,
1967; Yanagihara and Todd, 1980). This disease has aroused
much interest because of its association with sudden death
due to aneurysms and thrombotic occlusion of the coronary
arteries (Kato et al., 1975; Kawasaki, 1971).

Although multiple factors are likely to be involved in
the etiology of KS, several previous observations suggest
that immunoregulatory abnormalities are involved in the pathogenesis of this disease. First, the reported incidence of
KS is much higher in Japan than elsewhere in the world and
a disproportionate number of cases reported in the United
States occur in patients of Oriental background. Kato evaluated the frequency of HLA antigens in KS in Japan and found
HLA-BW22 to be statistically more common in patients with KS
as compared to controls (Kato et al. 1978). An increased
incidence of HLA-Bw51 has also been reported in Caucasian
children with KS (Krensky et al., 1981). The association of
an HLA phenotype with children who develop KS suggests the
possibility that immune responsiveness to certain unidentified
antigens genetically predispose to the development of this
disease. Second, the histopathologic findings in KS indicate
a panvasculitis with endothelial necrosis, immunoglobulin
deposition, and mononuclear cell infiltration into small and
medium-sized blood vessels (Hirose and Hamashima, 1978;
Landing and Larson, 1977). Despite the attention focused on

the occurrence of coronary arteritis in this disease, aneurysms of other medium-sized arteries also occur (Tanaka
et al., 1976). In addition, venulitis is a prominent finding
in autopsy studies of patients who have died from acute KS
(Fujiwara and Hamashima, 1978). Third, the acute phase of
KS is characterized by a deficiency of circulating suppressor/
cytotoxic T cells, increased numbers of activated helper T
cells and a marked increase in the number of activated B cells
spontaneously secreting IgG and IgM antibody (Leung et al.,
1982; Kuno-Saka, 1985). The antibody repertoire however, that
is activated in these patients is poorly defined. With few
exceptions, each of the immunoregulatory abnormalities resolve
during the convalescence phase of KS.

Since damage to the vascular endothelium is believed to
play an important role in the pathogenesis of KS, our laboratory recently examined the possibility that patients with
acute KS generated cytotoxic antibodies against vascular endothelial cells (Leung et al., 1976). Initial studies indicated
that neither sera from patients with KS nor sera from age-
matched controls had cytotoxic effects on cultured human umbilical vein endothelial (HUVE) cells. Since activated
helper T cells similar to those present in acute KS secrete
gamma interferon (γ-IFN), a potent inducer of new endothelial
cell surface antigens such as major histocompatibility complex
(MHC) class I and class II antigens (Pober et al., 1983), we
also examined the effects of sera from acute KS on HUVE cells
preincubated for 3-5 days with γ-IFN. We found that IgM antibodies in sera from patients with acute KS cause complement-
mediated killing of γ-IFN-treated endothelial cells. The
cytotoxic antibodies circulating during acute KS appear to be
directed against inducible antigenic determinants present on
γ-IFN-treated human vascular endothelial cells but not on
control or γ-IFN-treated autologous human dermal fibroblasts
nor on human vascular smooth muscle cells. Since γ-IFN induces the same level of class I or class II MHC antigen expression on fibroblasts, smooth muscle cells and endothelial
cells, the antigens recognized by acute KS sera are probably
not MHC determinants. This conclusion was further strength-
ened by the observation that when sera from acute KS sera was
absorbed with γ-IFN treated HUVE, B cells, monocytes, T cells
or erythrocytes only γ-IFN treated HUVE removed the cytotoxic
anti-endothelial cell activity (Leung et al., 1986).

The vascular lesion found during the acute phase of KS
is infiltrated with monocyte/macrophages as well as activated

T lymphocytes. Activated monocyte/macrophages secrete the mediators, interleukin-1 (IL-1) and tumor necrosis factor (TNF) which induce HUVE cells to express tissue factor-like procoagulant activity (Bevilacqua et al., 1984) and also induces HUVE cells to become more adherent for leukocytes (Bevilacqua et al., 1985). Concomitant with these functional changes in HUVE cells, TNF and IL-1 can induce HUVE cells to express a new surface antigen detected by the monoclonal a ti-body, H4/18 (Pober et al., 1986). All these IL-1or TNF ef-fects are more rapid (peak effect in 4-6 hours) than those mediated by γ-IFN, and are transient with loss of cell ex-pression by 24 hours, regardless of the continued presence or absence of IL-1 or TNF.

In a recent study, we investigated the possibility that cytotoxic antibodies to IL-1 or TNF-inducible endothelial cell surface antigens could also contribute to the vascular injury observed during the acute phase of KS (Leung et al., 1986). In these experiments we pretreated HUVE cells for 4 hours, 24 hours, or 72 hours with the mediators: interleu-kin-2, α-IFN, β-IFN, γ-IFN, IL-1 or TNF. Preincubation with α-IFN, β-IFN, or interleukin-2 for any length of time failed to render HUVE cells susceptible to lysis with acute KS sera. However, after 4 hours of incubation with IL-1 or TNF, endothelial cells did become susceptible to lysis with acute KS sera. This effect was not observed when the same cells were pre-incubated for 24 hours or 72 hours with IL-1 or TNF. In contrast, HUVE required 72 hours of incubation with γ-IFN before they became susceptible to lysis with acute KS sera (Leung et al., 1986).

The shorter incubation periods required for induction of target antigens by IL-1 and TNF suggested that these me-diators induced a different target antigen than that induced by γ-IFN. Indeed we have found that removal of cytotoxic activity to γ-IFN-treated HUVE cells by serum absorption experiments does not result in the loss of cytotoxic activi-ty against IL-1 or TNF-treated HUVE cell (Leung et al., 1986).

Vascular endothelial cells are thought to play an impor-tant role in maintaining the structural integrity of blood vessel walls. Most vasculitides, including acute KS, are characterized both by marked immune activation with increased secretion of mediators and polyclonal B cell activation. Our studies (Leung et al., 1986; Leung et al., 1986) suggest that antibodies directed to endothelial cell antigens inducible by

γ -IFN, IL-1, and TNF may represent a previously unrecognized mechanism for vascular injury in acute KS and potentially other vasculitides as well.

It has been reported that administration of intravenous gamma globulin (IVGG) in high doses, during the acute phase of KS, reduces the frequency of coronary artery aneurysms (Furusho et al., 1984; Newburger et al., 1986). The effect of high dose IVGG on the immunoregulatory imbalance observed during acute KS are of interest in attempting to unravel mechanisms by which IVGG prevents the development of coronary artery aneurysms in this disease. During an ongoing multi-center trial in the United States to study the effects of aspirin (ASA) alone versus ASA plus IVGG on the clinical outcome of KS, we studied the effect of these agents on the immunoregulatory abnormalities in acute KS (Leung et al., 1986). Peripheral blood mononuclear cells (PBMC) were obtained on day 1 and day 4 of treatment for enumeration of T cell subsets. Prior to therapy, the T cell subset distribution in each treatment group was similar. PBMC from both treatment groups demonstrated a significant decrease in their percentages of T cells in comparison to age-matched controls. This decrease in total T cells represented an absolute deficiency of circulating T lymphocytes because the mean value for the number of lymphocytes in the peripheral blood of patients with acute KS was lower than that obtained for age-matched controls. The mean lymphocyte counts in patients at enrollment were similar in the two treatment groups. The decrease of circulating T cells in acute KS reflected a significant decrease in both suppressor T cells and helper T cells. The decrease in suppressor T cells, however, was disproportionately greater than that observed with helper T cells. As a result, KS patients entered into this study had an abnormally increased ratio of circulating helper T cells to suppressor T cells. This ratio was 6.6 $\pm$ 5.2 in the ASA treated group and 8.0 $\pm$ 3.3 in the IVGG group compared to 2.4 $\pm$ 0.4 in age-matched controls (P < 0.01). More importantly, both groups had a highly significant elevation in their percentages of circulating activated helper T cells.

The T cell profiles obtained during this study differed from our previous observations in that we previously reported normal precentages of total T cells and helper T cells during acute KS (Leung et al., 1982). It should, however, be noted that the patients entering into the current treatment protocols were studied much earlier in the course of their illness,

i.e. patients studied during the IVGG trial were studied
within 10 days of the onset of fever whereas in our previous
study patients were studied up to 21 days after onset of
fever (Leung et al., 1982). Thus, this most recent study
indicated that both the helper T cell and the suppressor T
cell population may be reduced during the earliest phase of
acute KS.

After 4 days of treatment, the group treated with IVGG
plus ASA underwent a greater increase in their percentage of
T cells, helper T cells and suppressor T cells than did the
ASA treated group; these differences were, however, not statistically significant (p = 0.1) for changes in T cells and
helper T cells. Patients treated with IVGG + ASA did, however, have a significantly greater increase in their percentages of suppressor T cells (p<0.1) than did patients treated
exclusively with ASA. The most dramatic change in T cell
phenotype involved the percentage of circulating activated
helper T cells after treatment with IVGG. Between the first
and fourth treatment day, the percentage of activated helper
cells in patients treated with IVGG + ASA fell an average of
25.2% as compared to a rise of 1.5% (p<0.001) in children who
only received aspirin.

We also examined the level of spontaneous IgG and IgM
secretion by PBMC obtained on day 1 and day 4 of each treatment protocol. Prior to treatment spontaneous IgG and IgM
synthesis was significantly elevated in both treatment groups.
Following treatment with ASA plus IVGG there was a highly
significant decrease in spontaneous IgG and IgM synthesis
(p < 0.001). In contrast, after 4 days of treatment with ASA
alone, PBMC continued to secrete high levels of IgG and IgM
(p > 0.1) antibody.

Our results suggest that the infusion of high dose IVGG
has at least two beneficial effects in preventing vascular
injury during acute KS. First, it reduces T cell activation
and may therefore reduce the expression of inducible endothelial antigens by inhibiting mediator production. Second,
IVGG blocks B cell activation and therefore may inhibit the
production of anti-endothelial cell antibodies. Further
studies are in progress to correlate mediator production by
PBMC and serum anti-endothelial cell antibody titer with the
clinical course of KS.

REFERENCES

Bevilacqua MP, Pober JS, Majeau GR, Contran RS, Gimbrone MA
(1984). Interleukin-1 (IL-1) induces biosynthesis and cell
surface expression of procoagulant activity in human vascular endothelial cells. J. Exp. Med. 160:618.
Bevilacqua MP, Pober JS, Wheeler ME, Cotran RS, Gimbrone MA
(1985). Interleukin-1 acts on cultured human vascular endo-
thelium to increase adhesion of polymorphonuclear leukocytes, monocytes, and related leukocyte cell lines. J. Clin.
Invest. 76:2003.
Furusho K, Nakano H, Shinomiya K, Tamura T, Manabe Y, Kawarano
M, Baba K, Kamiya T, Kiyosawa N, Hayashidera T, Hirose O,
Yokoyama T, Baba K, Mori C (1984). High-dose intravenous
gammaglobulin for Kawasaki disease. Lancet ii:1055-1058.
Fujiwara H, Hamashima Y (1978). Pathology of the heart in
Kawasaki's disease. Pediatrics. 61:100-107.
Hirose S, Hamashima Y (1978). Morphological observations on
the vasculitis in the mucocutaneous lymph node syndrome.
Eur. J. Pediatr. 129:17-27.
Kato S, Kimura M, Tsuji K, Kusakava S, Asai T, Juji T,
Kawasaki T (1978). HLA antigens in Kawasaki disease. Pedi-
atrics. 61:252-255.
Kato H, Koike S, Yamamoto M, Ito Y, Yano E (1975). Coronary
aneurysms in infants and young children with acute febrile
mucocutaneous lymph node syndrome. J. Pediatr. 86:892-898.
Kawasaki T (1967). Acute febrile mucocutaneous syndrome with
lymphoid involvement with specific desquamation of the
fingers and toes in children: clinical observations of 50
cases. JPN. J. Allergol. 16:178-222.
Kawasaki T (1971). Acute febrile mucocutaneous lymph node
syndrome and sudden death. Acta. Pediatr. Jpn. (Overseas
Ed.). 75:433-434.
Krensky AM, Berenberg W, Shanley K, Yunis EJ (1981). HLA
antigens in mucocutaneous lymph node syndrome in New England.
Pediatrics. 67:741-745.
Kuno-Saka M (1985). Increase of Immunoglobulin - Bearing
Peripheral Blood Lymphocytes in Children with Kawasaki
Disease. Acta Pediatri. Jpn. 27:127-130.
Landing BH, Larson EJ (1977). Are infantile periarteritis
nodosa and fatal mucocutaneous lymph node syndrome the same?
Pediatrics. 59:651-662.
Leung DYM, Burns J, Newburger J, Geha RS (In press, 1986).
Reversal of immunoregulatory abnormalities in Kawasaki
Syndrome by intravenous gammaglobulin. J. Clin. Invest.

Leung DYM, Chu ET, Wood N, Grady S, Meade R, Geha RS (1983). Immunoregulatory T cell abnormalities in mucocutaneous lymph node syndrome. J. Immunol. 130:2002-2004.

Leung DYM, Geha RS, Newburger J, Burns J, Fiers W, LaPierre LA, Pober JS (1986). Two monokines, interleukin-1 and tumor necrosis factor, render cultured vascular endothelial cells susceptible to lysis by antibodies circulating during Kawasaki Syndrome. J. Exp. Med. 164:1958-1972

Leung DYM, Siegel RL, Grady S, Krensky A, Meade R, Reinherz EL, Geha RS (1982). Immunoregulatory abnormalities in mucocutaneous lymph node syndrome. Clin. Immunol. Immunopathol. 23:100-112.

Newburger JW, Takahashi M, Burns JC, Beiser AS, Chung KJ, Duffy CE, Glode MP, Mason WH, Reddy V, Sanders SP, Shulman ST, Wiggins JW, Hicks RV, Fulton DR, Lewis AB, Leung DYM, Waldman JD, Colton T, Rosen FS, Melish ME (1986). Treatment of Kawasaki Syndrome with intravenous gammagobulin. N. Engl. J. Med. 315:341-346.

Pober JS, Bevilacqua MP, Mendrick DL, LaPierre LA, Fiers W, Gimbrone MA (1986). Two distinct monokines, interleukin-1 and tumor necrosis factor, each independently induce biosynthesis and transient expression of the same antigen on the surface of cultured human vascular endothelial cells. J. Immunol. 136:1680.

Pober JS, Collins T, Gimbrone MA, Cotran RS, Gitlin JD, Fiers W, Clayberger C, Krensky AM, Burakoff SJ, Reiss CS (1983). Lymphocytes recognize human vascular endothelial and dermal fibroblast Ia antigens induced by recombinant immune interferon. Nature (Lond.). 305:726-729.

Tanaka N, Sckimoto K, Naoe S (1976). Kawasaki disease: relationship with infantile periarteritis nodosa. Arch. Pathol. Lab. Med. 100:81-86.

Yanagihara R, Todd JK (1980). Acute febrile mucocutaneous lymph node syndrome. Am. J. Dis. Child. 134:603-614.

Kawasaki Disease, pages 167–174
© 1987 Alan R. Liss, Inc.

IMMUNOLOGICAL ABNORMALITIES IN KAWASAKI DISEASE

Ko Okumura, Kazuhito Jujho and Yoshio Yanase

Department of Immunology, and Department of
Pediatrics, Juntendo University, School of
Medicine, Tokyo, Japan; and Department of
Pediatrics, Japanese Red Cross Medical Center,
Tokyo, Japan

INTRODUCTION

Many kinds of infectious diseases have been shown to
be associated with transient or chronic immunosuppression.
By using recently developed quantitative immunofluorescence
analysis, with monoclonal antibodies directed against the
cell surface antigens of human lymphocyte subsets, it may
be possible to specify more clearly any immunological dysfunction during human diseases. The present examination
was performed to study the alterations of lymphocyte subsets
in infectious diseases commonly encountered in childhood
and Kawasaki disease, which, on analysis of nation-wide
epidemiological studies in Japan (Yanagawa, et al., 1979),
appears to be some kind of infectious disease.

MATERIALS AND METHODS

1) Study population

The study population for single color analysis consisted of 13 patients with varicella, 5 with HFMD, 4 with
scarlet fever, 10 with measles, 20 with Kawasaki disease and
52 normal children matched to patients for age and sex.
They were selected from children seen at the Department of
Pediatrics, Japanese Red Cross Medical Center, Tokyo (Table
1). Each of the patients with an infectious disease had
typical clinical manifestations, and each of the 20 patients
with Kawasaki disease was hospitalized during the acute
febrile phase and fulfilled at least 5 major criteria. All

TABLE 1. Age distribution of patients with varicella, HFMD, scarlet fever, measles, Kawasaki disease and normal controls

Subjects Age	Varicella	HFMD	Scarlet fever	Measles	Kawasaki disease	Normal control
< 1 yr	1			1	6	7
1 yr	1	1		4	4	11
2 yr		1		1	4	6
3 yr	2	1			3	5
4 yr	4			2		7
5 yr	3	1	2		1	9
6 yr	1	1	2		1	3
7 - 13 yr	1			2	1	4
Total	13	5	4	10	20	52
Range of age	9mo-7yr5mo	1yr8mo-6yr1mo	5yr0mo-6yr10mo	8mo-8yr8mo	4mo-13yr2mo	4mo-13yr5mo
Mean ± SD	4.5 ± 1.9yr	3.6 ± 1.7yr	5.9 ± 0.7yr	3.3 ± 2.9yr	2.7 ± 2.9yr	4.1 ± 3.3yr

TABLE 2. Subset alterations as percentages of PBL in Kawasaki disease[a]

Subjects	Kawasaki disease (n=20)		Control (n=20)
Days of illness	≤ 7	27 - 32	
Leu-2a+ cells	18.2 ± 5.7	20.5 ± 5.8	19.8 ± 5.0
Leu-3a+ cells	29.6 ± 13.0b	42.0 ± 10.9	43.0 ± 9.4
Leu-4+ cells	43.2 ± 13.1b	58.3 ± 9.2	59.8 ± 9.1
Leu-7+ cells	15.4 ± 9.7	13.5 ± 8.1	13.0 ± 6.4
Leu-10+ cells	5.5 ± 2.9	6.1 ± 3.8	7.0 ± 3.3
2H7+ cells	10.4 ± 6.6	9.0 ± 7.3	11.4 ± 4.4
Leu-M3+ cells	13.4 ± 6.6c	12.4 ± 5.3	10.4 ± 5.3
HLA-DR+ cells	32.3 ± 8.9c	27.3 ± 8.9	29.7 ± 7.3
Leu-3a+ / Leu-2a+ ratio	1.81 ± 1.00b	2.25 ± 1.02	2.30 ± 0.69

[a] Data are expressed as means ± standard deviation.

[b] Significantly different from control (P < 0.001).

[c] Significantly different from control (P < 0.05).

20 patients with Kawasaki disease were treated by oral administration of 50mg/kg aspirin daily for at least one month. Four patients had coronary aneurysms, demonstrated by an echocardiagram, within 30 days after onset.

Subjects of the study for two color analysis were 15 children with Kawasaki disease (8 males and 7 females) aged between 4 months and 3.5 years (average, one year and 8 months) hospitalized at the Department of Pediatrics, Juntendo University. All subjects were given aspirin at a daily dose of 30-50 mg/kg after hospitalization. Some of them were additionally treated with dipyridamole (4~5 mg/kg/day). Of the 15 subjects, 13 showed no echocardio-graphic signs of coronary anuerysms one month after the onset of disease and were consequently handled as cases showing favorable progress. The remaining two patients had coronary aneurysms.

2) Monoclonal Antibodies

Fluorescein-conjugated monoclonal antibodies, termed Leu-2a, Leu-3a, Leu-4, Leu-7, Leu-10, Leu-M3 and HLA-DR, were purchased from Becton Dickinson Monoclonal Center (Mountain View, Calif.). A fluorescein-conjugated monoclonal antibody termed 2H7 which is known to react with B cell population was kindly provided by Dr. J.A. Ledbetter (Genetic Systems Corp., Seattle, Wash.). Leu-2a is directed at the suppressor/cytotoxic T cell subset; Leu-3a at the helper/inducer T cell subset; Leu-4 at total T cells; Leu-7 at natural killer/killer cells; Leu-10 at B cells and activated T cells; Leu-M3 at mature monocytes/macrophages; HLA-DR at B cells, monocytes/macrophages and activated T cells; and 2H7 at B cells.

3) Analysis of Stained cells with Flow Cytometry

Human peripheral blood mononuclear leukocytes (PBL) were prepared by centrifugation of heparinized venous blood on Ficoll-Isopaque (Ficoll-Paque; Pharmacia, Uppsala, Sweden) at room temperature and washed three times in ice cold MEM (Eagle MEM; Nissui, Tokyo, Japan). These cells were then stained for 40 minutes in microtiter plates on ice by reacting 5×10^4 target cells/well with saturation levels of directly fluorescein-conjugated monoclonal antibodies. Cells were then washed with MEM three times and analyzed, immediately using a fluorescence activated cell sorter (FACS-II; Becton-Dickinson, Mountain View, Calif.). After setting the forward light scatter gate on the lymphocyte

TABLE 3 Comparison of Percentage in Lymphocyte Subsets among Exanthematous Diseases compared with age-matched controls

Disease stage	Kawasaki D acute	Kawasaki D conv.	Scarlet F acute	Scarlet F e.conv.	Varicella acute	Varicella e.conv.	HFMD acute	HFMD e.conv.	Measles acute	Measles e.conv.
Leu-2a+ cells	-	-	-	↑	-	↑	-	↑	-	↑
Leu-3a+ cells	↓	-	↓	-	↓	-	↓	↑	↓	-
Leu-4+ cells	↓	-	↓	-	↓	-	↓	↑	↓	-
Leu-7+ cells	-	-	-	-	-	-	-	-	-	-
Leu-10+ cells	-	-	-	-	-	-	-	-	-	-
2H7+ cells	-	-	-	-	-	-	-	-	-	-
Leu-M3+ cells	↗	-	↑	-	↑	-	↑	-	-	-
HLA-DR+ cells	↗	-	↑	-	↑	-	↑	-	-	-
Leu-3a+/Leu-2a+ ratio	↓	-	↓	-	↓	↓	↓	↑	↓	-

conv. : convalescence　　　e.conv.: early convalescence　　- : unchanged

↑ : increased　　　↓ : decreased　　　↗ : slightly increased

cluster and monocyte cluster, 1×10^{4} cells were analyzed. Immunofluorescence staining with fluorescein conjugated mouse monoclonal non-specific IgG_1, IgG_2 and IgM (Becton-Dickinson Monoclonal Center, Mountain View, Calif.) was used as a negative control. Two color analysis was performed by FACS IV using FITC-conjugated monoclonal antibodies in combination with phycoerythrin (PE)-conjugated monoclonal antibodies. The numbers of cell populations were estimated from fluorescence-positive cells with background cells subtracted, and their proportions were expressed as percentages of the analyzed cells.

4) Statistical Analysis

The significance of the differences observed was evaluated by the paired t-test using multiple comparison of Bonferroni type. Data from all determinations were presented as the mean ± one standard deviation.

RESULTS

I. Single Color Analysis

In the acute phase of Kawasaki disease (Table 2), the percentages of Leu-3a^{+} and Leu-4^{+} cells were decreased (p<

3) Variation in HLA-DR positive cells

   In the percentage of Leu 3^+ HLA-DR$^+$ cells (Fig.3), no significant difference was noted between patients showing favorable progress and controls throughout the study period or between the three phases in patients showing favorable progress. On the other hand, both of the two patients who had coronary aneurysm showed a slightly larger percentage one week after the acute phase than in the acute phase.

   The percentage of Leu 2^+ HLA-DR$^+$ cells (Fig.4) registered for patients showing favorable progress in the acute phase was significantly larger than the figure for controls and the corresponding figure obtained one week later for the same patients ($p<0.05$). On the other hand, two patients who had coronary aneurysm showed a larger percentage of these cells one week after the acute phase than in the acute phase.

DISCUSSION

   Results of the present study indicate that the alterations in human lymphocyte subsets in the infectious diseases studies closely resemble one another, especially in the decrease of Leu-3a$^+$ (helper/inducer T) cells, Leu-4$^+$ (total T) cells and the increase of Leu-2a$^+$ (suppressor/cytotoxic T) cells. The decreased proportions of Leu-3a$^+$ cells and Leu-4$^+$ cells resulting in decreases in the Leu-3a$^+$/Leu-2a$^+$ ratio were common to all the infectious diseases examined. However, a distinct increase in the acute and convalescent percentages of Leu-2a$^+$ cells was not observed in Kawasaki disease, although the alterations in the percentages of Leu-3a$^+$ cells, Leu-4$^+$ cells and the Leu-3a$^+$/Leu-2a$^+$ ratio were similar to those in the infectious diseases examined. The proportion of Leu-M3$^+$ cells (monocytes) and HLA-DR$^+$ cells increased during the acute phase of scarlet fever, varicella, HFMD and Kawasaki disease, while no significant changes in measles were shown.

   In analyzing with the two-color immunofluorescence technique, an increased percentage of Leu-2$^+$15$^+$ (suppressor T) cells and an unchanged proportion of Leu-3$^+$8$^-$ (helper T) cells were observed in acute Kawasaki disease. In terms of activated T cells, a slight increase in the percentage of Leu-2$^+$ HLA-DR$^+$ cells was indicated, although no significant increase in the proportion of Leu-3$^+$ HLA-DR$^+$ cells was shown in the acute phase of Kawasaki disease.

It has been reported that a significant reduction in OKT8[+] cells has been found along with normal percentages of OKT3[+] (total T) cells and OKT4[+] cells and an increase in Ia-bearing OKT4[+] (activated T) cells during the acute phase of Kawasaki disease (Leung, et al., 1982). Since the data shown in this study was obtained from genetically homogenous patients in Japan, the direct comparison of these data with that of other races leaves some room for consideration.

At present, we can not account for the discrepancies between our data on lymphocyte subsets in Kawasaki disease and data previously published. However, from the data obtained in this study it is suggested that some kind of infectious agent is involved in the disease.

REFERENCES

Leung D Y M, Siegel R L, Grady S, Krensky A, Meade R, Reinherz E L, and R S Geha (1982). Immunoregulatory abnormalities in mucocutaneous lymph node syndrome. Clin. Immunol. Immunopathol. 23:100-112.

Yanagawa H, Shigematsu I, Kusakawa S, and T Kawasaki (1979). Epidemiology of Kawasaki disease in Japan. Acta Paediatr. Jpn. 21:1-10.

Kawasaki Disease, pages 175–184
© 1987 Alan R. Liss, Inc.

LYMPHOCYTE ABNORMALITIES AND COMPLEMENT ACTIVATION IN KAWASAKI DISEASE

Ronald M. Laxer*, Frederick M. Schaffer*, Barry L. Myones§, William J. Younts, Richard D. Rowe*, Laurence Rubin*, Leonard D. Stein*, Erwin W. Gelfand*, Earl D. Silverman*
*University of Toronto and § University of North Carolina.

INTRODUCTION

Immunoregulatory abnormalities have been reported in children with Kawasaki disease (KD) (1-8). These abnormalities include abnormal absolute numbers and percentages of T cells, B cells and T cell subsets, abnormal lymphocyte function, and the presence of circulating immune complexes. Results have varied from patient to patient and have also varied depending on the method of detection and the interval between diagnosis and testing.

We examined several parameters of immune function to evaluate a) the frequency of abnormalities of lymphocyte function and number, b) the presence of activation of the immune system and c) the presence of immune complexes and complement activation.

METHODS

A. Patients

All children were studied during the acute phase of their illness. The diagnosis of KD was based on the criteria established by the Japanese Mucocutaneous Lymph Node Syndrome Committee (9). After informed consent, patients were randomized to receive aspirin alone (100mg/kg/day) or aspirin plus intravenous immunoglobulin [Sandoglobulin] (1g/kg/day) for two days. All patients were seen within 9 days of their initial symptom.

B. Lymphocyte Studies

Lymphocyte studies were performed on study entry (Day 5-9 of disease) and 2-4 days later (Day 7-13 of disease). Peripheral blood mononuclear cells were separated by ficoll-hypaque density gradient centrifugation and T and B lymphocyte percentages were determined by indirect immunofluorescence using monoclonal antibodies to several T cell antigens [T11, T4, and T8] and to the B cell antigen B1 by standard techniques. B cell surface immunoglobulin (SIg) was detected on B cells by direct immunofluorescence. As a measure of T cell activation, numbers of Tac+ (T cell receptor for interleukin-2) and transferrin receptor positive cells were evaluated using mouse monoclonal antibodies. The soluble interleukin (IL-2) receptor was measured in serum in an ELISA assay by the method of Rubin et al (10).

C. Immunoglobulin Production

In vitro IgM, IgG and IgA production was evaluated by radioimmunoassay following culture with and without pokeweed mitogen (PWM) or Epstein-Barr Virus (EBV) for 7 and 14 days.

D. Immune Complex and Complement Studies

Serum levels of C3 and C4 were measured by nephelometry. Circulating immune complexes were measured by a fluid phase CIq binding assay. Values for CR1 (red blood cell C3b receptor) and complement activation products C3dg and C4d were measured on red blood cells by the method of Ross et al (11).

E. Statistics

Student's two-tailed paired t-test was used to compare differences of the means between groups.

RESULTS

A. Lymphocyte Studies

At study entry, there were no differences in lymphocyte

count and number of T11 positive cells between patients and normal controls. In addition, no changes in the above parameters were observed following the introduction of therapy. Eight of 9 patients had elevated T4/T8 ratios (> 2 standard deviations (SD) from the mean of the normal controls, Figure 1) which were due to a combination of increased percentages of T4+ cells and/or decreased percentages of T8+ cells (pretreatment T4+ range 21-63%, T8+ 4-16%). The trend in all patients was towards normal by Day 7-13 of disease regardless of their treatment (post-treatment T4+ range 30-50%, T8+ 12-30%). Two of 5 children treated with ASA alone still had an elevated T4:T8 ratio by day 7-13.

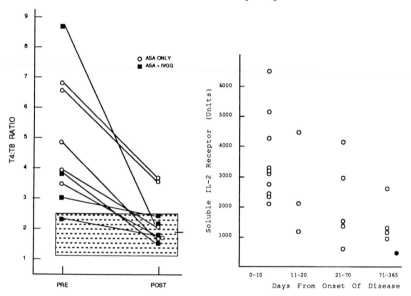

Fig 1. T4:T8 ratio measured pre (day 5-9) and post (day 7-13) therapy. Shaded area represents mean ± 2 SD,

Fig 2. Circulating soluble IL-2 receptor plotted against days from onset of KD [•= mean + 2 SD for adult controls].

None of the patients had an increased number of Tac+ cells nor did they express the transferrin receptor on T cells. Soluble IL-2 receptors have been noted in the serum of patients with Sezary Syndrome, Hodgkin's Disease, chronic lymphocyte leukemia and HTLV-1-associated T-cell leukemia (12). In view of the recent association of KD and retroviruses (13,14), we assayed for the presence of soluble IL-2

receptors in KD patient serum. Levels of circulating soluble
IL-2 receptor were raised in all patients measured early in
their disease (Figure 2), and reverted toward normal with
time. The means of the circulating IL-2 receptors remained
> 2 SD from the mean of normal adult controls for up to 1
year from diagnosis.

Five of 9 patients had percentage of B1 positive cells
that were > 2 SD from the mean of the normal controls
(Figure 3). These values returned to normal in all patients
within 4 days, regardless of the administration of IVGG.

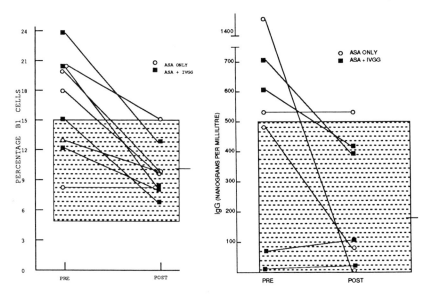

Fig 3. Percentage of B1+ cells
pre and post treatment. Shaded
area represents mean ± 2 SD
for controls.

Fig 4. Spontaneous IgG production pre and post treatment. Shaded areas represent
mean ± 2 SD for controls.

B. Immunoglobulin Production

It has been shown that spontaneous immunoglobulin production is elevated during the acute phase of KD (1) and
that it may relate to both increased T helper cell and decreased T suppressor cell function. We evaluated spontaneous
PWM, and EBV induced immunoglobulin production in our patients. Prior to treatment, 3/7 patients had spontaneous

IgM   production > 2 SD from the mean of the control, and
4/7 patients had pretreatment spontaneous IgG production
> 2 SD from controls (Figure 4). By day 7-13, all had norm-
al IgM and 6 of 7 had normal IgG production. This return
towards normal levels of spontaneous immunoglobulin production was independent of IVGG treatment. Co-culture of patient lymphocytes with either PWM or EBV did not increase
immunoglobulin production above that observed with normal
controls.

C. Immune Complex and Complement Studies

     Evaluation of immune complexes in KD have yielded vary-
ing results, depending upon the stage of disease when testing was performed and the method of testing (6-8). We measured circulating immune complexes in 13 patients during the
acute phase of KD using a Clq fluid phase radioimmunoassay
and failed to detect these complexes in any patients. We
also determined red blood cell (RBC) levels of complement
receptor 1 (CR1), the red blood cell receptor for C3d. Low
values for RBC bound CR1 have been described in two situations: (a) due to congential deficiencies of this receptor,
and (b) immune complex disease where the CR1 binds immune
complexes and is subsequently cleaved by cells in the
reticuloendothelial system. Six of 13 patients had RBC CR1
levels that were > 2 SD from the mean of normal controls
(< 310 molecules/RBC, Figure 5) during the acute phase of
their disease. Five of the 13 patients were retested one
year later, and the values rose in all 5; the means of the
early and late samples differed significantly (Figure 6,
P < 0.025), suggesting that the early deficiency of CR1
resulted from immune complex deposition on the RBC surface.

     To assess complement activation, we measured serum
levels of C3 and C4, as well as RBC bound C3dg and C4d. RBC-
C3dg and C4d levels represent a very sensitive measure of
complement activation (11). Levels of C3 and C4 were normal
or elevated in all children, and levels of RBC-C4d were
normal in all but 2. However, 11 of 13 had elevated levels
of RBC bound C3dg measured during the acute phase of their
disease (Figure 7). Levels of RBC-C3dg returned to normal
in all 5 patients re-evaluated one year later (Figure 8,
P < 0.005). A negative correlation (r=-.625) was observed
when RBC CR1 levels were plotted against C3dg during the

acute phase of disease, but not when these values were compared one year later.

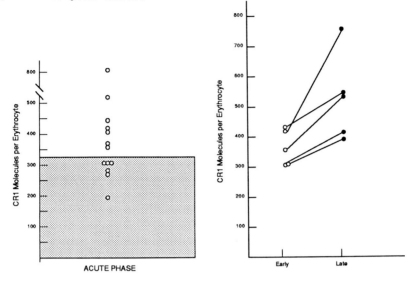

Fig 5. CR1 molecules per RBC in 13 children during acute phase of KD. Shaded areas represent values < 2 SD from mean of controls.

Fig 6. CR1 molecules per RBC measured in 5 children during the acute phase and one year after the onset of KD.

DISCUSSION

In this study we report immunologic abnormalities in patients with KD and the effect of IVGG on these abnormalities. We found normal percentages of total T cells as measured with a T 11 monoclonal antibody. We also found a significantly increased T4/T8 ratio which was primarily due to a decrease in percentage of T8+ cells. As opposed to Leung et al (4), we did not find any significant differences in these values between IVGG treated and untreated patients. However, 2/5 ASA treated patients still had abnormally elevated T4/T8 ratios 2-4 days after treatment, versus none of 4 IVGG treated patients. Previous studies have shown conflicting results. Leung et al have reported both normal

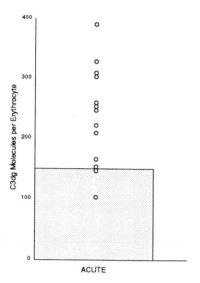

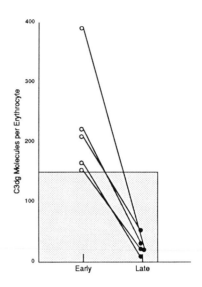

Fig 7. C3dg molecules per RBC measured in 13 children during the acute phase of KD. Shaded area represents mean ± 2 SD for controls

Fig 8. C3dg molecules per RBC measured in 5 children during the acute phase and one year after the onset of KD.

and diminished total T cell numbers in the acute phase of KD (1,3), and Barron et al showed an absolute lymphocytosis with an expansion of B and T cell subsets, the B cell subset affected to a greater degree than the T(5). The elevation of the percentage of Bl positive cells and increased spontaneous IgG and IgM production seen in our study is consistent with previous reports and with the reduction of suppressor cell numbers and function in the acute phase of disease (1,3,4). The return of both B cell numbers and function to normal correlated with the return of T4/T8 ratios toward normal as well.

We did not detect evidence of T cell activation as measured by the presence of either IL-2 or transferrin receptors on circulating T cells. Therefore, the previous report (3) of increased numbers of Ia positive T helper cells is unlikely to be the result of activation of T cells via the usual pathway which requires T cells to acquire both IL-2 and transferrin receptor prior to the expression of Ia. However, despite the normal number of T cells expressing the IL-2 receptor, we found elevated circulating levels of soluble IL-2 receptor which reverted towards normal with time.

The presence of soluble IL-2 receptor, despite its absence on circulating T cells, requires further explanation. One hypothesis is that IL-2 receptors originated from endothelial cells. Although there is no evidence to date to show this, IL-2 receptors are not limited to T cells, as previously thought, and have been found on the surface of activated B cells,   Langerhans epithelial cells in the skin and lung carcinoma cells (G. Mills, personal communication). Endothelial cells do express Ia on their surface (15), and may also be capable of expressing the IL-2 receptor. As KD is primarily a disease characterized pathologically by vasculitis, the endothelial cell must be more closely examined for evidence of "activation". An unlikely possibility is that we did not test the T cells early enough in their activation process and therefore missed the expression of Tac and transferrin receptors on the surface. A final possibility is that the IL-2 receptor is made and secreted by the T cell, but not expressed on the cell surface.

Evidence of complement activation was found in the acute phase in 11 of 13 children, likely resulting from activation of the complement cascade by immune complexes. All follow-up measurements of RBC-C3dg were normal, consistent with KD being an acute "one-hit" event with its long term consequences resulting from healing by scarring/fibrosis. We found C4d in only 2 patients. The failure to detect immune complexes by C1q binding, and lack of C4d in most patients may represent immune complexes that did not activate complement by the classical pathway, perhaps containing IgA or IgG 2/4 subclasses. Although not likely the primary inciting event, circulating immune complexes may play some role in the early inflammatory lesion seen in KD (16).

Further studies examining Kawasaki disease should focus on the endothelial cell and the role of complement activation in the pathogenesis of this inflammatory vasculopathy.

REFERENCES

1. Leung DYM, Siegel RL, Grady S, Krensky A, Meade R, Reinherz EL, Geha RS (1982). Immunoregulatory abnormalities in mucocutaneous lymph node syndrome. Clin Immunol Immunopathol 23:100-112.

2. Matsuoka Y, Yata J (1983). An immunological study on mucocutaneous lymph node syndrome: Activation of T_G suppressor cells. Acta Paediatr Jpn 25:192-197.

3. Leung DYM, Chu ET, Wood N, Grady S, Meade R, Geha RS (1983). Immunoregulatory T cell abnormalities in mucocutaneous lymph node syndrome. J Immunol 130:2002-2004.

4. Leung DYM, Burns J. Newberger J. Rosen FS, Geha RS (1985). Reversal of immunoregulatory abnormalities in Kawasaki syndrome by intravenous gammaglobulin. Clin Res 33:565A.

5. Barron KS, Lewis DE, DeCunto C, Blifeld C (1986). Immune abnormalities in children with Kawasaki syndrome. J Rheumatol 13:978.

6. Furuse A, Matsuda I (1983). Circulating immune complex in the mucocutaneous lymphnode syndrome. Eur J Pediatr 141:50-51.

7. Mason WH, Jordan SC, Sakai R, Takahashi M, Bernstein B (1985). Circulating immune complexes in Kawasaki syndrome. Pediatr Infect Dis 4:48-51.

8. Ono S, Onimaru T, Kawakami K, Hokonahara M, Miyata K (1985). Impaired granulocyte chemotaxis and increased circulating immune complexes in Kawasaki disease. J Pediatr 106:567-570.

9. The Japanese Kawasaki Disease Research Committee, Diagnostic Guidelines of Kawasaki Disease. 4th Revised Edition, Sept. 1984.

10. Rubin LA, Kurman CC, Fritz ME, Yarchoan R, Nelson DL (1985). Identification and characterization of a released form of the interleukin-2 receptor. In Oppenheim JJ, Jacobs DM (eds): "Leukocytes and Host defense". New York : Alan R. Liss, 95-102.

11. Ross GD, Yount WJ, Walport MJ, Winfield JB, Parker CJ, Fuller CR, Taylor RP, Myones BL, Lachmann PJ (1985). Disease-associated loss of erythrocyte complement receptors (CR1, C3b receptors) in patients with systemic lupus erythematosus and other diseases involving autoantibodies and/or complement activation. J Immunol 135:2005-2014.

12. Greene WC, Leonard WJ, Depper JM, Nelson DL, Waldmann TA (1986) The human interleukin-2 receptor: normal and abnormal expression in T cells and in leukemias induced by the human T-lymphotropic retroviruses. Ann Int Med 105:560-572

13. Shulman ST, Rowley AH (1986). Does Kawasaki disease have a retroviral etiology? Lancet II:545-546.
14. Burns JC, Geha RS, Schneeberger EE, Newburger JW, Rosen FS, Glezen LS, Huang AS, Natale J, Leung DYM (1986). Polymerase activity in lymphocyte culture supernatants from patients with Kawasaki disease. Nature 323:814-816.
15. Pober JS, Collins T, Gimbrone JR, Cotran RS, Gitlin JD, Fiers W, Clayberger C, Krensky AM, Burakoff SJ, Reiss CS (1983). Lymphocytes recognize human vascular endothelial and dermal fibroblast Ia antigens induced by recombant immune interferon. Nature 305:726-729.
16. Levin M, Holland PC, Nokes TJC, Novelli V, Mola M, Levinsky RJ, Dillon M, Barratt TM, Marshall WC (1985). Platelet immune complex interaction in the pathogenesis of Kawasaki disease and childhood polyarteritis. Br Med J 290:1456-1460.

Kawasaki Disease, pages 185–192
© 1987 Alan R. Liss, Inc.

IMMUNOPATHOLOGY OF THE SKIN LESION OF KAWASAKI DISEASE

Toshiaki Sugawara, Susumu Hattori* Sachiko Hirose*
Susumu Furukawa, Keijiro Yabuta and Toshikazu Shirai*

Department of Pathology* and Department of Pediatrics,
Juntendo University School of Medicine
2-1-1, Hongo, Bunkyo-ku, Tokyo 113, Japan

INTRODUCTION

One of the major clinical features at an acute phase of Kawasaki disease is polymorphous exanthema and induration of the skin (Kawasaki, 1967; Kawasaki et al., 1974). Morphologically, this lesion is typified by severe edema associated with the dilatation of small vessels in the papillary dermis. In the subcutaneous tissues, vasculitis develops with endothelial necrosis and subendothelial edema. Despite such an exudative nature of inflammation, there is a small number of infiltrating inflammatory cells, mostly mononuclear cells (Hirose and Hamashima, 1978). We characterized the cell surface phenotypes of the infiltrating inflammatory cells and changes in the epidermis of skin biopsy specimens from Japanese with Kawasaki disease. Also studied were the specimens from the site of BCG vaccination, where a marked, well circumscribed swelling of the skin is usually noted during the acute phase of the disease.

MATERIALS AND METHODS

We studied 9 children aged 1 to 7 years. All fulfilled the criteria for the diagnosis of Kawasaki disease. Skin biopsy specimens were obtained from the sites of either exanthema or BCG vaccination 4 to 10 days after onset of the disease. In one, the specimen was obtained on the 29th day, when the disease recurred. For comparative studies, skin specimens were also obtained from 2 children with measles.

Normal skin specimens were obtained at surgery from 6 age-
matched patients with congenital heart disease.

For immunofluorescence, cryostat sections were acetone-
fixed and stained either with fluorescein isothiocyanate
(FITC)-conjugated antibodies or with biotinylated antibodies
followed by avidin-FITC or avidin-phycoerythrin (PE). Double
staining of the tissues was carried out by staining first
with biotinylated antibodies and avidin-PE and secondary by
FITC-labelled antibodies. The specimens were examined under
a Zeiss incident-light fluorescence microscope. Immunohistochemical studies were also carried out in part by avidin-
biotin system, using peroxidase-labelled antibodies. The
antibodies used were those against fibrinogen, human immunoglobulin μ chain (Cappel Laboratories, Cochranville, PA),
Leu 2 (CD8), Leu 3 (CD4), Leu 4 (CD3), Leu 6 (CD1), Leu 14,
Leu M3 and HLA-DR (Becton Dickinson, Mountain View, CA).

TABLE 1. Cell surface phenotypes of infiltrating mononuclear
cells in the skin lesions of Kawasaki disease and measles

Case		Age (years)	Sex	Days from onset	T cell marker			B cell marker		LeuM3
					Leu4	Leu2	Leu3	Leu14	anti-μ	
KD[a]	1 MT[b] 1		M	7	+++[c]	+	+++	−	−	++
	2 MO[b] 1		F	9	+++	+	+++	−	−	++
	3 TH[b] 1		M	7	++	+	++	−	−	+
	4 HM 7		M	4	++	+	++	−	−	+
	5 RH 1		M	4	++	+	++	−	−	+
	6 MT 1		M	7	+	±	+	−	−	±
	7 ST 1		M	9	+	±	+	−	−	±
	8 MN[d] 1		M	29	+++	++	+++	−	−	++
	9 KS 5		F	10	++	+	++	−	−	+
Measles	10 YK 1		M	6	+++	++	++	−	−	+
	11 HA 1		M	8	+++	+++	+	−	−	+

a, Kawasaki disease.
b, Skin specimens were obtained from the site of BCG
vaccination.
c, +++,extensive; ++,moderate; +,a few; ±,occasional; −,none.
d, Recurrence of the disease.

RESULTS

The histology of the skin lesion of Kawasaki disease was characterized by severe edema in the papillary dermis and there was an associated marked dilatation of the capillaries. The number of inflammatory cell infiltrates was relatively small and were mainly composed of mononuclear cells and distributed mainly in the vicinities of superficial plexus of small vessels in the dermis and less in the papillary layer. A few infiltrates were also present in the epidermis. A mild liquefaction degeneration of keratinocytes was observed along the basal layer of the epidermis. Such changes were most extensive on the 4th day from the disease onset and gradually subsided thereafter, in keeping with the finding of Hirose and Hamashima (1978). The skin specimens obtained from the site of BCG vaccination (cases 1 to 3 in Table 1) of patients who had suffered from Kawasaki disease within approximately 10 months after vaccination showed similar histopathological changes. However, an extensive edema with fibrinogen exudation and an increase in mononuclear cell infiltrates were observed even on the 7th to 9th days from onset of the disease (Figs. 1 and 2). A patient with recurrence on the 29th day from the first onset of the disease (case 8) had a severe inflammatory skin lesion with increased mononuclear cell infiltration.

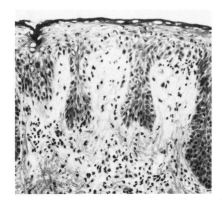 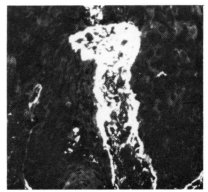

Figure 1. Extensive edema and mononuclear cell infiltration in the papillary dermis. Biopsy specimen from the site of BCG vaccination of case 1 (H & E).

Figure 2. Fibrinogen exudation at the papillary dermis of case 1 (FITC).

Results of the immunofluorescence investigation of the infiltrating mononuclear cells are summarized in Table 1. These cells were mainly comprised of Leu 4$^+$ T cells and Leu M3$^+$ macrophages. The majority of these T cells belonged to the Leu 3$^+$ subset and only a few Leu 2$^+$ cells were observed (Fig. 3). Double staining of the specimens with antibodies to Leu 3 and HLA-DR antigens demonstrated the presence of double-positive cells, mainly in the upper dermis and occasionally in the epidermal layer (Fig. 4). There were no T cells positive for both Leu 2 and HLA-DR. We found no B cells, as defined by the antibodies to human μ chain and Leu 14. There was no immunoglobulin deposition at the dermo-epidermal junction or along the vessel walls in the dermis.

The HLA-DR antigen was distributed intercellularly, in localized areas of the epidermis. The intensity and distibution of HLA-DR antigen were more extensive in the skin lesion at BCG vaccination (Fig. 5). An extensive expression of HLA-DR was also observed in a case with recurrence of the disease (case 8). Double staining of the skin specimens with antibobies to HLA-DR and Leu 6 revealed that the distribution of such intercellular HLA-DR extended beyond the distribution of Langerhans cells, as determined by staining

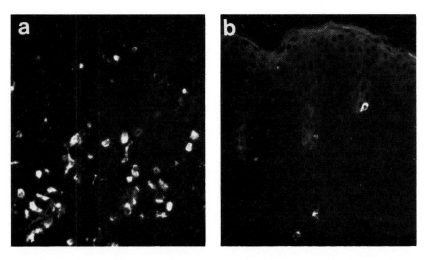

Figure 3. Leu 3$^+$ (a, FITC) and Leu 2$^+$ (b, PE) T cells, determined by double immunofluorescence staining of the same skin specimen of case 5.

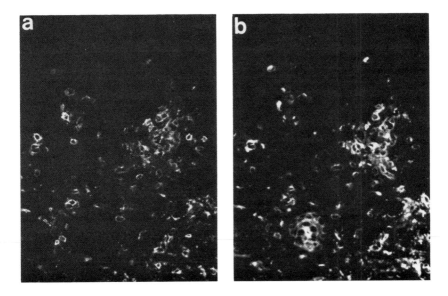

Figure 4. Double staining of the skin from case 9. (a) Leu 3 (FITC) and (b) HLA-DR (PE). Note the presence of double positive cells.

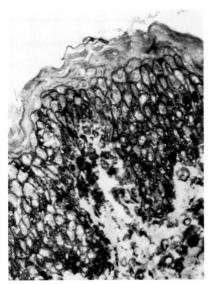

Figure 5. HLA-DR expression on the epidermal keratinocyte surface in case 3 (Peroxidase).

with anti-Leu 6 monoclonal antibodies (Harrist et al., 1983).
The number of Langerhans cells in the epidermis was similar
to that in the normal skin specimens.

The same immunofluorescence studies were carried out
on skin specimens obtained from patients with measles. As
compared with Kawasaki disease, an extensive mononuclear
cell infiltration was present mainly in the dermis. The
major population of such cells was Leu 2^+ T cells. Leu $M3^+$
macrophages were of much the same number seen in case of
Kawasaki disease. Histologically, a typical edema of the
papillary dermis in Kawasaki disease was not observed.

SUMMARY AND DISCUSSION

The skin lesion of Kawasaki disease was typified by
extensive edema associated with dilatation of small vessels
in the papillary dermis. Despite this exudative nature of
the inflammation, neutrophil emigration was slight and most
of the infiltrates were mononuclear cells. The site of BCG
vaccination showed a marked swelling. The histopathological
changes were basically similar to those described above,
although the inflammatory changes were more severe, exhibi-
ting exudation of fibrinogen and increase in mononuclear
cell infiltration. These mononuclear cells were mainly
comprised of macrophages and T cells and there were no or
few B cells. The major population of T cells belonged to
the Leu 3^+ helper/inducer subset. A large population of
these Leu 3^+ T cells was also HLA-DR$^+$, thereby probably
activated (Ko et al., 1979). Leu 2^+ T cells were negative
for HLA-DR antigen.

Expression of HLA-DR was also noted intercellularly in
localized areas of the epidermis in case of Kawasaki disease.
A typical example was observed at the site of BCG vaccination. Since the distribution of such HLA-DR antigen extended beyond that of Leu 6^+ Langerhans cells, the antigen
appeared to be expressed on the keratinocytes. It has been
reported that the expression of HLA-DR antigen on keratinocytes is found on several human dermatoses with lymphoid
infiltration, including delayed-type hypersensitivity
(Lampert et al., 1981; Lampert, 1984; Aiba and Tagami, 1984).
Although the mechanisms and the role of such Ia antigen
expression on keratinocytes are unknown, this phenomenon
appears to be linked to cellular immunity involving the

epidermis (Suitters and Lampert, 1982). It is possible that the infiltrating T cells stimulate the keratinocytes to produce Ia antigen via lymphokine such as γ-interferon. The γ-interferon is produced in mice by a group of helper T cells (T_H1) bearing L3T4 antigen, a murine counterpart of human Leu 3 (Mosmann et al., 1986) and acts to induce macrophage Ia expression (Steeg et al., 1982). Thus, the predominance of Leu 3^+ T cells in the skin lesion of Kawasaki disease may be related to the Ia expression on keratinocytes.

The similarity of skin lesion between Kawasaki disease and the delayed-type hypersensitivity has also been noted, on an morphological basis, e.g. extensive edema of papillary dermis, the presence of mast cells showing exocytotic degranulation at an early phase, and striking hypertrophy and occasional necrosis of vascular endothelial cells (Hirose and Hamashima, 1978; Dvorak et al., 1976). The extensive inflammatory changes at the site of BCG vaccination in patients with Kawasaki disease may be relevant.

The skin lesion of measles showed an extensive mononuclear cell infiltration, both in the dermis and epidermis, but lacked significant edema in the papillary dermis. The difference from the skin lesion of Kawasaki disease was evident in the predominance of Leu 2^+ cells in the infiltrating T cells. Transmissible agents have been implicated in the pathogenesis of Kawasaki disease (in this monograph). The agents, if any, would probably have to bear the potential to induce a skin lesion such as delayed-type hypersensitivity.

ACKNOWLEDGMENTS

We thank Drs. T. Kawasaki and Y. Yanase for cooperation and M. Ohara for critical reading of the manuscript.

REFERENCES

Aiba S, Tagami H (1984). HLA-DR antigen expression on the keratinocyte surface in dermatoses characterized by lymphocytic exocytosis (e.g. pityriasis rosea). Brit J Dermatol 111:285-294.
Dvorak AM, Mihm Jr MC, Dvorak HF (1976). Morphology of

delayed-type hypersensitivity reactions in man. Lab Invest 34:179-191.

Harrist TJ, Muhlbauer JE, Murphy GF, Mihm Jr MC, Bhan AK (1983). T6 is superior to Ia (HLA-DR) as a marker for Langerhans cells and indeterminate cells in normal epidermis: A monoclonal antibody study. J Invest Dermatol 80:100-103.

Hirose S, Hamashima Y (1978). Morphological observations on the vasculitis in the mucocutaneous lymph node syndrome. A skin biopsy study of 27 patients. Eur J Pediat 129:17-27.

Kawasaki T (1967). Mucocutaneous lymph node syndrome-clinical observation of 50 cases (in Japanese). Jpn J Allergol 16:178-222.

Kawasaki T, Kosaki F, Osawa S, Shigematsu I, Yanagawa S (1974). A new infantile acute febrile mucocutaneous lymph node syndrome (MCLS) prevailing in Japan. Pediatrics 54:271-280.

Ko HS, Fu SM, Winchester RJ, Yu DTY, Kunkel HG (1979). Ia determinants on stimulated human T lymphocytes. Occurrence on mitogen- and antigen-activated T cells. J Exp Med 150:246-255.

Lampert IA, Suitters AJ, Chisholm PM (1981). Expression of Ia antigen on epidermal keratinocytes in graft-versus-host disease. Nature 293:149-154.

Lampert IA (1984). Expression of HLA-DR (Ia like) antigen on epidermal keratinocytes in human dermatoses. Clin Exp Immunol 57:93-100.

Mosmann TR, Cherwinski H, Bond MW, Giedlin MA, Coffman RL (1986). Two types of murine helper T cell clone. I. Definition according to profiles of lymphokine activities and secreted proteins. J Immunol 136:2348-2357.

Steeg PS, Moore RN, Johnson HM, Oppenheim JJ (1982). Regulation of murine macrophage Ia antigen expression by a lymphokine with immune interferon activity. J Exp Med 156:1780-1793.

Suitters AJ, Lampert IA (1982). Expression of Ia antigen on epidermal keratinocytes is a consequence of cellular immunity. Br J Exp Path 63:207-213.

Kawasaki Disease, pages 193–207
© 1987 Alan R. Liss, Inc.

IMMUNE COMPLEXES IN KAWASAKI SYNDROME: A REVIEW

Lauren M. Pachman, M.D.[a], Betsy C. Herold, M.D.[a],
A. Todd Davis, M.D.[a], LeMing Hang, M.D.[b],
Jane G. Schaller, M.D.[c], Bruce Beckwith, M.D.[d],
Carlos M. Arroyave, M.D., Ph.D.[a], Maria S. Gawryl,
Ph.D.[e], Thomas Lint, Ph.D.[e], Stanford T.
Shulman, M.D.[a]

Department of Pediatrics, Children's Memorial
Hospital, Northwestern University Medical School,
Chicago, IL[a]; Scripps Clinic and Research
Facility, LaJolla, CA[b]; Tufts University,
Boston, MA[c]; University of Washington,
Seattle, WA[d]; Rush Presbyterian-St. Luke's Medical
Center, Chicago, IL[e]

This paper will review some general aspects of immune
complexes, some diseases in which they occur, methods of
measurement, and available data concerning immune complexes
in Kawasaki Syndrome. Immune complexes have been implicated
in experimental disease. The prototypic models are of serum
sickness (Germuth, 1953 and Dixon, 1958) in which administration of specific autologous antibody complexed to the
corresponding protein produced tissue injury in the host.
Circulating immune complexes comprise physiologic mechanisms
for the removal of exogenous and endogenous antigens and are
often eliminated without resultant tissue damage. Circulating immune complexes are found in normal subjects, demonstrate circadian and seasonal variations, and vary with the
type of food ingested, and level of exercise (Jans, 1982;
Paganelli, 1981).

Many different diseases have been found in which levels
of circulating immune complexes occur in excess of that
observed in healthy individuals. In some of these disorders,
including rheumatic, infectious, neoplastic and miscella-
neous diseases, elevated levels of immune complexes may
correlate with tissue injury (Table 1).

TABLE 1. Diseases Associated With Increased Concentrations of Circulating Immune Complexes.

Infectious diseases
Rheumatic diseases
Malignancy
Assorted acute and chronic conditions

Persistent infection	··········	Infectious agent
Autoimmunity	··········	Self-antigen
Extrinsic factors	··········	Environmental antigen

Mechanisms of immune complex production include an antibody response to a persistent infectious agent, a self-antigen, or an environmental stimulus. Multiple factors contribute to the biological activity and potential for producing pathological effects of these immune complexes (Table 2).

TABLE 2. Factors Affecting Immune Complex Biological Activity.

Immune Complex Size
    Antibody class and valence
    Antigen valence
    Concentration and affinity of antibody and antigen
Vascular Bed
Immunological Response

Size appears to be the most important factor. Large complexes are insoluble and are rapidly cleared by the reticulo-endothelial system, in contrast to smaller complexes which may continue to circulate and may not provoke an inflammatory response. Complexes of intermediate size are most often related to tissue injury. Complex size is determined by antibody and antigen valence, antibody affinity for antigen, as well as relative and absolute concentrations of antigen and antibody. Antigens that are univalent, together with bivalent antibodies, tend to form small immune complexes, while IgM antibodies and multivalent antigens tend to form larger complexes. In antigen excess, the antibody sites are saturated by individual antigen molecules, thus preventing cross-linkage and resulting in small complexes. Larger polymeric antigens with more than one site for binding antibody, however, may precipitate when antibody is in excess (Barnett, 1979; Theofilipoulos, 1979).

When considering the possibility of immune complex damage, the type of vascular bed is extraordinarily important. Immune complexes tend to be deposited in structures with specialized vasculature, like arterial walls, kidneys, skin, joints, and the choroid plexus, in which hydrodynamic factors such as filtration, increased luminal pressure and turbulence favor immune complex deposition. Depending on the subclass of immunoglobulin (IgG_1, IgG_2, IgG_3, IgG_4) complement will be fixed to a greater or lesser extent. Smaller or non-complement fixing immune complexes tend to be deposited in tissues and result in damage only if the permeability of local blood vessels is increased as a consequence of release of vasoactive amines. Immune complex deposition is enhanced by vascular permeability, which is increased by histamine and serotonin. Complement activation may promote the release of vasoactive amines and may proceed through the classical and/or alternative pathway. For example, the conversion of C5 to C5a and to a lesser extent, C3 to C3a, mediates leukocyte chemotaxis, but such activation does not seem to be necessary for tissue injury to occur. Until recently, reliable, sensitive indicators of complement activation have not been available and their application to immune complex diseases is just beginning. In fact, one needs to correlate the presence of immune complexes and some evidence of biological activity induced by these immune complexes to substantiate a hypothesis about their role as a causative agent in tissue injury. Immune complexes may also bind directly to platelets and cause release of their vasoactive amines. This effect is mediated by Fc receptors on platelet membranes which recognize subclasses of IgG but not other immunoglobulin isotypes. In addition, immune complexes may adhere to neutrophils, eosinophils, basophils, monocytes, and lymphocytes by virtue of receptors for Fc or various complement components. Activation of phagocytes may promote the release of hydrolytic enzymes as well as induce phagocytosis and degranulation. It is believed that complexes which also include IgM may induce enhanced antibody production, whereas IgG complexes may result in decreased IgG production. Immune complexes may moderate the proliferative response of B-cells to mitogen and inhibit T-cell helper activity and T-cell cytolysis.

TABLE 3.   Immune Complex Assays   -   Use Reported in Kawasaki Syndrome.

Cryoglobulins
Clq-Binding Assay (BA)
Clq-Solid Phase (SP)
Raji Cells
Platelet Aggregation
Monoclonal - RF
Staphylococcal Protein A
Complement Activation Products

Various methods (Table 3) of measuring immune complexes yield varying results. In Table 4, four representative diseases are compared using six different immune complex assays (Lambert, 1978). Most methods for detecting immmune complexes are unable to differentiate non-specific immuno-globulin aggregates from immune complexes containing antigen and antibody. Non-specific aggregation may occur during repetitive freezing and thawing, during the heating of serum samples or with evaporation and storage over time in porous containers. Because it is thought that the immune complexes themselves may be of varying sizes and composition at different times in the course of a a given disease, it is understandable that no single assay for immune complexes can be relied upon to provide assurance as to the presence or specificity of immune complexes in any disease (Endo, 1985; Kilpatrick, 1984).

TABLE 4. Immune Complex Detection in Disease (Percent Positive)[*].

Method	SLE	Vasculitis	RA	Leprosy
C1q-BA	78	76	83	74
C1q-SP	58	53	25	18
RAJI	91	65	71	89
KgB-SP	44	55	33	65
PAT	74	41	50	72
mRF-IA	25	53	71	30

[*] From Lambert, et al. (modified)

Cryoglobulins in sera precipitate on cooling and redissolve on warming. Cryoglobulins may be monoclonal, and are associated with multiple myeloma, cryoglobulinemia, malignant lymphoma, or with rare hyperviscosity syndromes. Cryoglobulins composed of IgG and IgM account for 75% of all cryoglobulins and are called precipitable rheumatoid factors, consisting of IgM directed against IgG. These complexes fix complement and are often associated with vasculitic syndromes. However, since other proteins and substances in sera may also precipitate when cooled, detection of cryoglobulins is not as specific or as sensitive as a test for immune complexes. When tested for cryoglobulins, sera should be collected, clotted, and centrifuged at 37°C and then refrigerated for 7 days to ensure that slow cold-precipitating proteins are detected.

There are several assays used to measure circulating immune complexes (Klein, 1981). Only those that have been applied to Kawasaki Syndrome will be discussed. In the C1q binding assay (C1q-BA) radiolabeled C1q, isolated from human sera and purified, is mixed with serum. The complexes bind to the labeled C1q in proportion to their concentration and then are precipitated with polyethylene glycol. However, there may be non-specific binding of C1q by various poly-anions, DNA, endotoxins, C-reactive protein, and heparin as well as by aggregated IgG and IgM (Theofilopoulos, 1979). In the solid-phase C1q assay (C1q-SP), C1q is coated on the surface of a tube and immune complexes that bind to immobilized C1q are measured by the addition of radiolabeled anti-IgG. Immune complexes of the IgG_4 subclass do not bind to complement. IgE and IgA may activate complement by the alternative pathway, but are not thought to bind directly to C1q; hence, this assay may fail to detect complexes that include IgG_4, IgA, and IgE.

The Raji cell lymphoblastoid line (RC) has receptors for C3 conversion products - C3b, C3d and other complement components including C1q. Complement fixing immune complexes will bind to the Raji cells and can be measured by the addition of radiolabeled anti-IgG. False positives may occur in the presence of IgG anti-lymphocyte antibody that reacts with Raji cell surface components. The C1q binding assay, both solid and fluid phase, as well as the Raji cell assay, all detect high molecular weight (2,000,000 daltons) complexes close to the equivalence zone, but not smaller complexes that may persist in the circulation (Krieger, 1985). Platelet aggregation may also be used to demonstrate immune complexes. Quantitation is obtained by recording the highest dilution of serum that produces the aggregation of a chosen sample of platelets. However, the presence of anti-platelet antibody, viruses, and enzymes may give false positive results, whereas rheumatoid factor and immune complexes with fixed complement inhibit platelet aggregation and decrease the sensitivity of the test. Monoclonal rheumatoid factors have a greater ability to precipitate immune complexes because they often have a greater binding affinity than does polyclonal rheumatoid factor, accounting for the greater sensitivity of the monoclonal rheumatoid factor assay in most situations. Rheumatoid factor assays will only detect IgG containing immune complexes, and rheumatoid factor in the test serum itself may interfere with the assay. Immune complexes may also be measured by the extent of the inhibition of binding of rheumatoid factor to IgG. Another protein which binds immune complexes is staphylococcal protein A via the Fc of IgG_1, IgG_2, and IgG_4, which has been used both for isolation of immune complexes and in inhibition assays.

TABLE 5. Summary of Immune Complex Data in Kawasaki Syndrome (Available in the English Language).

Author/Year	Method	Days After Onset	Percent Positive	Correlation with Coronary Artery Disease
Fossard/1977	PA	12	100	NT
Sawa/1979	RC, I-LA	14	41	
Weindling/1979	I-LA	14	100	NT
Elutheson[+]/1981	C1qBA	20-30	58	NT
Furuse/1983	C1qBA,	14	58,44	None
	Pro A.PT	30	16,33	
Miyata/1984	C1qBA	0-10	34	p<.05
Ono/1985		26-42	100	(Echo)
Mason/1985	C1qBA, RC	Variable	52,48	None (Echo)
Levin/1985	PA	10-30		p<.005
	IgA		85	(Echo)
	IgG			
Hashimoto/1986	C1qSP,	7, 25-35	3	None
	mRF,		3	(Echo)
	RBC Lysis		20	
Melish/1986	C1qBA, RC	30	50	None (Echo)
Mason[+]/1986	C1qBA, RC Anti-C3	Variable	69	None (Echo)

PA = Platelet Aggregation
RC = Raji Cell
I-LA = Inhibition Latex Agglutination
C1qBA = C1q Binding Assay
RBC = Complement Coated RBC
+ = abstract

C1q SPA = Solid Phase Assay
Anti C3 = $F(ab^1)_2$ Anti-C3 EIA
Prot A.PT = Staphylococcal Protein A. Precipitation Test
MRF=Monoclonal Rheumatoid Factor
NT = Not Tested

In reviewing the English-language literature concerning immune complexes in Kawasaki Syndrome (KS) (Table 5), a single patient (Fossard, 1977) was found to have a positive platelet agglutination test with a titer of 1:320 on day 12 with a low C4 and normal THC. In 1979, Sawa measured immune complexes using the Raji cell assay and an IgG latex agglu-

tination inhibition assay. Two weeks after onset of
symptoms, 41% of patients demonstrated immune complexes
(Sawa, 1979). A case report of a single child documented
inhibition of latex agglutination by presumed immune complexes in sera obtained about 14 days after disease onset
(Weindling, 1979). No coronary disease was noted.
Eluthesen (1981) reported that with the C1q BA, over 59% of
children with KS had immune complexes which appeared to be
maximal at 20-30 days after disease onset. In 1983, Furuse
used 2 assays, a C1q BA and staphylococcal protein A precipitation, to study 16 children with KS. Sera obtained at 14
days (acute phase) and 30 days after disease onset was
tested. Seven of 12 KS patients were positive for C1q and 4
of 9 were positive for staphyloccocal protein A in the acute
phase, 58% and 44% respectively. In 1984 and 1985,
(Miyata, 1984 and Ono, 1985) sera was tested from 32
children which had been obtained within 10 days of onset
(acute phase) and 26-42 days after onset (convalescent
phase). They used a C1q BA and showed that those KS children
with coronary aneurysms by echocardiography had higher
levels of circulating immune complexes (11/32) $p < .05$. All
14 with coronary disease had immune complexes detected by 50
days after onset of illness. Phagocytic activity was
decreased in patients with Kawasaki Syndrome, but this
decreased phagocytosis was not correlated with levels of
immune complexes. In 1985, Mason found that 42% of sera from
KS obtained at variable times after disease onset were
positive using a C1q solid phase assay, whereas the Raji-
cell assay RIA had 52% positive sera for immune complexes
two weeks after onset. By using one or both assays, 65% of
the 42 patients demonstrated the presence of immune complexes in their sera: with the C1q BA 52% were positive;
with the Raji cell assay, 48% were positive. He documented
that elevated serum immune complexes were present in all
stages of disease, but that they did not correlate with the
development of coronary artery disease. In 1985, Levin,
studying 19 children with Kawasaki Syndrome, found a factor
in KS sera that induced the aggregation and release of serotonin by normal platelets. This factor was of high
molecular weight with loss of activity at low pH, suggesting
that it was an immune complex. This factor rose concur-
rently with a rise in platelet count, contained IgG and IgA,
and was associated with the subsequent development of
coronary artery aneurysms. Coronary vessel disease was
correlated with platelet rise. IgA was present in 85% of
the immune complexes; IgG complexes were also elevated and

associated with platelet aggregating titer (p<.001). This observation was thought to indicate that immune complex vasculitis induced aggregation of platelets and release of serotonin. In 1986, Hashimoto, using paired sera from 30 KS patients drawn at day 7 and day 25-35, demonstrated that acute phase sera enhanced endothelial cell proliferation more than convalescent sera and more than sera from age-sex matched normal controls. Extensive search for immune complexes using a C1q solid phase assay (detects complement fixing complexes), monoclonal rheumatoid factors (detects IgG complement and non-complement fixing immune complexes) and red cell lysis in the presence of complement (detects C-3 bound complexes) were all essentially negative, 3%, 3%, and 20% respectively, suggesting that the promotion of proliferative endothelial cell activity was not an immune complex (Hashimoto, 1986). Melish commented in 1986 that the quantity of immune complexes in KS was lower than that found in SLE, but above that found in normal children, and that in her experience, their presence correlated neither with arthritis or coronary vessel disease. A recent abstract (Mason, 1986) reported that 29 children with KS had sera studied for immune complexes using 3 methods: Raji cell, C1q SPA, and anti-C3 ELISA. Immune complexes were present in 69% and their presence did not correlate with documented coronary vessel damage.

Therefore, published reports in the English literature indicate that variable results may be found when sera from children with Kawasaki Syndrome are tested for circulating immune complexes. It appears that complexes may be less frequent (detectable) in the very early phase of the disease (prior to 10-14 days post-onset). Those who have identified complexes appear to have done so in the third to fourth weeks of the disease.

In an attempt to clarify whether complexes played a role in producing the pathologic changes observed in Kawasaki Syndrome, we sought evidence of deposition of immunoglobulin in myocardial, endocardial and coronary tissue. We studied heart tissue from 6 children with fatal coronary artery disease of Kawasaki Syndrome (KS) and 8 age/sex/date-of-death and location matched controls using blocks containing the appropriate tissue and avidin-biotin complex staining techniques (Robb, 1981). Deposition of kappa, lambda, mu and gamma was found in the myocardium and in the coronary vessel walls.

TABLE 6.   Summary of Immunohistochemical Staining.

	Coronary		Myocardium		Endocardium	
	IgM	IgG	IgM	IgG	IgM	IgG
Controls	1/8	2/8	2/8	3/8	0/8	1/8
Kawasaki	6/6+	6/6++	5/6+++	5/6	2/6	3/6

+ = p<0.01   ++ = p<0.02   +++ = p<0.05

    IgG and IgM were both deposited in the coronary
myocardium and endocardium of the Kawasaki Syndrome children
more than in the control children, with the myocardium the
most significant for IgM, p<0.05 (Herold, 1985).
Furthermore, when 25 children with KS were studied for the
presence of cryoglobulins (Table 7), 10 of 25 had cryoprecipitants. These cryoprecipitants correlate with the
development of coronary artery abnormalities detected by
echocardiography (p=0.04) (Herold, unpublished observations).   Analysis of the cryoprecipitates showed only IgG
and IgM.   These studies were done prior to the utilization
of IV gammaglobulin as a study modality to assess its effect
on the development of coronary artery disease.   Mason
suggested recently that the administration of aspirin or IV
gammaglobulin does not alter the presence of immune
complexes (Mason, 1986).

TABLE 7.   Correlation of Cryoprecipitates with Echocardiographic Findings.

	Coronary Artery Abnormality Present	Coronary Artery Abnormality Absent
Positive Cryoprecipitates	7	3
Negative Cryoprecipitates	4	11

p = 0.04

In the laboratories of Drs. Gawryl and Lint we have very preliminary data which has employed a double sandwich enzyme-linked immunoabsorbent assay for the quantitation of the terminal complement complex in human sera (Gawryl, 1987). In this assay, the plate is coated with goat anti-human C-9, followed by rabbit antihuman C-5 and horseradish peroxidase conjugated goat anti-rabbit IgG. In sera obtained 4-17 days after onset, there is no consistent increase in the terminal complement complex in KS children vs. age/sex matched controls (Table 8).

TABLE 8.   Terminal Complement Complex (TCC), C5b-9 (ug/ml) in Kawasaki Syndrome Sera Obtained 4-17 Days Post-Onset

Patient	Kawasaki Syndrome	Sex/Age Control
1	< 0.3	< 0.3
2	< 0.3	12.1
3	< 0.3	5.6
4	< 0.3	< 0.3
5	< 0.3	< 0.3
6	8.2	< 0.3
7	< 0.3	< 0.3
8	< 0.3	< 0.3
9	< 0.3	4.3
10	< 0.3	< 0.3
Mean	1.09	2.41

* Adult Normal < 0.3 ug/ml TCC

However, in sera obtained from 6 children 18-31 days after onset there was a significant rise in terminal complement activation (p<.025) (Table 9). All 6 were paired to sera displayed in Table 8 and showed a relative increase over time of terminal complement activation.

TABLE 9. Terminal complement complex (TCC), C5b-9 (ug/ml) in Kawasaki Syndrome Sera Obtained 18-31 Days Post-Onset.

Patient	Kawasaki Syndrome	Sex/Age Controls
1	290.0	< 0.3
2	7.9	< 0.3
3	6.0	ND**
4	10.6	< 0.3
6	26.0	6.9
10	5.9	5.7
Mean	57.7 (p<.025)	2.7+

* Adult Normal < 0.3 ug/ml
** ND = Not done

In summary, we conclude from these studies that sera of patients with Kawasaki Syndrome may contain cryoprecipitates of the IgG and IgM classes and these cryoprecipitates appear to be more frequent in individuals who develop coronary artery abnormalities. A number of investigators have identified the presence of immune complexes in Kawasaki sera, reaching a peak at 24-30 days after onset of fever, but the relationship of these circulating immune complexes to both terminal complement complex activation and development of coronary artery damage remains to be determined. The presence of IgG and IgM deposition in the myocardium and coronary vessel walls suggests that these complexes may play a role in the pathogenesis of tissue damage, or they may be deposited there as a result of increased localized vascular permeability.

REFERENCES

Barnett EV, Knutson DW, Abrass CK, et al (1979). Circulating immune complexes: Their immunochemistry, detection and importance. Ann Intern Med, 91:430-440.

Dixon FJ, Vazquez JJ, Weigle WO, et al (1958). Pathogenesis of serum sickness. Arch Pathol 65:18-28.

Eluthesen K, Marchette N, Melish M, et al (1981). Circulating immune complexes in Kawasaki disease. Presented at the 21st Interscience Conference on Antimicrobial Agents, November 4.

Endo L, Corman LC, Panush RS (1983). Clinical utility of assays for circulating immune complexes. Med Clin North Am 69:623-636.

Fossard C, Thompson RA (1977). Mucocutaneous lymph-node syndrome (Kawasaki disease): probable soluble-complex disorder Br Med J 1:883.

Furuse A, Matsuda I (1983). Circulating immune complex in the mucocutaneous lymphnode syndrome. Eur J Pediatr 141:50-51.

Gawryl MS, Simon MT, Eatman JL, Lint TF (1987). An enzyme-linked immunoabsorbant assay for the quantitation of the terminal complement complex from cell membranes or in activated human sera. J Immunol Methods (In press).

Germuth FG (1953). A comparative histologic and immunologic study in rabbits of induced hypersenstitivity of the serum sickness type. J Exp Med 97:257-282.

Hashimoto Y, Yoshinoya S, Aikawa T (1986). Enhanced endothelial cell proliferation in acute Kawasaki Disease (Muco-cutaneous lymph node syndrome). Pediatr Res 20:943-946.

Herold B, Pachman LM, Davis AT, et al (1985). Immune complexes (IC) in the serum and cardiac tissue of children with Kawasaki syndrome (KS). Arthritis Rheum 28:S57.

Herold B, Hang L, Schaller J, et al: Immune complexes in the cardiac tissue of children with Kawasaki Syndrome (Manuscript in preparation).

Herold B, Davis AT, Arroyave C, et al: Cryoprecipitates in Kawasaki Syndrome: Correlation with coronary artery aneurysms (Manuscript in preparation).

Jans H, Dybkjaer E, Halberg P (1982). Circulating immune complexes in healthy persons. Scand J Rheumatol 11:124-198.

Kilpatrick DC, Weston J (1985). Immune complex assays and their limitations. Med Lab Sci 42:178-185.

Klein M, Liminovitch K (1981). The significance and limitations of current methods for detecting immune complexes. J Rheum 8:188-191.

Krieger G, Kneba M, Bolz I, et al (1985). Binding characteristics of three complement dependent assays for the detection of immune complexes in human serum. J Clin Lab Immunol 18:129-134.

Lambert PH, et al (1978). A WHO collaborative study for the evaluation of eighteen methods for detecting immune complexes in serum. J Clin Lab Immunol 1:1-15.

Levin M, Holland PC, Nokes TJC, et al (1985). Platelet immune complex interaction in pathogenesis of Kawasaki disease and childhood polyarteritis. Br Med J 290:1456-1460.

Mason WH, Jordan SC, Sakai R, et al (1985). Circulating immune complexes in Kawasaki syndrome. Pediatr Infect Dis 4:48-51.

Mason W, Jordan S, Sakai R (1987). The effect of gamma globulin (GG) infusions on levels of circulating immune complexes (CICs) in patients with Kawasaki Syndrome (KS). (In press).

Melish ME (1986). Intravenous immunoglobulin in Kawasaki syndrome: a progress report. Pediatr Infect Dis 5:S211-215.

Miyata K, Kawakami K, Onimaru T, et al (1984). Circulating immune complexes and granulocyte chemotaxis in Kawasaki disease. Jpn Circ J 48:1350-1353.

Ono S, Onimaru T, Kawakami K, et al (1985). Impaired granulocyte chemotaxis and increased circulating immune complexes in Kawasaki Disease. J Ped 106:567-570.

Paganelli P, Levinsky RJ Atherton DJ (1981). Detection of specific antigen within circulating immune complexes: Validation of the assay and its application to food antigen-antibody complexes formed in health and food allergic subjects. Clin Exp Immunol 46:44-53.

Reeback JS, Silman AJ, Holborow EJ, et al (1985). Circulating immune complexes and rheumatoid arthritis: a comparison of different assay methods and their early predictive value for disease activity and outcome. Ann Rheum Dis 44:79-82.

Robb JA (1981). A new enzyme immunolectin tissue stain. Diagnostic Med 4:87-95.

Sawa F (1979). Circulating immune complexes in MCLS. Acta Paed Jap 83:493-498.

Theofilopoulos AN, Dixon FJ (1979). Biology and detection of immune complexes. Adv Immunol 28:89-228.

Weindling AM, Levinsky RJ, Marshall WC (1979). Circulating immune complexes in mucocutaneous lymph-node syndrome (Kawasaki Disease). Arch Dis Child 54:241-242.

virological and bacteriological examinations and the remaining parts were fixed for light and electron microscopic studies. The synovial fluid and fluid from the blisters were smeared on glass for microscopic observation. The smears and sections from biopsy specimens were stained with Gimsa, Hematoxylin and Eosin stains. Direct and indirect immunofluorescent staining techniques, using FITC conjugated antibody, were also used. For the indirect immunofluorescent stain, we examined the same samples with neutralized anti-serum by using antigen and also unimmunized rabbit serum to exclude non-specific changes.

As with the controls, biopsy specimens from other various diseases, namely, cervical lymph node from a malignant lymphoma patient, mesenteric lymph nodes from patients with a pancreatic cyst, duodenal benign tumor, myoma uteri, skin biopsy specimens from exanthema of a malignant lymphoma patient, Osler's node from an infective endocarditis patient, and synovial fluid from two juvenile rheumatoid arthritis patients, were examined with the same methods and techniques as were used in this study.

RESULTS

1. Circulating immune complexes (CICs)

Raji cell assay : CICs were detected in 50 of 67 cases (75% of the cases), when FITC-conjugated anti-human IgG rabbit serum was used. (Fig. 1) In the initial phase of the illness lower titer levels were found. However, these titer levels gradually increased with time. Immune complexes reached a peak level at about the 30th day of illness and high IC titer levels continued for some time, before gradually decreasing. 16 of 20 cases with coronary aneurysms were positive for CICs. Furthermore, the CICs were detected during the early days of the illness. In 3 of the 20 cases, CICs were still detectable after more than one year. In one case without aneurysm two relapses occured. During both relapses, CICs were detectable in high titer in the initial stage of the relapse.

Clq EIA : In 11 of 36 cases (31% of the cases), positive titers were detected. A similar time course was

Figure 1.   IgG   circulating   immune   complex (Raji cell assay)

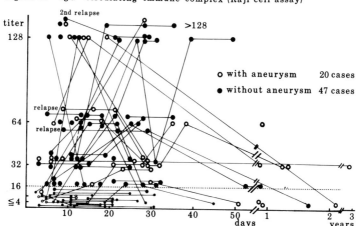

Note: A titer of 16 or greater is considered positive.

noted, i.e. a gradual increase in titer level with a peak between the 20th and 30th day of illness.

2. IgG soluble immune complex in serum and exudate

We compared ICs in sera with those in exudate. (Table 1) In the first case, the serum showed a titer of 1 : 16, but the titer in pericardial fluid was 1 : 128, by the Raji cell assay. Furthermore, C1q EIA was 1.5 mcg/ml in sera, as compared to a high value of 16.2 mcg/ml in pericardial fluid. Thus, IC titer levels in exudates from different body compartments were much higher than IgG IC levels, and these high titer levels were also detectable in the initial stage of the illness.

3. Antigen moiety of the CICs

The antigen moiety of the CICs was investigated by use of the Raji cell assay, in order to find a clue to the etiology of this disease. At first, we postulated that there may be a relationship between the hepatitis B virus surface antigen (HBs-Ag) and Kawasaki disease, because there was a previous report which described periarteritis nodosa associated with HBs-Ag (Gocke et al., 1970). However, in all specimens of HBs-Ag negative sera from 23 Kawasaki disease patients, we were unable to demonstrate HBs-Ag as the antigen moiety of the CICs.

Table 1   Soluble immune complex in serum and exudate (MCLS)

Pt. No.	Age	Sex	Day of illness	Immune complex titer IgG	
				serum	exudate
1	3	M	24	16	128 pericardial fluid
2	5	M	12	16	128 synovial fluid
3	3	F	12	4	128 synovial fluid
4	5	M	11	4	64 synovial fluid
5	3	F	7	4	80 vesicular fluid
6	1	F	5	128	64 vesicular fluid

Note : A titer of 16 or greater is considered positive.

1) Mite-antigen and CICs

Using the Raji cell assay with FITC conjugated anti-rabbit IgG goat serum incubated with anti-mite rabbit serum, we discovered that 28 of 38 cases (74% of the cases) were positive, indicating the presence of mite antigen.

2) P. acnes antigen and CICs

Cross antigenicity to P. acnes was found in the CICs in 27 of 63 cases (43% of the cases). In order to exclude non-specific changes, we examined the same specimens with neutralized anti-P. acnes (agglutinin-absorbed) serum or with non-immunized rabbit serum, and we received negative results. In the control group, P. acnes antigen was not detected in the CICs from juvenile rheumatoid arthritis patients nor from systemic lupus erythematosis patients.

4. Immune complex study of biopsy specimens

We examined the antigen found in biopsy specimens in two series of investigations. At first, we intended to detect the mite antigen, after P. acnes was isolated from the cervical lymph nodes and blood samples of Kawasaki disease patients. We tried to detect P. acnes antigen in the inflammatory sites of Kawasaki disease patients by using an indirect immunofluorescent stain combined with anti-P. acnes rabbit serum.

1)mite antigen in biopsy specimens (Table 2)

IgG or IgM immunoglobulins were detected in all specimens from Kawasaki disease patients. In the complement component, either C3 or C4 was detected in three of four synovial fluid smears, in one of seven smears from skin blister specimens, and in two of the three skin rash specimens. Mite antigen was demonstrated in twelve of the eighteen specimens from Kawasaki disease patients; however, it was not detected in any of the specimens from the control group.

Table 2 MITE ANTIGEN in BIOPSY SPECIMEN

		No.	Sex	Age	Day of illness or Diagnosis	IgG	IgM	C₃	C₄	Mite antigen
synovial fluid	KD.S	1	F	3	12	+	−	−	−	−
		2	F	10	24	+	+	−	+	−
		3	M	5	11	+	+	+	−	+
		4	F	3.7	17	+	+	−	+	+
	control	1	F	4	J.R.A.	+	−	−	−	−
		2	M	2.5	J.R.A.	+	N.D.*	−	N.D.	−
lymph node	KD.S	1	M	6	11	+	−	−	−	+
		2	M	0.5	7	+	−	−	−	+
	control	1	M	56	Pancreas cyst	−	−	−	−	−
		2	F	31	Duodenal benign tumor	−	−	−	−	−
		3	F	36	Myoma uteri	−	−	−	−	−
axillar aneurysm	KD	1	F	0.3	52	+	−	−	−	±
		2	M	0.3	71	+	−	−	−	±
blister	KD.S	1	F	3	7	+	−	−	−	+
		2	F	1	5	+	−	−	−	+
		3	F	2	7	+	+	−	−	+
		4	F	1	7	+	−	−	−	+
		5	M	3.6	6	+	+	−	−	−
		6	M	6	7	+	+	+	−	+
		7	F	0.8	33	−	+	−	−	−
skin	KD.S	1	M	2	5	+	−	−	−	+
		2	F	0.8	4	+	−	+	+	+
		3	M	0.9	5	+	−	+	+	+
	control	1	M	8	infective endocarditis	+	+	+	N.D.	−

* Not Done

2) P. acnes antigen in biopsy specimens (Table 3)

In both cases for the two patients with arthritis, P. acnes antigen, complement and immunoglobulin were detected in synovial fluid smears. In only one case, P. acnes antigen was detected in the rash specimen, but neither immunoglobulin nor complement was detected in this specimen. P. acnes antigen was detected in two of the three smears made from specimens of skin blisters. However, we could not find P. acnes antigen in the lymph node specimens. Seven out of eleven specimens from Kawasaki disease patients gave positive indications for the P. acnes antigen.

Table 3 Propionibacterium acnes ANTIGEN in BIOPSY SPECIMEN

		No.	Sex	Age	Day of illness or Diagnosis	IgG	IgM	C_3	C_4	P.acnes A strain*
synovial fluid	MCLS	1	F	4	10	+	−	+	−	+
		2	F	3.7	17	+	+	−	+	+
	control	1	M	2.5	J.R.A.	+	N.D.**	−	N.D.	−
lymph node	MCLS	1	M	0.9	5	−	+	+	N.D.	−
		2	M	4	5	−	+	+	−	−
	control	1	F	7	Malignant lymphoma	−	+		N.D.	−
blister	MCLS	1	M	3.6	6	+	+	−	−	+
		2	M	6	7	+	+	+	−	+
		3	F	0.8	33	−	+	−	−	−
skin	MCLS	1	M	0.10	5	−	−	−	N.D.	+
		2	M	2	5	+	−	−	−	−
		3	F	0.8	4	+	−	+	+	−
	control	1	F	7	Malignant lymphoma	−	−	−	N.D.	−
		2	M	8	infective endocarditis	+	+	+	N.D.	−

* Isolated from MCLS patient's lymph node

** Not Done

In all, we examined twenty-three specimens from twenty-three patients with Kawasaki disease and eight control specimens from patients with various other disease. Both immunoglobulin and complement showed positive immunofluorescent staining in nine patients with Kawasaki disease (39% of the patients). Only immunoglobulin was detected in thirteen of the specimens from Kawasaki disease patients i.e. in 57% of the patients. In only one specimen from a Kawasaki disease patient (4% of the total patient population), neither immunoglobulin nor complement was detected. Six specimens were investigated to determine the presence of both mite antigen and P. acnes antigen in the same specimen. These six specimens were : one of the five synovial fluid smears, three of the seven smears from skin blister specimens, and two of the five specimens of skin rash. Both antigens were detected in the same smear in the one synovial fluid smear, and in one of the smears from a skin blister specimen. We subsequently confirmed that the P. acnes antigen was one of the major components of the mite antigen, as determined by the micro-Ouchtalony method.

DISCUSSION

We studied the role of immune complexes in Kawasaki disease by serially determining the titer of soluble immune complexes in sera and exudates, and we investigated the antigen moiety of the immune complexes in order to find a clue to the etiology of this disease. In addition, we examined biopsy specimens for the presence of mite antigen and P. acnes antigen in the biopsy specimens, and also for the presence of IgG and IgM immunoglobulins and complement in the biopsy specimens. Circulating immune complexes were demonstrable in 50 of 67 cases (75% of the cases). The titers of soluble immune complexes from the pericardial effusion specimen, and from synovial fluid and vesicular fluid specimens were higher, in comparison with paired sera. Neither of the classes of immunoglobulin nor complement was detected in one of the skin rash biopsy specimens. A high incidence of P. acnes antigen was demonstrated in all of the biopsy specimens. Although we could not detect immune complex directly in the biopsy specimens, the fact that we detected immune complexes in these specimens may indicate that immune complexes play an important role in the inflammatory process in Kawasaki disease. Since P. acnes was isolated from cervical lymph node lesions and from the blood samples of Kawasaki disease patients, and cross antigenicity to P. acnes was detected in the biopsy specimens from Kawasaki disease patients, one should not neglect the possibility that P. acnes, i.e. (Propionibacterium acnes), may be the etiological agent causing Kawasaki disease.

Reference

Fujimoto T, Kato H, Ichinose E, and Sasaguri Y (1982). Immune Complex and Mite Antigen in Kawasaki disease. Lancet II : 980-981.

Gocke DJ, Hsu K, Morgan C, Bombardieri S, Lockshin M and Christian CL (1970). Association between polyarteritis and Australia antigen. Lancet II : 1149-1153.

Kato H, Fujimoto T, Inoue O, Kondo M, Koga Y, Yamamoto S, Shingu M, Tominaga K and Sasaguri Y (1983). Variant Strain of Propionibacterium acnes : A clue to the aetiology of Kawasaki disease. Lancet II : 1383-1388.

Kato H, Koike S, Yamamoto M, Ito Y, and Yano E (1975). Coronary aneurysm in infants and young children with acute febrile mucocutaneous lymph node syndrome. J Pediat 86 : 892-898.

Kawasaki T, Kosaki F, Okawa S, Shigematsu I and Yanagawa H (1974). A new infantile acute febrile mucocutaneous lymph node syndrome (MLNS) prevailing in Japan. Pediatrics 54 : 271-276.

Tung KSK, Woodroffe AJ, Ahlin TD, Williams Jr RC and Wilson CB (1978). Application of the solid phase Clq and Raji cell radioimmune assays for detection of circulating immune complexes in glomerulonephritis. J Clin Invest 62 : 61-72.

Yata J and Sawa F (1977). Demonstration of serum immune complex by Raji cell assay. Clin Immunol 9 : 1001-1006. (Jpn)

Kawasaki Disease, pages 219-226
© 1987 Alan R. Liss, Inc.

IMMUNE COMPLEXES AND CYTOTOXICITY

Wilbert Mason and Stanley Jordan

Childrens Hospital of Los Angeles, Los Angeles,
California (WM), Cedars-Sinai Medical Center,
Los Angeles, California (SJ)

INTRODUCTION

Numerous clinical and pathological manifestations of
Kawasaki disease (KD) have suggested the illness might be
an immunologically mediated disorder (Melish, 1986; Landing
and Larson, 1977). Indeed, a number of immunologic abnormalities have been described during KD including the presence of immune complexes (ICs) in the sera of patients with
the illness (Fossard and Thompson, 1977). ICs were detected
by either Raji cell radioimmune or Clq solid phase assays in
69% of sera specimens from patients with KD seen at Childrens Hospital of Los Angeles (Mason et al, 1985). (Fig. 1)
These observations were consistent with the findings of a
number of other investigators (Corbeel et al, 1977; Eluthesen et al, 1981). The most striking histopathologic finding
in KD is a panvasculitis with monocytic infiltration of the
walls of medium to small blood vessels associated with immunoglobulin deposition and endothelial necrosis. (Fig. 2)
The concomitant findings of ICs in serum of patients with a
severe vasculitis suggests the possibility that there might
be a cause and effect relationship between the two.

In this presentation we will briefly review the
biological effects of immune complexes, especially cytotoxic
mechanisms of injury and what evidence exists regarding cytotoxicity of ICs in KD.

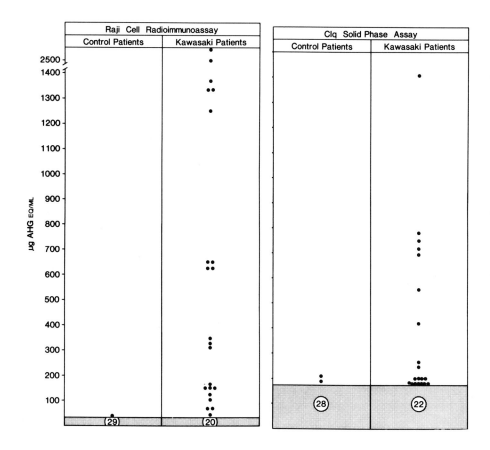

Figure 1. Detection of circulating immune complexes by
RC-RIA and Clq-SPA methods in sera from patients
with KD and normal control sera. Serum samples with normal
levels are enumerated in the shaded areas. (Normal levels:
RC-RIA 31.69 ug AHG eq/ml; Clq-SPA 34.32 ug AHG eq/ml.)
The difference in distribution between control and KS patient sera is highly significant at the 0.005 level.

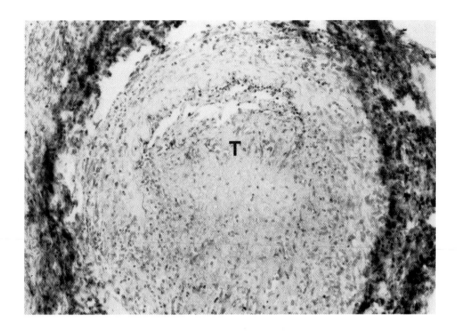

Figure 2. Cross section of a thrombosed coronary artery from a 16 week old child who died with Kawasaki syndrome. Thrombus is indicated (T) centrally. Darkly stained material in the adventitia and media of the artery is tissue stained for immunoglobulin (IgG).

BIOLOGY OF IMMUNE COMPLEXES

Antigen-antibody complexes take on properties that are not inherent to either antigen or antibody alone. These include the ability to react with complement and with cellular Fc and complement receptors (Theofilopoulos and Dixon, 1980). Several factors influence the biological activity of ICs including the nature of the antigen and the nature of the antibody and, more importantly, the ratio of the two reactants (Aguado and Theofilopoulos, 1985). In antigen excess polyvalent antigens form very small ICs, usually with a single antibody molecule divalently attached to two antigen molecules. Such ICs cannot fix complement or initiate the inflammatory response. Alternatively, ICs formed in abundant antibody excess tend to be large, due to lattice formation, insoluble and are rapidly phagocytised from the circulation. They fix complement and thus have the potential to initiate the inflammatory response but because they are so rapidly cleared, their inflammatory potential is limited. The ICs with the greatest potential to cause disease are those formed at slight antigenic excess (Dixon, 1963). These are of intermediate size and are soluble but not rapidly phagocytized. They circulate widely and are large enough to fix complement so the potential for disseminated inflammatory response is present.

Under normal circumstances complement acts to prevent ICs from forming large lattices and precipitating in tissues. It also allows for attachment of the complement fixed-IC to red blood cell (RBC) receptors specific for C3b, termed CR1 receptors. The RBC then transports the IC to reticulo-endothelial cells for removal from the circulation (Schifferli et al, 1986).

In pathological circumstances, ICs are deposited in tissues augmented by an increase in the permeability of blood vessels caused by the release of vasoactive amines, such as serotonin, by aggregated platelets. The multifaceted effects of ICs operating through complement activation leads to the discharge of lysosomal enzymes by neutrophils and macrophages and the induction of phagocytic cell opsonization and ingestion (Aguado and Theofilopoulos, 1985).

EFFECTS OF IMMUNE COMPLEXES ON CYTOTOXICITY

ICs may influence cytotoxicity through the action of complement or cellular mediators:
1. Complement activation. Cells can be lysed directly by the assembly of the terminal attack sequence of complement following its activation by ICs bound to the cell membrane. Alternatively, cell death may occur indirectly in a bystander fashion when there is activation of complement in the fluid phase.
2. Cell mediated cytotoxicity. IC may inhibit cytotoxicity by blockade of cell mediated cytotoxicity by lymphocytes and macrophages. Alternatively, ICs formed in antibody excess can "arm" non-immune "killer" or K-cells which in turn become cytotoxic against target cells coated with the antigen in question (Perlmann et al., 1972), so called antibody dependent cell cytotoxicity.

Disease or conditions where one or more of these cytotoxic mechanisms have come into play as a result of IC deposition include acute and chronic serum sickness, the Arthus reaction, systemic lupus erythematosus and glomerulonephritis.

CYTOTOXICITY OF IMMUNE COMPLEXES IN KD

Until very recently relatively little data directly or indirectly implicating IC-mediated cytotoxicity in KD was available. In 1984, Niwa and Sohmiya suggested that there was a marked increase in oxygen intermediate generation induced by activated polymorphonuclear leukocytes (PMNs) in the early stage (i.e. the first 5 days) of KD. When PMNs from KD patients were incubated with ^{51}Cr-labled endothelial cells, the release of ^{51}CR was markedly elevated implicating oxygen intermediates in the endothelial cell damage. The authors speculated that ICs, known to be present in the early stages of KD, might potentiate the generation of oxygen intermediates by PMNs which, in turn, cause endothelial cell necrosis in KD.

A separate study (Levin et al, 1985) associated the rise in circulating platelets in KD with the appearance in the circulation of a factor that induced platelet aggregation and serotonin release in normal platelets. This factor was of high molecular weight and its activity was lost at low pH, features that were suggestive of an IC. Moreover, the authors demonstrated appearance of ICs in the circulation as the platelet count increased. From these observations the authors proposed that following the initial (probably infective) phase of KD an immune complex vasculitis ensued when antibodies to the inciting agent appeared in the circulation. The ICs then caused platelet aggregation and the release of serotonin which increased vascular permeability and facilitated further deposition of ICs in tissues. Direct evidence of cytotoxicity was not offered in this study, however.

Recently, reports from Japan and the United States showed that intravenous administration of immunoglobulin within the first 10 days of KD ameliorated the symptoms and significantly decreased the prevalence of coronary artery abnormalities. Investigations at our institutions failed to show any significant decline in the

occurence of ICs in the sera of KD patients following immunoglobulin therapy or a lower incidence of ICs compared to
a group of KD patients who received aspirin alone (Mason et
al, 1986). In addition, we were unable to demonstrate any
correlation between the presence of clinical parameters
(i.e. fever, myocarditis or coronary artery abnormalities)
and the presence of ICs. Finally, the sera of 12 patients
with KD were examened using an ELISA assay for antiendothelial cell antibodies which have been found in the sera of
patients with other systemic vasculitic diseases. No correlation between the presence of antiendothelial cell antibodies and ICs could be shown. These, albeit, indirect observations suggested that ICs were not implicated in the
pathogenesis of the vasculitis in KD.

The most significant observations to date regarding the
role that ICs might play in the induction of cytotoxic effects on vascular endothelium was recently reported by Leung
et al (1986) who hypothesized that vascular damage in KD was
initiated by circulating antibodies directed to vascular
endothelium. They assayed sera of patients in the acute and
convalescent phases of KD and age matched controls for complement dependent cytotoxic activity against ^{111}In-labelled
human umbilical vein endothelial (HUVE) cells. Sera from KD
or control patients failed to induce cytotoxicity of cultured endothelial cells (EC) under standard conditions. However, when EC were preincubated with gamma interferon, complement – mediated killing of HUVE cells was observed. Their
studies further demonstrated that the serum factor responsible for the cytotoxicity was IgM antibody directed against
inducible antigenic determinants present on δ-IFN – treated
human vascular EC. Significantly, they showed that the observed cytotoxic effects were not mediated by ICs since none
of the tested sera in the study were positive for IC and
certrifugation of the sera did not remove the antiendothelial cell activity. In addition, formation of IC by heat
treatment did not result in an increase in endothelial cell
cytotoxicity.

CONCLUSIONS

1. ICs can produce cytotoxicity by complement activation or cell mediated mechanisms in certain in vitro systems
and pathologic states.
2. With respect to KD, there is no clear cut relationship thus far demonstrated between the presence of IC and

cellular cytotoxicity.

    3. Demonstrable endothelial cell cytotoxicity in KD seems to be related to serum factors other than ICs.

REFERENCES

Aguado MT, Theofilopoulos AN (1985). Immune complexes in human and experimental disease. In Gupta S, Talal N (Peds): "Immunology of rheumatic diseases", New York and London: Plenum, pp 493-513.

Corbell L, Delmotte B, Standaert L, Casteels-VanDael M, Eeckels R (1977). Kawasaki disease in Europe. Lancet 1:797.

Dixon FJ (1963) The role of antigen-antibody complexes in disease. Harvey Lect 58:21-52.

Eluthesen K, Marchette NJ, Melish ME, Hick RM (1981). Circulating immune complexes in Kawasaki's disease: detection by Clq bending assay. Presented at 21st Interscience Conference on Antimicrobial agents and chemotherapy.

Fossard C, Thompson RA (1977). Mucocutaneous lymph-node syndrome (Kawasaki disease): probable soluble-complex disorder. Br Med J 1:883.

Landing BH, Larson EJ (1977). Are infantile periarteritis nodosa with coronary artery involvement and fatal mucocutaneous lymph node syndrome the same? Comparison of 20 patients from North America with patients from Hawaii and Japan. Pediatrics 59:651-662.

Leung DYM, Collins T, Lapierre LA, Gelia RS, Pober JS (1986). Immunoglobulin M antibodies present in the acute phase of Kawasaki syndrome lyse cultured vascular endothelial cells stimulated by gamma interferon. J Clin Invest 77:1428-1435.

Levin M, Holland PC, Nokes TJC, Novelli V, Mala M, Levensky RJ, Dillon MJ, Barratt TM, Marshall WC (1985). Platelet immune complex interaction in pathogenesis of Kawasaki disease and childhood polyarteritis. Br Med J 290:1456-1460.

Mason WH, Jordon S, Sakai R, Takahashi M (1986). The effect of gamma globulin infusions on levels of circulating immune complexes in patients with Kawasaki syndrome. Presented at 26th Interscience Conference on Antimicrobiol Agents and Chemotherapy.

Melish ME (1986). Intravenous immunoglobulin in Kawasaki syndrome: a progress report. Pediatr Infect Dis 5:5211-5215.

Niwa Y, Sohmiya K (1984). Enhanced neutrophilic functions in mucocutaneous lymph node syndrome, with special reference to the possible role of increased oxygen intermediate generation in the pathogenesis of coronary thromboarteritis. J Pediatr 104:50-60.

Perlmann P, Perlmann H, Biberfeld P (1972). Specifically cytotoxic lymphocytes produced by preincubation with antibody - complexed target cells. J Immunol 108:558-561.

Schifferli JA, Ng YC, Peters DK (1986). The role of complement and its receptor in the elimination of immune complexes. N Engl J Med 315:488-495.

Theofilopoulos AN, Dixon FJ (1980). Immune complexes in human disease. Amer J Path 100:531-569.

Kawasaki Disease, pages 227-237
© 1987 Alan R. Liss, Inc.

PLATELET IMMUNE COMPLEX INTERACTION IN THE
PATHOGENESIS OF KAWASAKI DISEASE

Michael Levin
Philip C. Holland
Valerio Novelli
Departments of Immunology and Infectious Disease
Institute of Child Health and The Hospital For
  For Sick Children
Great Ormond Street, LONDON, WC1N 1EH

INTRODUCTION

It is not surprising that there has been interest in the role of platelets in the pathophysiology of Kawasaki disease as thrombocytosis is a characteristic feature of the disorder, and coronary artery thrombosis is the most important complication. The role of platelets in thrombosis is familiar to everyone, but less well known is their function as inflammatory cells (Nachman and Polley, 1979).

Platelets can be activated by many different stimuli including: contact with subendothelial tissues; immune complexes of IgG and IgE subclasses which bind to Fc receptors on the platelet; platelet activating factor released from leukocytes; adrenalin, serotonin and thromboxane A_2; and several toxins or enzymes released by bacteria and viruses. In response to any of these stimuli, platelets aggregate and release their granule contents, in an energy dependent process analagous to neutrophil degranulation. Many of the substances released by platelets have important inflammatory properties: serotonin increases vascular permeability, and has mitogenic and vasoactive activity; adrenalin and thromboxane A_2 are potent aggregating and vasoconstrictive agents; platelet factor 4 neutralizes heparin, as does beta thromboglobulin, which also inhibits prostacyclin synthesis; platelet derived growth factor stimulates proliferation of subendothelial tissues and is chemotactic for smooth muscle cells, and a variety of proteolytic enzymes are able to degrade or damage vascular connective tissue and membranes (Gordon, 1981).

While release of these inflammatory substances from platelets probably contributes to vascular damage in many diseases, of most relevance to Kawasaki disease is the evidence that platelets play an important role in the pathogenesis of immune complex vasculitis (Cochrane, 1971). In a series of studies in the 1960's, C.G. Cochrane and others studied the role of platelets in a rabbit model of serum sickness vasculitis, which is similar to the vasculitis of Kawasaki disease in affecting predominantly the coronary arteries, and other extraparenchymal muscular arteries (Cochrane and Hawkins, 1967). One to two weeks after injection of foreign protein into the rabbits, high molecular weight antigen antibody complexes appeared in the circulation. These complexes interacted with platelets either directly or by triggering release from leukocytes of platelet activating factors, and caused platelet activation and release of vasoactive and inflammatory mediators (Kniker and Cochrane, 1968). The platelet derived mediators (of which, in the rabbit, serotonin and histamine are the most important), increased vascular permeability and allowed the immune complexes to deposit in the subendothelial tissues. The pathogenic importance of the platelets was confirmed by prior depletion of platelets with antiplatelet antibody, which greatly diminshed the vascular damage, as did injection of histamine and serotonin antagonists (Kniker and Cochrane, 1968; Cochrane 1971).

Immune complexes have been detected in the acute phase of Kawasaki disease in several studies (Kusakawa and Heiner, 1976; Fossard and Thompson, 1977). Futhermore, several published studies also suggest that platelet activation occurs in Kawasaki disease: platelets are hyperaggregable in both acute and convalescent phases of the illness (Shirahata, et al, 1983; Yamada, et al, 1977), circulating platelet aggregates have been detected (Shirahata, et al, 1983) and raised plasma concentrations of platelet derived factors such as beta thromboglobulin (Shirahata, 1983), platelet factor 4 (Shirahata, 1983), and thromboxane A_2 (Inamo, 1983) indicate that platelet release has occurred.

It is thus possible that an interaction between immune complexes and platelets similar to that occurring in the rabbit vasculitis model may occur in Kawasaki Disease. In order to establish the mechanisms of platelet activation in Kawasaki Disease, we have studied a series of 19 children fulfilling the diagnostic criteria for Kawasaki Disease who were admitted to the Hospital For Sick Children, Great Ormond Street, London (Levin, et al, 1983).

METHODS

The presence of serum factors which aggregate platelets was detected by a modification of the platelet aggregating titre (PAT) test of Penttinnen and Myllyla (Penttinnen and Myllyla, 1968). Serial dilutions of patients' or control serum were added to washed group-O platelets in microwells, and aggregation detected macroscopically after overnight incubation. Plasma factors which induce platelet aggregation were detected by mixing patients' or control plasma with washed normal platelets, and observing aggregation in a Payton dual channel aggregometer.

To identify factors causing platelet granule release, platelets from a healthy group-O donor were labeled with C^{14} serotonin. The amount of C^{14} serotonin released following mixing of the platelets with either Kawasaki or control plasma was then quantified by beta counting.

To characterize the platelet aggregating factors, plasma or serum from children with Kawasaki disease was fractionated by sucrose density gradient ultracentrifugation, and the individual fractions were tested for aggregating activity using the PAT test and aggregometry. As we suspected that the platelet aggregating factors might be immune complexes, immune complexes were precipitated from serum with 2% polyethylene glycol, and the concentrations of IgM, IgA, and IgG in the precipitates were quantified using an ELISA.

RESULTS

All 19 patients developed thrombocytosis in the second and third week of the illness, as the fever and mucous membrane changes began to subside. After reaching a peak in the third and fourth week of the illness (often exceeding 1,000 x 10^9/L), the platelet count fell rapidly in the fifth week and then declined gradually toward normal (Figure 1).

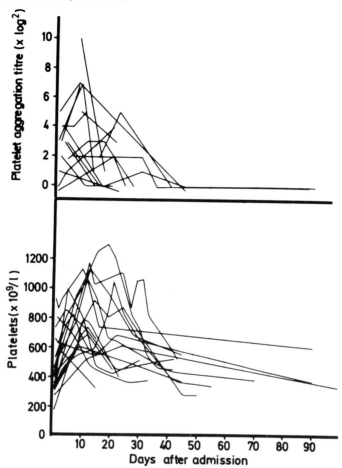

FIGURE 1. Time course of platelet count (bottom) and platelet aggregating titre (top) after admission in patients with Kawasaki disease.

The peak platelet count was significantly higher in those who developed coronary artery aneurysms (detected by cross sectional echocardiography) than in those who did not (p < 0.005 using students t-test) (Figure 2).

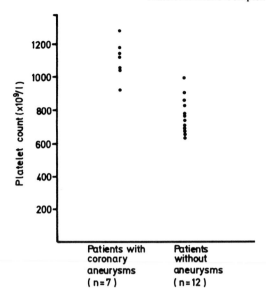

FIGURE 2: Peak platelet count in patients with and without coronary artery aneurysms detected on cross sectional echocardiography.

The rise and subsequent fall in platelet count was associated with a similar rise and fall in serum platelet aggregating activity detected by the PAT test (Figure 1). There was a significant correlation between the platelet count and the platelet aggregating titre (p < 0.001 using Spearman Rank test).

Plasma from the Kawasaki disease patients also aggregated washed normal platelets when mixed in the platelet aggregometer, whereas, no aggregation was observed on mixing control plasma with normal platelets. The aggregation was diminished by calcium chelation with EDTA, and completely inhibited by prostacyclin in a concentration of 10 nanomoles/liter (Figure 3).

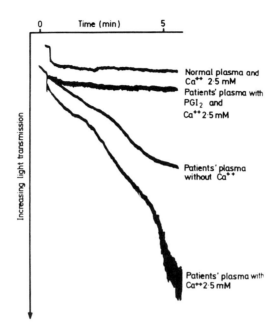

FIGURE 3:   Aggregation on addition of plasma from normal
control   and   patients   with   Kawasaki   disease   to   washed
normal platelets.

When Kawasaki disease plasma was mixed with normal
platelets previously labeled with C14 serotonin, 20 to 70
percent of the serotonin was released from the platelets,
whereas, release did not occur on mixing normal plasma
with labeled platelets.

When KD serum or plasma was fractionated by Sucrose
density gradient ultracentrifugation at pH7, all the platelet
aggregating activity was found in the high molecular
weight fractions (above that of IgM).   However, when the
fractionation was performed following acidification of the
plasma to pH3, no aggregating activity was detected in any
fraction (fractions tested after readjusting the pH to 7)
(Figure 4).

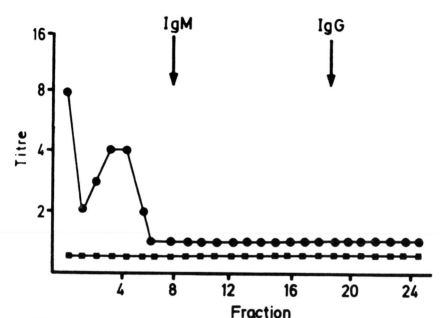

FIGURE 4: Fractionation of serum from patients with Kawasaki disease by sucrose density gradient ultracentrifugation. IgM and IgG were used as molecular weight markers. Aggregating activity was detected in fractions 1 through 6 separated at pH 7 (dots). No aggregation was detected in fractions prepared at pH 3 (squares).

The relatively high molecular weight of the aggregating factor and the loss of activity following fractionation at low pH suggest that the factor is an immune complex. This was supported by the highly significant correlation between the platelet aggregating titre and the presence of IgG immune complexes, detected by PEG precipitation (p < 0.001, Spearman rank correlation) (Figure 5).

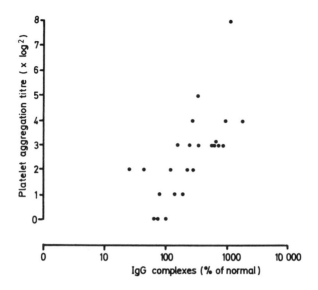

FIGURE 5: Correlation between platelet aggregating titre and IgG immune complexes in patients with Kawasaki disease (p < 0.001; Spearman Rank correlation).

SUMMARY

We have shown that the thrombocytosis which occurs in the 3rd and 4th week of Kawasaki disease is associated with the appearance in the circulation of platelet aggregating factors detected by the PAT test. These factors induce aggregation and serotonin release from normal platelets. The aggregation can be blocked by EDTA and Prostacyclin. The aggregating factor appears to be of high molecular weight, and its activity was lost following fractionation at low pH. The platelet aggregating activity was significantly associated with the presence of IgG immune complexes, and these features suggest that IgG immune complexes are responsible for the platelet aggregating activity.

DISCUSSION

The appearance in the 2nd and 3rd week of Kawasaki disease of platelet aggregating immune complexes, which induce serotonin release from platelets, is reminiscent of the events occurring in rabbit serum sickness vasculitis (Cochrane, 1971). It seems likely that the release from platelets of vasoactive and inflammatory mediators may contribute to the vascular damage by increasing vascular permeability and facilitating deposition of immune complexes in the vessel wall.

It is perhaps paradoxical that thrombocytosis rather than thrombocytopenia is associated with the presence of platelet aggregating immune complexes, as platelets are normally rapidly cleared from the circulation following activation. However, immune complexes are known to impair reticulo-endothelial function and to delay the clearance of damaged red blood cells or colloidal carbon aggregates (Haakenstad and Mannik, 1974; Lockwood, et al, 1979). The rise in platelet count may, therefore, be a reflection of reticulo-endothelial blockade by immune complexes.

The time course of the thrombocytosis and appearance of platelet aggregating immune complexes, occurring in the 3rd week of the illness, when the fever and systemic manifestations are often improving suggests that Kawasaki disease may have at least two pathophysiological phases. We would suggest that the initial febrile phase, when lymphadenopathy and mucocutaneous manifestations are prominent, is most compatible with an infectious etiology. In the 3rd week of the illness IgG antibody to the initiating agent is produced, and the resulting antigen-antibody complexes may initiate the 2nd phase of the illness, an immune complex vasculitis, during which platelets are aggregated by the immune complexes, and by releasing mediators of inflammation, contribute to the vascular damage.

While identification of the causative infectious agent is obviously the major research priority, the involvement of platelets in the pathogenesis of the vascular and thrombotic lesions may offer areas for therapeutic intervention. Plasmapheresis to remove immune complexes or the administration of immunoglobulin to modulate the size or solubility of immune complexes have already been utilized with beneficial effects. Platelet inhibiting drugs, such as prostacyclin and Dipyridamole, or drugs which antagonize mediators released from platelets (such as the serotonin inhibitor, Kentanserin) may lessen both the vascular damage and the likelihood of coronary artery thrombosis.

ACKNOWLEDGEMENT

Figures 1 through 5 were reproduced from Levin et al, 1985 with kind permission of the British Medical Journal.

REFERENCES

Cochrane CG (1971). Mechanisms involved in the deposition of immune complexes in tissues. J Exp Med 134:755-758.

Cochrane CG, Hawkins D (1967). Studies on circulating immune complexes. III. Factors governing the ability of circulating complexes to localize in blood vessels. J Exp Med 127:137-154.

Fossard C, Thompson RA (1977). Mucocutaneous lymph-node syndrome (Kawasaki disease): probable soluble complex disorder. Br Med J i:883.

Gordon JL (Ed.) (1981). Platelets In Biology and Pathology. 2. Research Monographs in Cell and Tissue Physiology. Vol 5. Elsevier/North Holland Biomedical Press. Amsterdam, New York.

Haakenstad AO, Mannik M (1974). Saturation of the reticulo-endothelial system with soluble immune complexes. J Immunol 112:1939-1948.

Inamo Y (1983). Studies on plasma thromboxane B-2 levels in patients with Kawasaki disease: as an indicator of coronary aneurysm formation. Acta Pediatrics Japonica 25:154-159.

Kusakawa S, Heiner DC (1976). Elevated levels of immunoglobulin E in acute febrile mucocutaneous lymph node syndrome. Pediatr Res 10:108-111.

Kniker WT, Cochrane CG (1968). The localization of circulating immune complexes in experimental serum sickness. J Exp Med 127:119-135.

Levin M, Holland PC, Nokes TJC, Novelli V, Mola M, Levinsky R, Dillon MJ, Barratt TM, Marshall WC (1985). Platelet immune complex interaction in the pathogenesis of Kawasaki disease and childhood polyarteritis. Brit Med J 290:1456-1460.

Lockwood CM, Worlledge S, Nicholas A, Cotton C, Peters DK (1979). Reversal of impaired splenic function in patients with nephritis or vasculitis by plasma exchange. N Engl J Med 300:524-530.

Nachman RL, Polley M (1979). The platelet as an inflammatory cell. Trans Am Clin Climatol Assoc 90:38-43.

Penttinnen K, Myllyla G (1968). Interaction of human blood platelets, viruses, and antibodies. I. Platelet aggregation test with micro equipment. Annales Medicinae Experimentalis et Biologiae Fenniae 46:188-192.

Shirahata A, Nakamura I, Asakura A (1983). Studies on blood coagulation and antithrombotic therapy in Kawasaki disease. Acta Paediatrica Japonica 25:104-115.

Yamada K, Shirahata A, Shinakai A, Meguro T (1977). Hematological studies on acute febrile mucocutaneous lymph node syndrome with special reference to the platelet--the thrombus formation and etiology of MCLNS. Acta Paediatrica Japonica 81:1263-1271.

Kawasaki Disease, pages 239-250
© 1987 Alan R. Liss, Inc.

COAGULATION ABNORMALITIES IN KAWASAKI DISEASE

Kaneo YAMADA, Akira SHIRAHATA[*] and Minoru INAGAKI[**]

Department of Pediatrics, School of Medicine, St. Marianna
University, Kanagawa, Department of Pediatrics, University of
Occupational and Environmental Health, Kitakyushu[*] and Depart-
ment of Pediatrics, Keio University, Tokyo,[**] Japan

At first, the authors have to mention that the study of
coagulation in the following review includes the study of
the factors of coagulation itself, and also platelets and
the factors of fibrinolysis. The purposes of studying coagulation, platelets and fibrinolysis in Kawasaki disease
are provided in the following three items.

The first purpose is to investigate the state of hypercoagulability in Kawasaki disease. By researching the grade
and duration of the state of hypercoagulability, we can at-
tain information that is useful in developing a program of
therapy. The second purpose is to find a valuable indicator
for the grade of the disease among the many examinations of
coagulation. Especially of value would be an indicator that
would signify the developement of an aneurysm at an early
stage. The third purpose is to aid in the discovery of the
etiology, which remains unknown. Among the three purposes
in this extensive study of coagulation, works on the first
and second purposes have been carried out, while the search
for the etiology continues to produce no results. The most
common work relating to the first and second purposes has
been consisting of the activation of platelets.

Activation of platelets

Since 1977 many workers have reported platelets being
activated in Kawasaki disease by using various methods of
assay (Table 1). These methods have included platelet aggregation, spontaneous platelet aggregation, the assay of
the von Willebrand Factor, platelet adhesion, βthrombo-

globulin (βTG), production of malondialdehyde (MDA) and the conversion of arachidonic acid to TXB_2.

TABLE 1. Studies on activation of platelets in Kawasaki disease (Part 1)

Items	Authors	Remarks
Platelet aggregation	K. Yamada, et al. 1977, 1978 T. Yokoyama, et al. 1980 Mukaiyama 1982	Increased for 6 months
Spontaneous platelet aggregation (Wu & Hook method)[6]	A. Shirahata, et al 1979	Demonstrated for 6 months Increased especially in thrombocytosis
von Willebrand factor	M. Yasui, et al. 1979 M. Shinozaki, et al. 1979	Increased in early stage
Platelet adhesion (Baumgartner's method)	M. Inagaki, et al. 1982	Increased for 3 months
βThromboglobulin (βTG) Platelet factor 4(PF4)	A. Shirahata, et al. 1983	Increased for 6 months
Production of Malondialdehyde (MDA)	N. Yoshino, et al. 1983	Increased in early stage
Conversion rate of arachidonic acid to thromboxane B_2 (TXB_2)	T. Hidaka, et al. 1983	

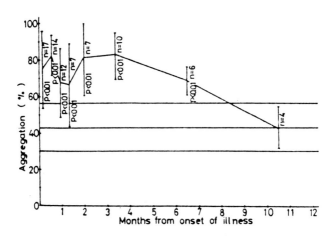

Figure 1. Changes in platelet aggregation induced by 2 X 10^{-6} M ADP

Figure 1 shows the level of platelet aggregation, induced with 2 mM of ADP, during the course of Kawasaki disease as first demonstrated by us in 1977, 1978. The rate of platelet aggregation greatly increased during the 3 weeks from the onset of the disease, followed by a moderate increase for more than 6 months. Aspirin and other anti-platelet agents were not administered to patients during the investigation because, at the time, these agents were not widely used in Kawasaki disease therapy. Using the Wu and Hook method, Shirahata et al. reported that the rate of spontaneous platelet aggregation increased for more than 6 months from the onset of Kawasaki disease. He and his group first carried out the study of βTG and PF4, indicating that platelet activation continues for a long time. Inagaki was also successful in finding the hypercoagulable state by using the method of Baumgartner.

TABLE 2. Studies on activation of platelet in Kawasaki disease (Part 2)—— Relation with abnormal levels of laboratory examinations and development of aneurysm

Items	Authors	Remarks
βTG PF4	J. Burns, et al. 1984 T. Nakamura 1985	Significant relation with high level in first 2-3 weeks and developement of aneurysm.
Thromboxane B_2	Inamo, et al. 1982	Relation with increased level for early stage and CA involvement in later period.
	M. Taki, et al. 1983	Poor response by OKY 046, ASA in aneurysm cases.

Table 2 shows the recent studies on the activation of platelets in Kawasaki disease. These investigations have begun to be carried out with observations of the coronary artery, using the two dimensional echogram. According to Burns' results on the level of βTG, seven of twenty-four patients (29%) during the first three weeks had elevated βTG as defined by a value of 43 ng/ml, the upper end of the range for the control group. Four of seven patients subsequently developed coronary artery aneurysms.

The previous results of PF4 and βTG, shown in Table 1, demonstrated that the abnormality in βTG sustained a little longer than those that were assayed by Burns et al. In Shirahata's group, Nakamura carried out further investigations on βTG, PF4, and also on an assay of circulatory platelet aggregates (CPA), based on the Wu and Hook method for spontaneous platelet aggregation assay. According to his results, in patients where the marked coronary involvement still can be observed 60 days into the illness, there existed abnormal levels of βTG, PF4 and CPA more frequently during the first 14 days. This is in comparison to other patients in whom the coronary involvement disappeared at 60 days, or didn't appear perfectly at all. He also demonstrated that aspirin was effective in reducing the frequency of abnormally high levels of βTG, PF4 and low levels of CPA in the acute stage of Kawasaki disease, compared with other antiplatelet agents, such as flurbiprofen or dipyridamole. Inamo & Ohkuni earlier reported that the plasma level of thromboxane B_2 was generally high in the initial stage of patients with Kawasaki disease, and especially high in patients that developed aneurysms in later periods. Recently in our group, Taki et al. demonstrated that in patients who have already developed any severe coronary artery abnormality, the high levels of TXB_2 and βTG were not perfectly responsive to the single administration of aspirin.

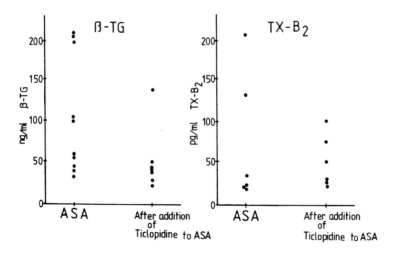

Figure 2. Effect of combination therapy with ASA and Ticlopidine on β-TG, TXB_2

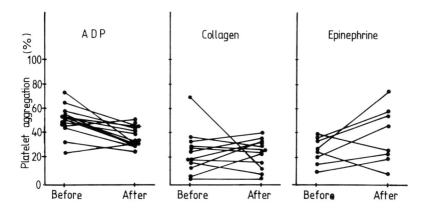

Figure 3. Effect of combination therapy with ASA and
Ticlopidine on platelet aggregation

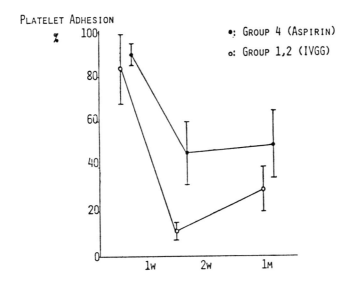

Figure 4. Changes of platelet adhesion during IVGG therapy

Also in our group, Ohyama et al. demonstrated that a combination therapy of 3 mg/kg of aspirin and 5 mg/kg of Ticlopidine
appeared to be effective in reducing the abnormal levels of
βTG and TXB_2 (Fig. 2), along with decreasing the rate of
ADP induced platelet aggregation (Fig. 3). With the results

of a single administration of Ticlopidine already reported
by Nakano et al., we expected stronger antithrombotic effects
of combination therapy in the patients with severe coronary
artery abnormality. Under the present combination therapy,
the patients sometimes demonstrated hemorrhagic tendencies,
such as ecchymosis or epistaxis.

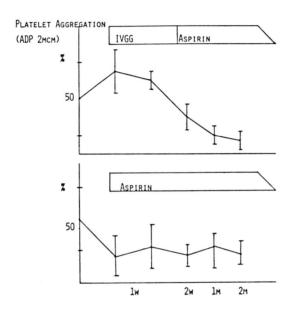

Figure 5. Changes of platelet aggregation during IVGG therapy

The study of changes in platelet functions during the
therapy of intravenous gammaglobulin(IVGG, Furusho, Newburger)
was carried out by Inagaki et al.(1984). As shown in Fig.4,
the platelet adhesion by Baumgartner's method was more suppressed during the therapy of IVGG, than with the administration of aspirin or flurbiprofen alone. The mean + SD rate
of platelet adhesion was lowered to 12.5 + 25.1% with administration of 400 mg per kg of IVGG four days. The adhesion
rate of patients treated with aspirin or flurbiprofen was
46.5 + 13.2%. The changes in platelet aggregation during
the administration of IVGG were also demonstrated by Inagaki
et al. Eight patients who were treated by IVGG showed a mild
decrease in platelet aggregation(ADP 2mM) during the therapy.
This is in comparison to enhanced platelet aggregation when
no therapy was given to the patients (Fig. 5). These results

indicate that suppression through the therapy of IVGG, followed by the administration of ASA, seems the most apparent
and stable.

Coagulation Factors in Kawasaki disease

The level of fibrinogen increases during the acute
stage of Kawasaki disease, while that of Factor XIII increases during the recovery stage (Fig. 6). Other workers
have found that Factor VIII C (VIII C) and Factor VIII
related antigen (VIII R: AG) increases during the acute
stages. An increase of Factor VIII, fibrinogen and α_1 antitrypsin (α_1 AT) in the early stage of the disease represents
a pattern of acute phase reaction. An increase in the level
of factor XIII in the recovery stage represents a pattern
of wound healing, from injury caused by inflammation.

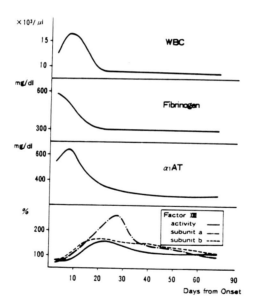

Figure 6. Fibrinogen, Factor XIII in Kawasaki disease
          (The patterns of WBC, α_1 AT illustrated together)

These data on coagulation factors demonstrate the phenomenon
of acute inflammation. Recently, increased levels of circulating anticoagulants in Kawasaki disease were reported by
Shirahata et al. As shown in Table 3, the level of circu-

lating anticoagulants was found to be high in the acute stage
of some patients with Kawasaki disease, this being related
to the development of coronary artery involvement in later
periods. The examination of circulating anticoagulants is
possible only through the usage of a kaolin partial thrombo-
plastin time (KPTT). The importance of the results of these
simple and rapid examinations is that they may provide prognostic information prior to any coronary artery involvement.

TABLE 3. Circulating anticoagulants in acute stage of Kawasaki
disease

Patient	Age	C A (abnormalities)	APTT	KPTT	A.a.	Circulating anticoagulants
1	8/12	+	40.2	58.6	43.1	−
2	1	±	36.4	68.0	49.3	±
3	2	−	34.7	55.9	49.4	±
4	3	−	28.8	54.0	47.3	−
5	2	+	34.8	72.6	50.9	+
6	4	−	29.4	54.1	52.5	+
7	10/12	−	37.9	84.8	48.3	−
8	1	+	25.8	55.8	49.1	±
9	2	−	31.8	55.4	45.8	−
10	5	−	32.5	59.5	48.5	−
11	1	+	30.3	69.0	51.0	+
12	1	−	44.5	81.7	56.5	+
Control			30.3	41.2	41.2	

A.a.: Anticoagulant activity by assay of KPTT

Factors of fibrinolysis

Regarding Kawasaki disease, reports on factors of fibrinolysis are few. Increased levels of FDP, and the pro-
longation of euglobulin lysis time can be found in some of
the patients with Kawasaki disease, offering suspicion that
DIC is involved in the acute stage of some patients. The
results of our recent investigation on tissue plasminogen
activators (TPA) revealed that two peaks of TPA can be found
in the course of Kawasaki disease. The first peak can be
found within 1-2 weeks and the second peak within 3-4 weeks.
The significance of each peak will be studied in the future (Moriuchi et al.).

Summary of Studies on Coagulation in Kawasaki disease

Based on the results of investigations which have been carried out by many workers, we would like to talk about the useful monitors that can tell whether or not the patient is likely to develop significant coronary involvement (Table 4). Among the laboratory examinations that have reported the presence of abnormalities, the most significant in offering a prognosis are underlined. These are thromboxane B_2, thromboglobulin, and platelet factor 4. The circulating anticoagulants and the tissue plasminogen activator are to be included in a future study.

TABLE 4. Laboratory examinations for coagulation study in Kawasaki disease

	Acute stage 0-2weeks	Severe stage 1-3or4weeks	Recovery stage 3weeks-
Fibrinogen	↑↑		
Factor Ⅷ R:AG	↑↑		
Factor Ⅷ R:VF	↑↑		
Factor Ⅶ C	↑↑	↑↑~↑	
Factor ⅩⅢ (A and S)			↓↓
Circulating anti-coagulants	↑↑	↑	
Platelets	↑	↑↑	
Platelet aggregation		↑↑	↑
Malondialdehyde(MDA)	↑		
Thromboxane B₂	↑↑		
β-thromboglobulin(βTG)	↑↑	↑↑	↑
Platelet Factor4(PF4)	↑↑	↑↑	↑↑
Tissue plasminogen activator(TPA)	↑↑	↑↑	↑
Elastase like protease(ELP)	↑↑	↑	
ESR	↑↑	↑	
CRP	↑~↑↑	↑↑	
α-Antitrypsin(α-AT)	↑~↑↑	↑	

Summary of pathogenesis of thrombosis in Kawasaki disease and comments on therapy

Fig. 7 illustrates the mechanism by which the activation of platelets takes place and shows the effects of antiplatelet agents in Kawasaki disease. It is suspected that an etiological factor that causes Kawasaki disease activates the platelets by altering the endothelium and mesothelium and/or by aneurysms in which blood flow is disturbed. The possible direct influence of etiological factors on the

platelets has also been considered. These mechanisms are
all connected to inflammation and the immune complex, each
of which are caused by Kawasaki disease. Although the mechanisms that result in platelet activation in this disease
are partially suppressed by conventional antiplatelet agents,
they are not enough to suppress platelet adhesion to the subendothelium.

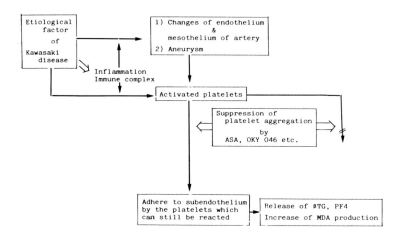

Figure 7. Scheme for activation of platelets and suppression
of antiplatelets.

As I have already mentioned, the addition of another
antiplatelet agent, such as Ticlopidine to aspirin reduced
the abnormally high levels of βTG and PF4. This has been
shown in the patients with any severe abnormality of the
coronary artery, where the level could not be reduced by a
single administration of aspirin. The final goal for the
prevention of thrombus formation in Kawasaki disease is to
reduce inflammation to the minimum. By reducing the incidence of coronary artery abnormalities, the frequency of
thrombus formation can be minimized. To this point, high
doses of gammaglobulin therapy will be expected.

REFERENCES

Burns J, Glode M, Clarke H, Wiggins J, Hathaway W (1984).
    Coagulopathy and platelet activation in Kawasaki syndrome:
    Identification of patients at high risk for development of

coronary artery aneurysms. J. Ped 105:206-211.

Furusho K, Sato K, et al. (1983). High-dose intravenous gammaglobulin for Kawasaki disease. Lancet II 1359.

Hidaka T, Nakano M, Ueda T, Komatsu Y and Yamamoto M (1983). Increased synthesis of thromboxane A_2 by platelets from patients with Kawasaki disease. J. Pediat 102:94-96.

Inagaki M, Yamada Y, et al. (1982). Inhibitory effects of various kinds of antiplatelet agents on platelet adhesion to subendothelium. Blood & Vessel 11:415-417.

Inagaki M and Yamada K (1984). Effect of gammaglobulin on platelet interaction to the vessel wall in Kawasaki disease. The first US-JAPAN Workshop on Kawasaki Syndrome in Hawaii.

Inamo Y and Ohkuni M (1983). Thromboxane in Kawasaki disease. Pediatrics of Japan 24:581-587.

Moriuchi H, et al.(1987). Tissue plasminogen activator in Kawasaki disease, Tokyo, to be reported.

Mukaiyama H (1982). Studies on platelet in mucocutaneous lymphnode syndrome (MCLS)—— platelet function —. Jap J. Clinical Hematology 23:447-456.

Nakamura T (1985). Studies on activation of platelets in Kawasaki disease. Acta Paed Jap 89:1845-1860.

Newburger JW, Takahashi M, Burns JC, et al.(1986). The treatment of Kawasaki syndrome with intravenous gammaglobulin. N. Engl J. Med 315:341-347.

Ohyama Y, Kurokawa Y, Moriuchi H, Yamada K, et al.(1984). Combination therapy with Ticlopidine and aspirin for patients with coronary abnormalities in Kawasaki disease. 87th Pediatric Congress of Japan.

Seto S, Nakano H, et al.(1984). Antiplatelet therapy for coronary artery involvement in Kawasaki disease, especially for treatment by Ticlopidine. Japanese J. Pediatrics 47:1035-1040.

Shinozaki M, Ohkubo I, et al.(1979). Factor VIII in patients with Kawasaki disease (MCLS) — Possible role of VIII:C, VIII: RAGN and VIII: vWf in thrombus formation in coronary arteries — . Acta Paed Jap 83:170-178.

Shirahata A, Yamada K, et al.(1979). Studies on aspirin administration in acute febrile mucocutaneous lymph node syndrome (MCLS), based on the antithrombotic effect of aspirin. Acta Paed Jap 83:365-373.

Shirahata A, Nakamura T and Asakura A (1983). Studies on blood coagulation and antithrombotic therapy in Kawasaki disease. Acta Paed Japa 25:180-191.

Shirahta A, et al.(1986). Circulating anticoagulants in Kawasaki disease. 28th Congress of Clinical Haematology,

Akita.

Taki M, Inagaki M, et al.(1983). Effect of OKY-046 on platelet aggregation and adhesion. The Medicine and Pharmacological Science 6:1836.

Tomita Y, Inagaki M, Taki M, Meguro T and Yamada K (1982). Clotting activity and immunological antigen level of factor XIII in Kawasaki disease. Pediatric Oncology No 17, 52-55.

Wu KK and Hook JC (1974). A new method for the quantitative detection of platelet aggregate in patients with arterial insufficiency. Lancet II:924-926.

Yamada K, Shinkai A, Meguro T and Shirahata A (1977). Hematological study on MCLS with special reference to the platelet — thrombus formation and etiology in MCLS. Acta Paed Jap 81:1263-1271.

Yamada K, Meguro T, et al.(1978). The platelet functions in acute febrile mucocutaneous lymph node syndrome and a trial of prevention for thrombosis by antiplatelet agent. Acta Haematol Jap 41:113-124.

Yasui M, Kin T, et al. (1979). Platelets, fibrinogen, factor VIII related antigen and factor XIII in Kawasaki disease. Nara Med J. 30:235-241.

Yokoyama T, Kato H and Ichinose E (1980). Aspirin and platelet functions in Kawasaki disease. Kurume Medical Journal 27:57-61.

Yoshino N, Akatsuka J, et al.(1983). MDA generation and aggregation of platelets in MCLS. Acta Haematol Jap 46:555.

Kawasaki Disease, pages 251–255
© 1987 Alan R. Liss, Inc.

GENETIC ANALYSIS OF KAWASAKI DISEASE

Takehiko Sasazuki[1], Fumiki Harada[1] and Tomisaku Kawasaki[2]

1. Department of Genetics, Medical Institute of Bioregulation, Kyushu University, 3-1-1 Maidashi, Higashi-ku, Fukuoka 812, Japan

2. Department of Pediatrics, Japan Red Cross Medical Center, 4-1-22 Hiroo, Shibuya-ku, Tokyo 150, Japan

INTRODUCTION

Kawasaki disease (KD) is an acute febrile illness primarily affecting young children. Sudden death occurs due to coronary arteritis accompanied by aneurysms and thrombotic occlusion. The etiology and pathogenesis are unknown. As the disease is extraordinarily prevalent among the Japanese living in Japan, either environmental or genetic factors, specific to the Japanese, may be involved. Since an epidemic in Hawaii revealed that children of Japanese ancestry were at the highest risk (Dean et al., 1982), and since a statistical association between KD and HLA has been reported (Kato et al., 1978: Klensky et al., 1981), genetic factors might be involved in the pathogenesis of KD. To estimate the possible heritability of KD, we performed a study on twins and utilized the affected sib-pair method (Thomson and Bodmer, 1977) to test a genetic model for the susceptibility to KD.

AFFECTED SIB-PAIR METHOD

We examined HLA-A-B-C-DR of 23 families with 63 members where two siblings were affected with KD.

Out of 23 affected sibpairs, four shared two HLA haplotypes identical by descent, 12 shared one HLA haplotype identical by descent and seven shared no HLA haplotype. The distribution of HLA haplotypes shared by the affected sib-pairs did not significantly differ from the random distribution (Table 1).

Table 1. Distribution of Shared HLA Haplotypes in Affected Sib-Pairs with KD

No. shared HLA haplotype	Observed	Random expected	χ^2
Two	4	5.75	0.533
One	12	11.50	0.022
None	7	5.75	0.272
Total	23	23.00	0.827

Note: df = 2 , $P > 0.6$

Furthermore, an analysis of 23 probands did not confirm the statistical association between KD and any HLA specificities. Thus, there were negative findings in both association and linkage between KD and HLA (Sasazuki et al., 1984).

TWIN STUDY

In April 1984, we mailed questionnaires to pediatricians of 954 hospitals all over Japan and obtained data on 108 twins from 575 hospitals (60.3%), up to the end of June 1984. Of these 108, 15 were concordant for KD (13.9%) and 93 discordant (86.1%). We estimated the relative proportion of monozygous (MZ) and dizygous (DZ) twins by the method of Weinberg (Weinberg, 1902). The twin concordance was found in 14.1% of the MZ twins and 13.3% of the DZ twins, with no statistical difference (Table 2).

Table 2. Twin Concordance for KD

Twins	Concordant Pairs (%)	Discordant Pairs (%)	Total Pairs
MZ	11 (14.1%)	67 (85.9%)	78
DZ	4 (13.3%)	26 (86.7%)	30
Total	15 (13.9%)	93 (86.1%)	108

Note: P = 0.594 (by Fisher's direct method)

The male / female ratio was 1.4 and did not differ from the usual slight male predominance. The sex ratio of concordant twins was 1.5 and that of discordant twins was 1.3. The difference was not so significant as to negate the sex effects on the twin concordance. These data suggested that genetic factors would be not involved in the pathogenesis of KD (Harada et al., 1986).

Out of 30 patients in 15 concordant twins, four (13.3%) had been involved in coronary arteritis accompanied by aneurysms. A MZ twin was concordant for coronary aneurysm and two DZ twins were discordant (Table 3). This suggests a possibility that genetic factors might be involved in the pathogenesis of coronary aneurysm with KD. The interval of onsets in both affected pairs were usually within 2 weeks.

Table 3. Twin Concordance for Coronary Aneurysm in Both Affected Pairs with KD

Twins	Concordant pairs for coronary aneurysm	Discordant pairs for coronary aneurysm	Total
MZ	1	0	1
DZ	0	2	2
Total	1	2	3

Note: P = 0.33 (by Fisher's direct method)

GENETIC EPIDEMIOLOGY

Since KD occurs mostly in nursing infants, twins arround that age are expected to have been similarly exposed to putative environmental factors involved in the pathogenesis in KD. However, the observed concordance of 13.9% in all twins, regardless of zygosity, is extremely low compared with that of other acute febrile disease such as measles (Figure 1).

Figure 1. Twin Concordance for Various Diseases

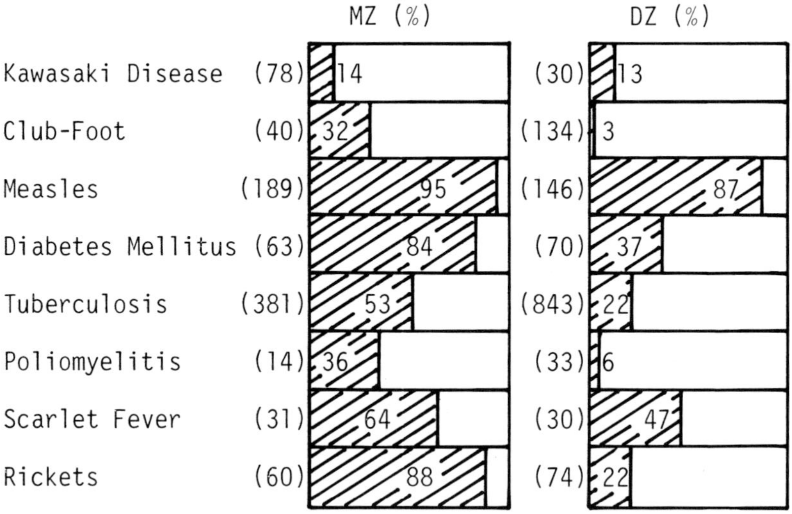

	MZ (%)	DZ (%)
Kawasaki Disease	(78) 14	(30) 13
Club-Foot	(40) 32	(134) 3
Measles	(189) 95	(146) 87
Diabetes Mellitus	(63) 84	(70) 37
Tuberculosis	(381) 53	(843) 22
Poliomyelitis	(14) 36	(33) 6
Scarlet Fever	(31) 64	(30) 47
Rickets	(60) 88	(74) 22

Note: Modified data in "Principle of Human Genetics (Stern, 1973)"

Thus, the virulence of environmental factors , infectious or toxic agents, might be either extremely weak or highly complex, so that it would be taken into account that the genetic difference had not been observed in our study. On the other hand, the concordance of 13.9% in all twins is significantly higher than that of 1-2% in siblings (Yanagawa and Shigematsu, 1983). It suggests that putative precipitating agent(s) should expose children at critical age to develop KD. In conclusion, we found no evidence to support the idea of genetic link in children with KD.

REFERENCES

Dean AG, Melish ME, Hicks R, et al. (1982). An epidemic of Kawasaki syndrome in Hawaii. J Pediatr 100: 552-557.

Kato S, Kimura M, Tsuji K, et al. (1978). HLA antigens in Kawasaki disease. Pediatrics 61: 252-255.

Harada F, Sada M, Kamiya T, et al. (1986). Genetic analysis of Kawasaki syndrome. Am J Hum Genet 39: 537-539.

Sasazuki T, Harada F, Sada M, et al. (1984). Kawasaki disease (Mucocutaneous Lymph Node Syndrome), In Albert ED, Baur MP, Mayr WR (eds). "Histocompatibility Testing 1984" Berlin: Springer-Verlag, pp402-403.

Stern C (1973). "Principle of Human Genetics"(3rd ed). San Francisco: Freeman WH and Company.

Thomson G, Bodmer WF (1977). The genetics of HLA and disease association, In Christianssen TB, Feachel TM, Barndorff-Nielsen O (eds),"Measuring Selection in Natural Population" Berlin: Springer-Verlag, pp545-564.

Weinberg W (1902). Beitrage zur Phygiologie und Pathologie der Mehrlingsgeburten beim Menshen. Arch F Ges Physiol 88: 346-430.

Yanagawa H, Shigematsu I (1983). Epidemiological features of Kawasaki disease in Japan. Acta Paediatr Jpn 25: 94-107

Kawasaki Disease, pages 257–273
© 1987 Alan R. Liss, Inc.

A PATHOLOGICAL ANALYSIS OF KAWASAKI DISEASE
-WITH SOME SUGGESTIONS OF ITS ETIO-PATHOGENESIS-

Masahisa Kyogoku, M.D.

Department of Pathology, Tohoku University School
of Medicine, Seiryo-machi, Sendai, Japan 980

INTRODUCTION

The key to open the door to the hidden room of etiology
or pathogenesis of any disease does exist in the "site" of
disease. Intimate analytical observations of the
pathological picture of disease must let us know something.
Therefore, in this paper we are going to remind you the
characteristic pathological picture of Kawasaki disease
especially of their various target organs such as skin,
heart, kidney, lymph nodes, stressing on their peculiarities, in which could be hidden some clues to find the still-
unknown etiology of Kawasaki Disease (KD). Several animal
models of arteritis, induced and spontaneous, to be useful
to confirm some hypothetic points about KD, will be also
presented.

1)EARLY DERMATOPATHOLOGICAL FINDINGS:

In their first week of illness, the only available
pathological specimen is biopsied skin tissue (Hirose et al
1978, Kyogoku et al 1985), where (1) the edema of papillary
layer of dermis, (2) perivascular infiltration of
granulocytes and monohistiocytes, (3) swelling of
endothelial cells, with such a large nucleus and nucleoli
(Fig 1), (4) IgG deposition on vascular wall, (5) activation
of Langerhans' cells, (6) liquefactions of basal squamous
cells are the common pathological features. Marked
deposition of immunoglobulin, fibrinoid necrosis,
leucocytoclastic vasculitis, granulomas and arteritis, which

are usual and characteristic of various immunological
diseases, especially in   immune complex diseases, have
never been observed. If you could imagine some hitherto-
known diseases with similar histopathological features it
must be that of some toxemic or viremic status.

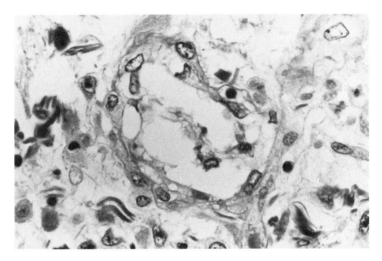

Fig 1.   Endothelial damage in the early stage of KD

2) CARDIAC CHANGE IN THE 2ND WEEK:

In the second week a number of autopsy cases and few
lymph node biopsy material were available.

The early pathological feature of the heart of KD is
that of diffuse interstitial pancarditis (Hamashima 1973,
1977, Tanaka et al 1976, Fujiwara et al 1978a, 1978b, Amano
et al 1979a, 1979b, 1980, Kyogoku et al 1985, Kageyama et al
1986). By our observation the infiltrated cellular
components are the mixture of Leu M1 positive granulocytes
and Leu M3 positive monohistiocytes and earlier after onset,
higher the rate of granulocytes.
The inflammation gradually concentrates to the
surrounding tissue of arteries and here the Leu M1 positive
granulocytes are leading them in their front row, seeming to
destroying the arterial wall mostly from their adventitial
side. But in some place where the inflammation is very much
advanced, granulocytes gathered on the intima to destroy the
endothelium and internal elastic lamina introducing plasma

insudation from luminal side (Fig 2a,b). IgG was transiently positive around such site mostly on the muscle cells and some histiocytes but C3, C4 deposit has not been confirmed.

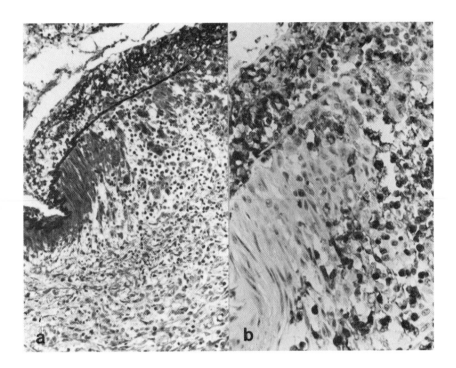

Fig 2. In the 2nd week, granulocyte infiltration not only in adventitial side but also in the intima is characterstic, which destroy the media and internal elastic lamina. (a)Elastica Masson   (b)Leu M1

3) VASCULAR CHANGES IN THE 3RD TO 5TH WEEK:

The cellular composition changed rapidly along the disease course. In the 3rd to 5th week Leu M1 positive granulocytes disappeared and mononuclear cells with peculiar shape, Leu M3 positive, acid phosphatase containing and HLA-DR positive monohistiocytes took majority (Fig 3). Leu 4 positive T cells, mostly Leu 3a positive Th cells were also emerging in the site, although not so much in number. Immunogloblin deposition and B-plasma cell infiltration has not been revealed so much. A characteristic edematous

dissociation of medial smooth muscle cells is a typical
feature of this stage (Fig 4). The situation is same in
other organs including kidney, where usually glomeruli were
free of immune complex deposition.

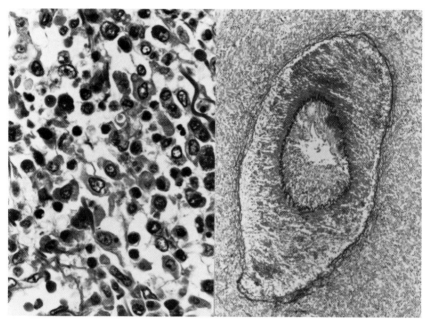

Fig 3. In the 3rd week, the
majority of the cells infiltrating around the artery
are mono-histiocyte with
peculiar shape.

Fig 4. This is a typical
pathological feature of
KD arteritis with char-
cteristic edematous dis-
sociation of media with-
out fibrinoid degeneration.
Intimal thickening is
already marked.

In these weeks, the active interstitial inflammation
over the body has almost completely disappeared and the
inflammation in chronic state seemed to be concentrated on
the arterial wall, where fibrocellular intimal thickening
was most distinctive features (Fig 5). The cell components
of the thickened intima were mostly activated myocytes,
which had proliferated in the media and immigrate through
the perforated internal elastic lamina (Fig 6). These
activated intimal myocytes produce mostly hyaluronic acid

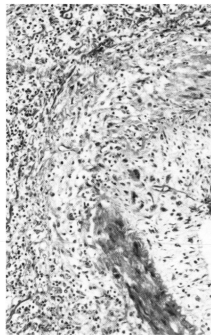

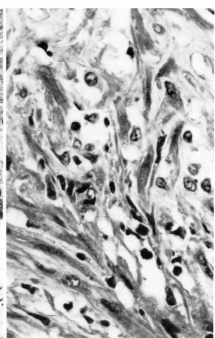

Fig 5. KD arteritis in 5th week. Granulomatous pan-arteritis with marked fibro-cellular intimal thickening.

Fig 6. Activated myocytes are immigrating from media to the intimal side (upwards).

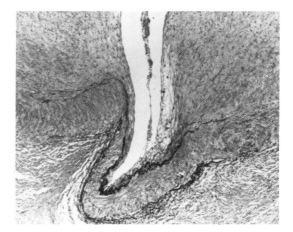

Fig 7. KD coronary aneurysma with marked intimal thickening leaving apparently "normal" arterial lumina between them.

for much longer time comparing with adult cases. Plasma component sequestrated in the thickened intima seemed to accelerate the intimal thickening. Aneurysmal formation, thrombus formation does not only accelerate the intimal thickening but also cause sudden death through acute infarction during these weeks of illness (Fig 7).

4) LPS ARTERITIS AND INTIMAL THICKENING:

In order to get some information to clarify the histopathogenesis of such an unusually mucopolysaccharide rich intimal thickening, following experiment has been performed by us. According to our ideas that probably the granulocyte infiltration on the arterial wall in the 1st week of illness will be responsible for such a peculiar intimal thickening, we wrapped the exposed femoral artery of

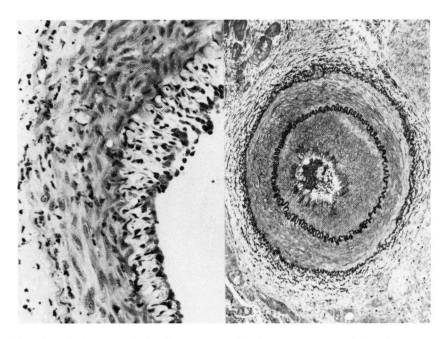

Fig 8. LPS arteritis in infant rabbit, granulocyte infiltrated not only in the advetitia but on the endothelia (2nd day).

Fig 9. LPS arteritis in infant rabbit. Twelve weeks after experiment, marked intimal thickening was observed.

rabbit with oxycellulose which was immersed with 0.5mg of
LPS, an famous granulocyte inducer. But it does not mean
LPS might be a causative agent of KD. We used it as just a
nonspecific granulocyte inducer. A couple of days after
application, granulocytes gathered not only in its
adventitial side but also just on the endothelium, which
subsequently induces marked intimal thickening (Fig 8). The
immigration of proliferated and activated myocytes occurred
through the fenestration of internal elastic lamina. If
the elastic lamina has been destroyed by granulocytes the
speed and grade of intimal thickening was much more
accelerated. Difference between infant and adult rabbit
was remakable. The degree and speed of intimal thickening
of infant rabbit was always accelerated than adults and
contained much more amounts of mucopolysaccharides in their
matrix (Fig 10). (Fujiyama et al 1986a,1986b)

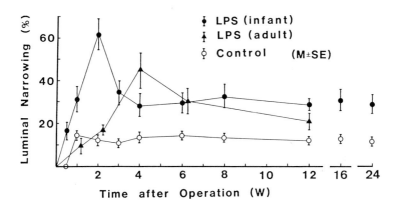

Fig 10. Time course of intimal thickening in LPS
arteritis in infant and adult rabbits.

5)IN VITRO STUDIES ON THE SMOOTH MUSCLE PROLIFERATION:

Further in vitro studies using cultured myocytes
revealed that (1) LPS itself had not so much effect on the
proliferation but also destruction of myocytes, (2)
granulocyte effect was just a destructive one and never
showed any proliferative effects even in their very diluted
condition, (3) culture sup of mono-macrophage had a
inhibitory effect if diluted, but showed rather stimulative

tendency when it was concentrated, (4) plasma component (full of platelets) contained very strong growth factor (Fig 11), (5) lysate of smooth muscle cells also had strong proliferating effects (Fig 12).

In this LPS experiment, in case the medial damage was so much advanced, the arterial wall has been distended to form true aneurysms, and in such case there was no tendency of intimal thickening (Kato et al unpublished data).

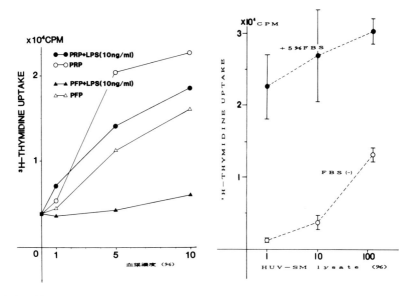

Fig 11. Blood plasma compo-nents with full of platelets (PRP) contains very strong growth factor. LPS complete-ly abolish the platelet free plasma (PFP) growth factor.

Fig 12. Muscle cell lysate also shows strong growth activity with and without fetal calf serm.

These experimental results seem to tell us that:
1) Arterial tissue of <u>young</u> individuals has more tendency of intimal proliferation, which mainly consisted of activated myocyte producing more mucopolysaccharide than adults, and retained for a long time.
2) Granulocyte inflltration on the arterial wall can stimulate the intimal thickening through: (1) releasing

various myocyte-proliferating factors from platelet, fibrin and even muscle cells itself in consequence of their enzymatic destruction; (2) destroy the endothelium and elastic lamina, letting the immigrating activated myocyte to move towards intimal side more freely.

6) WHAT'S STUDIED FROM HISTOPATHOLOGY OF KD AND LPS ARTERITIS MODEL

Histopathology of arteritis in KD is different from that of Kussmaul-Maier type PN, in which the fibrin deposit in the intima-media area with medial degeneration and segmental, stage-mixed arteritis are characteristic. On the contrary, arteritis of KD, started with endothelial swelling and degeneration causing interstitial edema, and after transient infiltration of granulocytes leads to the quite characteristic arteritis with infiltration of peculiar mono-histiocytes and edematous dissociation of medial muscle cells. Usually the histopathological feature is in the same stage all over the body, which means KD arteritis is a kind of "one hit" disease preferentially attacks the endothelium and finally involves the whole arterial wall leaving severe cicatrical arteritis with marked intimal thickening, which seemed to be introduced by strong myocyte-proliferating factors derived from platelets and degenerated myocytes. Accelerated mucopolysaccharide production in the infant is another important factor. There is no evidence of immune complex disease.

7) HISTOPATHOLOGY OF LYMPH APPARATUS IN KD

Another important histopathological feature for the study of etiopathogenesis will be that of lymph apparatus; thymus, lymph nodes, spleen and intestinal lymph follicle. Dr. Tanaka already reported that the histopathological pictures of swollen lymph node in the 1st week was that of "necrotizing lymphadenitis" (Kageyama et al 1986). In the following weeks the thymus was atrophic especially in its cortex, but not so marked as other serious systemic infections or viremias. All of the lymph apparatus were hyperplastic in T and B of both area in the 2nd to 3rd week of illness. Usually follicular proliferation and hyperplasia was remarkable in such stage, but various karyolytic foci were noticeable mostly in their B zone (Fig

13). Then the T cell start to disappear leaving edematous scanty cellular zones and empty periarterial sheath. The follicles with giant germinal center were still remarkable, but in such germinal center, there was no evidence of still active B cell proliferarion and subsequent immunoglobulin production. In some case, few number of immunoblast has seen mostly in the sinus, but never been so marked as in case of infectious mononucleosis.

About the histopathology of lymph apparatus, we felt that this is a picture of lymphoproliferation and subsequent destruction, at the beginning of B cells and then T cells, though its grade is not so remarkable as the usual EBV infections in the adults.

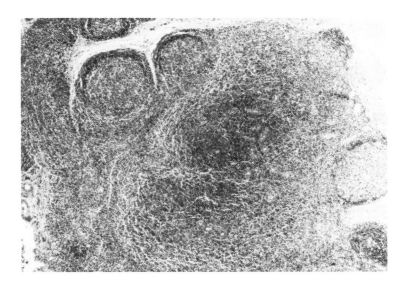

Fig 13. Swollen lymph node in KD (3rd week) Hyperplasia of T and B zones are remarkable, but cell components are already disappearing leaving the frame work.

8) ANIMAL MODELS WITH RETROVIRUS INDUCED ARTERITIS

Concerning the recent hot debate about retrovirus in KD (Leung et al 1983, Burns et al 1986, Shulman et al 1986), I want to introduce to you two strains of mice which develop vasculitis spontaneously in relation to murine retrovirus.

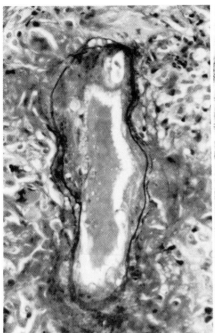

Fig 14. Necrotizing
(Kussmaul-Maier type)
arteritis in SL/Ni
mouse

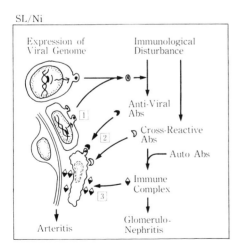

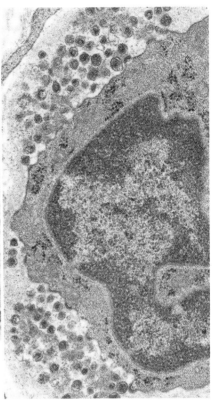

Fig 15. C type retrovirus
is budding from the cyto-
plasmic membrane of arte-
rial myocytes

Fig 16. Schematic diagram
of histopathogenesis of
necrotizing (Kussmaul-
Maier type) arteritis of
SL/Ni mouse

One is SL/Ni mouse, which was bred in Japan by Dr.
Nishizuka and its reports have already been seen in J.
Immunology and several publications (Nishizuka et al 1975,
Kyogoku et al 1977, 1980, 1987, Yoshiki et al 1979, Nose et
al 1980, 1986, Miyazawa et al 1987). This strain of mouse
suffers from Kussmaul-Maier type "necrotizing fibrinoid
arteritis" with 30% incidence (Fig. 14). In this animal, C
type, ecotropic retrovirus particles are budding from the
cytoplasmic membrane of smooth muscle cells of the arterial
wall (Fig. 15) and antibody against this virus particle,
exclusively against its envelope antigen GP70, attacks the
viral particles together with the virus-budding muscle
cells to destroy it with the aid of complement. And after
following immune complex insudation, typical fibrinoid
necrotizing arteritis completed (Fig. 16). Usually
endothelial cells are free. This animal also develops
lymphoid cell hyperplasia at 2 months of age, at the same
time as vasculitis appeared. According to recent studies
made by Dr. Hiai of Aichi Cancer Center, at least two kinds
of retrovirus seemed to be concerned; one is endogenous and
the other is exogenous which probably is transmitted on
delivery from maternal side (Hiai et al 1982).
    The major differences between SL/Ni vasculitis and KD
are: 1) SL/Ni vasculitis is that of Kussmaul-Maier type
polyarteritis (fibrinoid type) occurring in their
adolescence after the appearance of a great amount of
immune complexes to form typical lupus nephritis. 2) No
evidence of diffuse interstitial inflammation in SL/Ni
mouse, probably because virus kept away from endothelium.
    Another strain of mouse is famous MRL/Mp-lpr/lpr mouse,
which also develops arteritis spontaneously with 30%
incidence. The pathology of this arteritis is that of
"granulomatous type" (Fig. 17). This animal also develops
endogenous retrovirus dependent lymphoid hyperplasia in
their adolescence and forms an enormous amount of GP70
immune complex in their circulation. This type of
arteritis has been caused by the destruction of the
arterial wall by activated macrophages under the influence
of proliferating T cells. Such an angry macrophage ingests
a great amount of IC (Fig. 18) and releases various kinds of
destructive agents in the vicinity to destroy not only the
vascular wall but also the joint and other organs (Fig. 19)
(Kyogoku et al 1987, Nose et al 1986, 1987).
    The difference between MRL/lpr arteritis and KD are: 1)
MRL/lpr arteritis occurred in their adolescence after an

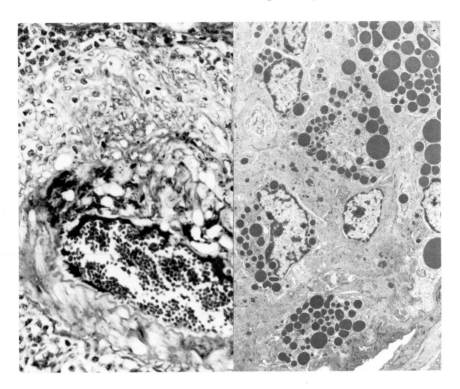

Fig 17. Granulomatous arteritis in MRL/Mp-lpr/lpr mouse

Fig 18. Dense body inclusions
(immune complex) are
evident in the cytoplasm
of peculiar macrophage
infiltrated into the site
of arteritis

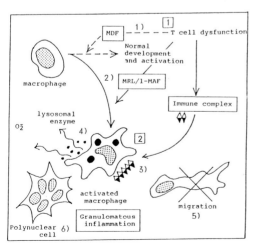

Fig 19. Schematic diagram
of pathogenesis of
granulomatous destructive
arteritis of MRL/Mp-lpr/
lpr mouse

appearance of a great amount of GP70 IC in circulation which can form lupus nephritis, too. 2) No evidence of contagious suspicions.

These two strains of animal model seem to be telling us that retrovirus can induce vasculitis, directly or indirectly in either way, although the epidem' logy and type of arteritis is different from KD.

Information from the famous "equine infectious anemia," which virus is a contagious RNA virus and can introduce arteritis, is also quite useful to evaluate the retrovirus theory of KD.

9) SUMMARY

As a conclusion, reviewing the pathological findings of KD and several animal models it will be clear that:

1) Kawasaki Disease is a systemic disease that attacks infants of <u>immature</u> immunological and angio-structural background.
2) The nature of the disease is that of "<u>one-hit</u>" type which attacks infants with some deranged biological conditions. The fate and grade of the disease depend merely on the grade of the hit in the first week of illness. The following is just a course of adaptation and repair of the injured sites.
3) The disease starts from the initial seroexudative inflammation, and through its transient granulocyte-leading stage, comes to the final (lymph) mono-histiocyte dominant interstitial inflammation, which seems to concentrate to the arterial wall.
4) The grade of granulocyte infiltration, the high potentiality of the mesenchymal cells and the growth factor derived from aggregated platelets and destroyed muscle cells seem to decide the fate of arterial lesion.
5) This is a disease which is different from a usual infection, or immune-complex induced disease. But from a pathological point of view, it "could" be caused by some "toxic substance including some virus," proliferated in the blood stream or endothelium of the infants with somewhat deranged defense mechanisms.

6) The information from two strains of mice, SL/Ni and MRL/Mp-lpr/lpr, which develop arteritis with a participation of retrovirus, will be useful to evaluate the retrovirus theory of KD.

ACKNOWLEDGEMENT

A part of these studies has been supported by Grant in aid from (1) Ministry of Education and (2) Ministry of Health and Welfare of Japanese Government and (3) Japanese Heart Association. The efforts of Miss Yuko Ishigaki in preparation of the manuscript are greatly appreciated.

REFERENCES

Amano S, Hazama F and Hamashima Y (1979a). Pathology of Kawasaki desease: Pathology and morphogenesis of the vascular changes. Jap Circ J 43:633-643
Amano S, Hazama F and Hamashima Y (1979b). Pathology of Kawasaki desease: Distribution and incidence of the vascular lesions. Jap Circ J 43:741-748
Amano S, Hazama F, Kubagawa H, Tasaka K, Haebara H and Hamashima Y (1980). General pathology of Kawasaki disease on the morphological alterations corresponding to the clinical manifestations. Acta Pathol Jpn 30:681-694
Burns JC, Geha RS, Schneeberger EE, Newburger JW, Rosen FS, Glezen LS, Huang AS, Natale J and Leung DYM (1986). Polymerase activityin lymphocyte culture supernatants from patients with Kawasaki disease. Nature 323:814-816
Fujiwara H and Hamashima Y (1978a). Pathology of the heart in Kawasaki disease. Pediatrics 61:100-107
Fujiwara H, Kawai C and Hamashima Y (1978b). Clinicopathological study of the conduction system in 10 patients with Kawasaki disease. Am Heart J. 96:744-750
Fujiyama J, Ogata H, Sawai T and Kyogoku M (1986a). Experimental studies on the factors to determine the prognosis of arteritis. J Jap Assoc PedeatCircul (Jpn) 2:230-237
Fujiyama J, Sawai T and Kyogoku M (1986b). Role of myointimal cells in intimal thickening of arteritis in Kawasaki desease. The Heart (Jpn) 18:907-913
Hamashima Y , Kishi K and Tasaka K (1973). Rickettsia-like bodies in MCLS. Lancet 819:42
Hamashima Y (1977). Kawasaki disease. Tr SocPathol Jpn

(Jpn) 66:59-92

Hiai H, Ikeda H, Kaneshima H et al (1982). Slvr-1: a new epistatic host gene restricting expression of endogenous ecotoropic virus in SL/Ni mice distinct from Fv-4. Proc Jap Cancer Assoc (Jpn) 41:335

Hirose S et al (1978). Morphological observations on the vasculitis in the MCLS-A skin biopsy study of 27 patients. Eur J Pediat 129:17-27

Kageyama K, Aoyama Y, Hatakeyama S, Hotch M, Kawakami M, Kyogoku M, Naoe S, Saito K, Shimizu K, Sumiyoshi A, Tanaka N, Takemura T and Yutani C (1986). Kawasaki disease among the Japanese-A pathological study. Asian Medical Journal 29:133-156

Kato M and Kyogoku M. unpublished data

Kyogoku M (1977). Studies on SL/Ni mouse, Animal models of PN in Shiokawa Y (ed) "Vascular lesions of collagen diseases and related conditions", Tokyo: U of Tokyo Press, pp356-366

Kyogoku M (1980). Pathogenesis of vasculitis in SL/Ni mice in Fukase M (ed) "Systemic Lupus Erythematousus" Tokyo: U of Tokyo Press, pp281-294

Kyogoku M, Fujiyama J and Sawai T(1985). Reexamination of KD Pathology -Facts and Hypothesis- Pediatric Medicine (Shoni-Naika) (Jpn) 17:731-737

Kyogoku M, Nose M, Sawai T, Miyazawa M, Tachiwaki O and Kawashima M (1987). Immunopathology of murine lupus-overview, SL/Ni and MRL/Mp-lpr/lpr, in Kawamata J and Melby EC Jr (eds) " Animal Models: Assessing the scope of their use in biomedical research", New York: Alan R Liss, pp95-130

Leung DYM, Chu ET, Wood N, Grady S, Meade R and Geha RS (1983). Immunoregulatory T-cell abnormalities in MCLS, J Immunol 130:2002-2004

Miyazawa M, Nose M, Kawashima M and Kyogoku M (1987). Lysis of vascular smooth muscle cells by anti-ecotropic murine leukemia virus natural antibodies and the pathogenesis of spontaneous arteritis in SL/Ni mice, J Exp Med (Submitted)

Nishizuka Y, Shisa M and Taguchi O (1975). Experimental studies on polyarteritis nodosa, Tr Soc Pathol Jpn(Jpn) 64:108

Nose M, Kawashima M, Yamamoto K and Kyogoku M (1980). Role of immune complex in the pathogenesis of arteritis in SL/Ni mouse: possible effect as accelerator rather than as initiator. in Shiokawa Y, Abe T and Yamauchi Y (eds) "New Horisons of Rheumatoid Arthritis", Amsterdam: Excerpta Medica, pp109-115

Nose M and Kyogoku M (1986). Lupus mice and arteritis, The Ryumachi (Jpn) 26:116-125

Nose M, Tachiwaki O and Kyogoku M (1987). Macrophage functions and their regulation in MRL/1 lupus mice in Wigzell H and Kyogoku M (eds) " New Horizons in animal models for autoimmune disease", New York: Academic Press, in press

Shulman ST and Rowley AH (1986). Does Kawasaki disease have a retroviral eiology? The Lancet 8506: 545-546

Tanaka et al (1976). Kawasaki disease, Relationship with infantile PN, Arch Path Lab Med 100:81-86

Yoshiki T, Hayasaka , Fukatsu R, Shirai T, Itoh T, Ikeda H and Katagiri M (1979). The structural proteins of murine leukemia virus and the pathogenesis of necrotizing arteritis and glomerulonephritis in SL/Ni mice. J Immunol 122:1812-1820

Kawasaki Disease, pages 275–276
© 1987 Alan R. Liss, Inc.

DISCUSSION:

PATHOGENESIS OF KAWASAKI DISEASE

Dr. H. Murata (Tokyo) inquired of Dr. Lehman about
several aspects of the Lactobacillus casei animal model,
including a) the incidence of coronary arteritis (75-100%
depending upon how diligently one seeks evidence of
inflammation); b) whether living L. casei had been used
(not as effective in producing lesions and with a slower
time course); and c) age susceptibility of animals (both
old and young animals develop characteristic changes). Dr.
S. Naoe (Tokyo) asked whether Dr. Lehman's model demonstrates renal artery or small vessel arteritis (only in
autoimmune strains of mice) and whether there is much
lot-to-lot variation in the inducing cell wall material
(apparently not).

Dr. D. Leung (Boston) commented on the apparent differences among the immunologic data in Kawasaki Disease from
different laboratories. He ascribed at least some of the
differences to the fact that Laxer studied patients on two
occasions 7-13 days apart while he studied them 4 days
apart. Dr. K. Okumura (Tokyo) indicated that 4 or 5
different laboratories in Japan have assessed helper and
suppressor cell numbers without finding decreased
suppressor (CD8) cells. He asked whether this was a
finding peculiar to those with Japanese ethnicity. Dr.
Marchette (Honolulu) reported that depressed CD8 cells were
seen early in Kawasaki Disease in Japanese-Americans in
Hawaii. Dr. F. Rosen (Boston) asked whether CD8
polymorphism existed in Japanese. Dr. T. Tada (Tokyo)
responded that there are a small number of families in Nara
and Kyushu in which CD8 expression is lacking although

suppressor cell function is intact.

Dr. L. Pachman (Chicago) asked if there was any prognostic significance to any immunologic findings. Dr. Laxer (Toronto) indicated that data were insufficient. Dr. Leung reported that there was no increase in the depressed number of CD8 cells in those few children who developed coronary lesions despite gamma globulin therapy. He suggested that looking at IL-1 and gamma interferon production might be more important.

Dr. G. Koren (Toronto) asked for suggestions as to how steroids might worsen the outcome of Kawasaki Disease. Dr. M. Levin (London and Denver) suggested that the presence of immune complexes may correspond with reticuloendothelial system blockade and that steroids might further depress RES function. Dr. Leung asked how circulating immune complexes, present especially during the third week of illness, could be related to the pathogenesis of coronary lesions that apparently have their onset earlier. Dr. Levin speculated that a toxin or other factor might initiate coronary damage with immune complexes contributing to subsequent damage.

Kawasaki Disease, pages 277–286
© 1987 Alan R. Liss, Inc.

CARDIOVASCULAR INVOLVEMENT IN KAWASAKI DISEASE:
EVALUATION AND NATURAL HISTORY

Hirohisa Kato

Department of Pediatrics, Kurume University
School of Medicine, Kurume 830, Japan

INTRODUCTION

At the begining of the cardiology session, I would
like to summarize about the overall cardiovascular
problems in Kawasaki disease, particularly on the
cardiovascular spectrum and natural history which are the
most important clinical issues in Kawasaki disease. About
19 years ago, when Dr. Kawasaki first reported this
disease (Kawasaki, 1967), the prognosis was thought to be
good. However, the first nation-wide survey in Japan
clarified that 1.7% of the patients died from acute
cardiac failure, and all autopsies showed coronary
arteritis accompanied by aneurysms and thrombotic
occlusion (Japan Research Committee on Kawasaki disease,
1971). In those days most pediatricians considered that
Kawasaki disease was complicated with coronary arteritis
only in rare instances which may be fatal, because of the
great contrast in prognosis between these rare fatal cases
and the large number of non-fatal cases which were quite
asymptomatic.

In 1973, we performed coronary angiography in 13
cases who had survived from Kawasaki disease when they
were quite asymptomatic (Kato et al., 1975). In many
instances abnormal findings such as coronary aneurysms
were noted which suggested that coronary arterial lesions
in Kawasaki disease are not limited to fatal cases and
that subclinical or asymptomatic coronary aneurysms are
seen quite often in the survivor. Since 1973, we have
employed the coronary angiography as the routine

examination because it was the only way to evaluate coronary aneurysms accurately at that time (Kato et al., 1982). So far, we have experienced 1009 cases over fourteen years. With the introduction of echocardiography in 1979 the evaluation was made by both coronary angiography and two-dimensional echocardiography (2-D echo) to clarify the sensitivity of 2-D echo. Since 1983, the patients have been selected for angiography when they had abnormal findings by serial 2-D echo studies. Of all patients, 210 or 20 % were diagnosed as having coronary aneurysms. From our experience, we summarize in this article the cardiovascular problems, particularly the cardiovascular spectrum, natural history and the recommended management for Kawasaki disease.

1. CARDIOVASCULAR SPECTRUM AND EVALUATION FOR CORONARY ARTERY LESIONS.

Kawasaki disease is a systemic vasculitis syndrome which involves the medium and small-sized arteries, and particularly the coronary artery (Fujiwara, 1978). It is also accompanied by acute inflammation of multisystem organs. Cardiovascular lesions are composed of aneurysms in the coronary artery or other peripheral arteries, myocarditis, valvulitis and pericarditis. The cardiovascular spectrum of Kawasaki disease is summarized in Table 1. The inflammation is characterized by a self-limited nature. However, the coronary aneurysms may progress to cause sudden death or ischemic heart disease due to thrombotic occlusion in some cases. Therefore, the evaluation for coronary aneurysms in the acute stage of illness is the most critical problem in the management of this disease.

Most children who have Kawasaki disease are free of cardiac symptoms and demonstrate no specific manifestations on chest roentogenogram or electrocardiogram, even if they have coronary aneurysms. Several trials to predict coronary aneurysms have appeared (Asai, 1983; Nakano, 1986). Factors to predict aneurysms appear to be i) boys under 1 year of age, ii) fever lasting longer than 2 weeks, iii) an elevated erythrocyte sedimentation rate persisting for more than 4 weeks, and iv) palpable axillary arterial aneurysms. While only 2 % of the patients had palpable axillary arterial aneurysms, the presence of this physical finding always accurately predict the finding of coronary aneurysms. However, it is usually difficult to diagnose presence of coronary aneurysms from clinical presentations or routine cardiac examinations (Kato and Ichinose, 1984).

Recently, 2-D echo has become the most useful non-invasive method to evaluate coronary aneurysms. The right and left main coronary arteries and the peripheral right coronary artery can be visualized by 2-DE. The normal echocardiographic findings show the main coronary artery to be less than 3mm in diameter in infants and less than 4mm in young children. Normal 2-D echo reveals a uniformity of the coronary artery diameter with less dense echo in the arterial wall. The peripheral right coronary artery can be visualized by the subxiphoid approach. By using 2-DE we have correctly diagnosed aneurysms of the left main coronary artery with 98% sensitivity and 95% specificity. The evaluation for right coronary artery aneurysms was less sensitive. False negative diagnoses were mainly due to the presence of isolated small peripheral coronary aneurysms, which appeared in rare instances. Large but normal coronary artery (dominancy) may be assumed to be only mild dilatation in some cases. From echocardiographic studies, it became evident that coronary dilatation appeared at around the 10th day of illness, and more than half of the patients revealed mild coronary dilatation in this period. However, most of those revealed transient dilatation and regressed within 3 to 5 weeks of illness. Thus, coronary aneurysms have developed in about 20 % of all patients. Obstructive lesions in the coronary artery are difficult to evaluate by 2-DE in many instances. However, high frequency transducer can provide an evaluation of such lesions. Massive thrombus formation can be evaluated by serial 2-DE studies in some patients where there are large aneurysms in the main coronary arteries (Ichinose et al., 1985).

Coronary angiography is the most accurate method to define the presence or absence of coronary arterial lesions in Kawasaki disease. From 1973, we have employed coronary angiography as a routine examination. We have designed special catheters for selective coronary angiography for children, which consist of three different sizes; for infants, toddlers, and for school children. Using these catheters we have performed coronary angiography safely and satisfactorily even in infants.

Our indications for angiography at present time are the presence of abnormal 2-DE findings, the presence of ischemic symptoms or findings, valve regurgitation or evidence of cardiac dysfunction, and intracoronary thrombolytic treatment.

A coronary artery lesion is the most important lesion in Kawasaki disease. However aneurysms in other arteries were observed in 2 % of our patients. Axillary, iliac or renal artery aneurysms were frequently observed, and in a few patients intramammarian arteries were also involved. We were able to palpate the axillary aneurysms by daily physical examination.

We have experienced acute mitral regurgitation in 11 cases (1.1%). In most of the patients this disappeared eventually after a few months to several years. The etiology of this condition may be considered to be valvulitis or papillary muscle dysfunction caused by myocarditis or ischemia. Mitral regurgitation caused by valvulitis or myocarditis appears in the acute stage of the illness and papillary muscle dysfunction caused by ischemia may occur in any stage of illness and usually reveals severe mitral regurgitation. Aortic regurgitation may appear in rare instances. Recently, we have performed Doppler echocardiography in each case which suggested the incidence of valvular regurgitation, particularly the tricuspid or mitral valve, is much higher than previously appreciated.

CORONARY ARTERY		
transient dilatation in acute stage	201/432	(46.5%)
coronary aneurysms	210/1009	(20.8%)
ANEURYSMS OTHER THAN CORONARY ARTERY		
axillary, iliac, renal etc.	20/1009	(2.0%)
MITRAL REGURGITATION	11/1009	(1.1%)
AORTIC REGURGITATION	0/1009	(0%)
PERICARDITIS or PERICARDIAL EFFUSION		
including mild effusion by ECHO	169/673	(25.1%)
MYOCARDITIS		
probably more than half of the patients		(? %)
MYOCARDIAL INFARCTION	13/1009	(1.3%)
FATAL CASES	6/1009	(0.6%)

1973—1986.9 KURUME UNIV.

Table 1. CARDIOVASCULAR SPECTRUM in KAWASAKI DISEASE

Pericarditis including mild pericardial effusion detected by echocardiogram appeared in 25 % of the patients who were in acute phase, and was mostly subclinical and disappeared within 1 or 2 weeks. Massive pericardial effusion or cardiac tamponade was also rare, appearing in only 3 out of 1009 patients. Pericardiocentesis was performed in two patients. Bloody pericardial effusion was examined and found to contain many neutrophils and higher levels of immune complex than those in serum. There have been no reports on its progression to chronic or constrictive pericarditis.

Relatively mild myocarditis was observed in many patients who were in the acute phase, especially in the first and second weeks of illness, regardless of the presence of coronary aneurysms. Gallop rhythm, distant heart sound, ST-T changes or decreased voltage of R waves in electrocardiograms may suggest the presence of myocarditis. In many instances cardiac enzyme levels such as the creatine phosphokinase did not change significantly. Cardiomegaly or decreased ejection fraction of the left ventricle caused by myocarditis were noted in some patients. It generally followed an acute course to resolution, seldom developing into a chronic condition or to cardiomyopathy.

2. MYOCARDIAL INFARCTION OR SUDDEN DEATH IN KAWASAKI DISEASE

We have analysed 104 fatal case reports which were collected through a nationwide survey in Japan in 1984 (Kato et al., 1985). More than half had died within 2 months of illness; however about 20 % of them revealed a comparatively late death after more than 1 year of illness. Almost all cases revealed a sudden onset of cardiogenic shock. The main cause of death was acute myocardial infarction. Eighteen percent of the patients died of congestive heart failure. Five patients died from rupture of coronary aneurysms. Five patients without coronary aneurysms died probably due to myocarditis or arrhythmias.

We also analysed 195 cases with myocardial infarction (Kato et al., 1986). This was found to occur mostly within the 1st year of illness. In more than half of the patients it occurred during sleep or at rest. The main

symptoms of acute myocardial infarction were shock,
unrest, vomiting, abdominal pain, and chest pain. Chest
pain was more frequently recognized in the survivors and
in the older children. Asymptomatic myocardial infarction
was seen in 37 %. Twenty-two percent died at the first
attack. Sixteen percent of the survivors from the first
attack were confronted with a 2nd attack. From the
coronary angiographic studies in the patients with
myocardial infarction, most of the fatal cases had the
obstruction in the left main coronary artery or in both
the right main coronary artery and the anterior descending
artery. In such cases coronary bypass surgery may be
necessary (Hirose et al., 1986). In survivors, one vessel
obstruction, particularly in the right coronary artery,
was frequently recognized. Even if the patients can
survive acute myocardial infarction, about half of the
patients have various types of complications such as
ventricular dysfunction, mitral regurgitation or
arrhythmias, and these may occur even in those who had
asymptomatic myocardial infarction.

3. NATURAL HISTORY OF CORONARY ANEURYSM AND FOLLOW-UP

The natural history of Kawasaki disease and the fate
of coronary aneurysms is of considerable interest for
pediatricians. We have performed coronary angiography in
a routine examination since 1973, and have been conducting
follow-up coronary angiographic studies in 171 cases who
had previously had coronary aneurysms. The follow-up
angiography was performed about one or two years after the
first angiography (Kato et al., 1982). All cases have
been followed for more than 2 years, with the longest
follow-up being 14 years. One of the most exciting
findings regarding the coronary lesions in Kawasaki
disease has been the dramatic regression of aneurysms.
Ninety-nine (58%) of 171 patients with documented coronary
aneurysms on initial angiography (within 1 to 3 months
after onset of disease) had completely normal findings at
the 2nd angiography. Obstruction, stenosis, or
irregularity of the arterial wall was not seen in those
whose aneurysms had fully regressed. This suggests
coronary aneurysms in Kawasaki disease show a strong
tendency to regression within one or two years. None of
the patients with regression of coronary aneurysms
revealed cardiac symptoms in the long-term follow-up
periods, and their electrocardiogram, exercise stess

testing, thallium myocardial scintigraphy and left ventricular function were all within normal limits.

In contrast, the other 72 patients had abnormal findings at the 2nd coronary angiography such as obstructive lesions or persistent aneurysms of the coronary artery. Some of these patients have demonstrated various cardiac symptoms such as sudden death or myocardial infarction and cardiac dysfunction.

We investigated various factors which could effect the prognosis of coronary aneurysms (Ichinose, 1986). By multivariate analysis, the most important factor to predict the prognosis was the size of coronary aneurysms. By discrimination analysis, the risk factors for coronary aneurysms to develop to ischemic heart disease were aneurysm diameter more than 8mm, shape being of large diffuse or saccular type, prolonged fever over 21 days, treatment by steroid rather than by aspirin, and age at onset being over 2 years. Thus, giant coronary aneurysm has serious problem in the prognosis, because it is likely to produce massive thrombus formation and to develop to ischemic heart disease. The incidence rate of giant coronary aneurysms is 26 % in the patients with coronary aneurysms, and is 5.5 % among all Kawasaki disease patients in our series.

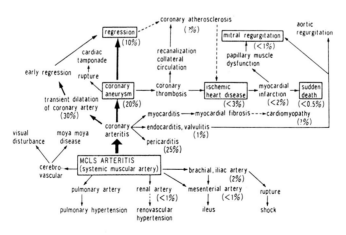

Fig.1. CARDIOVASCULAR SPECTRUM and NATURAL HISTORY

4. LONG-TERM PATHOLOGY AND PREMATURE ATHEROSCLEROSIS.

The pathological mechanisms of regression of aneurysms are marked proliferation of intima without massive thrombus formation which consists of rich, smooth muscle cells, and well regenerated endothelium covering a superficial thrombus (Sasaguri and Kato, 1982). Hemodynamic forces may regulate to make the adequate lumen of such arteries. It is uncertain whether intimal thickening eventually leads to obstructive lesions. However, from our long-term follow-up study of the patients who had regressed aneurysms, we believe that it does not progress to occlusion if massive thrombus formation is absent.

Pathology in patients several years later from the onset demonstrates calcification, deposits of protein-like materials and hyalinized degeneration in the thickened intima, which are similar to atherosclerotic lesions. Organization of massive thrombus or intimal thickening are likely to develop to atherosclerotic changes, and other coronary atherosclerotic risk factors such as hyperlipemia, smoking or hypertension may accelerate these conditions. Kawasaki disease may be a long-term coronary risk factor and in the near future, the advanced cardiovascular problem may be handled in the field of adult cardiology.

REFERENCES

Asai T, (1983). Evaluation method for the degree of seriousness in Kawasaki disease. Acta Paediatr Jpn 25:170-175

Fujiwara H, Hamashima Y(1978).: Pathology of the heart in Kawasaki disease.
Pediatrics 61:100-105

Hirose H, Kawashima Y, Nakano S, Matsuda H, Sakakibara T, Hiranaka T, Imagawa H, Osawa M, Harima R(1986): Long-term results in surgical treatment of children 4 years old or younger with coronary involvement due to Kawasaki disease.
Circulation 74(suppl I):77-81

Ichinose E, Kato H, Inoue O (1985): Intracoronary thrombolytic therapy in Kawasaki disease and the usefulness of two-dimensional echocardiography in detecting intracoronary thrombi. J Cardiography 15:79-85

Ichinose E, Inoue O, Kato H.(1986). Fate of coronary aneurysm in Kawasaki disease: Analysis of prognostic factors. In Doyle EF, Engle MA, Gersony WM, Rashkind WJ, Talner NS (eds): "Pediatric cardiology" New York: Springer-Verlag, pp 1099-1101

Japan Research Committee on Kawasaki disease (1971), Report of fatal cases of Kawasaki disease. Japanese Ministry of Health and Welfare

Japan Research Committee on Kawasaki disease (1984). Report of subcommittee on standardization of diagnostic criteria and reporting of coronary artery lesions in Kawasaki disease. Japanese Ministry of Health and Welfare

Kato H, Koike S, Yamamoto M, Ito Y, Yano T. (1975). Coronary aneurysms in infants and young children with acute febrile mucocutaneous lymph node syndrome. J Pediatr 86:892

Kato H, Ichinose E, Takechi T, Yoshioka F, Suzuki K, Rikitake N. (1982). Fate of coronary aneurysms in Kawasaki disease: Serial coronary angiography and long-term follow-up study. Am J Cardiol 49:1758

Kato H, Ichinose E (1984). Cardiovascular involvement in Kawasaki disease. Act Paediatr Jpn. 26:132-145

Kato H, Ichinose E, Yanagawa Y, Kawasaki T. (1985). Clinical analyses of 104 fatal cases in Kawasaki disease. Shonika 26:1017-1021

Kato H, Ichinose E, Kawasaki T. (1986). Myocardial infarction in Kawasaki disease: Clinical analyses of 195 cases. J Pediatr 108:923-927

Kawasaki T (1967). Acute febrile mucocutaneous syndrome with lymphoid involvement with specific desquamation of the fingers and toes in children. Jpn J Allerg 16:178-222

Nakano H, Ueda K, Saito A. (1986). Scoring method for identifying patients with Kawasaki disease at high risk of coronary artery aneurysms. Am J Cardiol 58:739-743

Sasaguri Y, Kato H (1982). Regression of aneurysms in Kawasaki disease: A pathological study. J Pediatr 100:225-231

Kawasaki Disease, pages 287–297
© 1987 Alan R. Liss, Inc.

PREDICTION OF PATIENTS WITH A HIGH RISK OF CORONARY ARTERY
ANEURYSM IN KAWASAKI DISEASE: INDICATION FOR IMMUNOGLOBULIN
THERAPY

Hiroyuki Nakano

Division of Pediatric Cardiology, Shizuoka Children's Hospital, Shizuoka, Japan

INTRODUCTION

The prognosis of Kawasaki disease varies mainly in ac-
cordance with the severity of the coronary artery lesion,
which is the most serious complication of the illness. Although several treatment modalities (Kato et al., 1979; Kijima et al., 1982) have been tried in an effort to prevent coronary aneurysm, satisfactory results have not been obtained.
Recently, Furusho and his associates (Furusho et al., 1983)
proposed the use of large doses of immunoglobulin for Kawasaki disease, and subsequent reports have supported the efficacy
of immunoglobulin therapy (Furusho et al., 1984; Newburger
et al., 1986). Immunoglobulin, however, is expensive and it
has potential adverse effects such as infection and allergic
reactions. Moreover, taking into consideration that the incidence of coronary artery complications is low with usual
aspirin therapy, it is not practical to give large doses of
immunoglobulin to all patients with Kawasaki disease (Feigin
and Barron, 1986). We believe that a better policy is to
identify patients with a high risk of coronary aneurysm
during the early phase of the illness, and to give immunoglobulin therapy selectively to these high-risk patients
(Nakano et al., 1986). The purpose of this study was to de-
vise a scoring method for evaluating the severity of Kawasaki
disease in terms of coronary artery involvement on the basis
of clinical and early laboratory findings.

SEVERITY OF CORONARY ANEURYSM IN KAWASAKI DISEASE

Coronary artery lesions develop in approximately 20% of

patients with Kawasaki disease, with a broad spectrum of varying degree ranging from transient slight coronary dilatation to giant coronary aneurysm. It is clinically important to determine the course of these lesions and to study the relation between coronary artery disease and prognosis or cardiac function. The evaluation of severity of coronary aneurysm was also a prerequisite for the present study as a predictor of coronary risk.

As reported previously, we have quantitatively classified the severity of coronary aneurysms remaining after Kawasaki disease into 4 grades (Table 1) based on observations of the clinical course of coronary lesions on repeated coronary angiograms (Nakano et al., 1985). Mild coronary aneurysms with a maximal diameter of less than 4.0 mm (grade I) usually regressed to normal within a short time, while most giant aneurysms with a maximal diameter greater than 8.0 mm (grade III) either progressed to become obstructive coronary lesions or persistent large aneurysms. Almost all myocardial infarctions following Kawasaki disease were seen in patients with giant coronary aneurysms which had developed in the early stage of the illness (Nakano et al., 1986). The course of grade II aneurysms with a maximal diameter of between 4.0 and 8.0 mm varied depending on the initial coronary diameter, but all were eventually reduced in size. Using this classification, we were able to predict the course and prognosis of coronary artery disease from angiographic findings shortly after onset of the illness. Although this angiographic grading may be applicable to echocardiographic evaluation, slight dilatation of the coronary artery is often difficult to identify accurately with this modality (Feigin and Barron, 1986).

TABLE 1. Classification of Severity of Coronary Artery Aneurysm Following Kawasaki Disease

Grade	Severity	Maximal coronary diameter
0	Normal	3.0 mm or less
I	Mild	4.0 mm or less
II	Moderate	4.0 - 8.0 mm
III	Severe	8.0 mm or more

CORONARY ANEURYSMS WITH ASPIRIN THERAPY

Between May 1977 and October 1985, there were 165 patients with Kawasaki disease who were admitted to our hospital within 7 days of disease onset. The main treatment modalities during the acute febrile period included aspirin alone in 78 patients, glucocorticoid in 35 patients, and immunoglobulin in 52 patients. Because the occurrence of coronary artery lesions is considered to be affected by the various agents used, only the clinical information obtained for patients who received aspirin as a standard treatment (Kato et al., 1979) formed the data base of the therapeutic study. As seen in Table 2, a total of 19 patients (24.3%) given aspirin therapy had coronary aneurysms, and the severity of these lesions was as follows: slight coronary dilatation of grade I was seen in 3 patients (3.8%), moderate-sized aneurysms of grade II in 14 (17.9%) patients, and giant aneurysms of grade III in 2 (2.6%) patients.

TABLE 2. Incidence of Coronary Artery Aneurysm with Aspirin Therapy

Grade	Patients	%	Risk group
0	59	75.7	Low
I	3	3.8	
II	14	17.9	High
III	2	2.6	
Total	78	100.0	

PREDICTION OF DEVELOPMENT OF CORONARY ANEURYSMS

From data on the 78 patients who received aspirin therapy, we devised a method of predictive scoring to assess the likelihood of development of coronary artery lesions on the basis of early clinical and laboratory findings (Nakano et al., 1986). First, patients were divided into 2 groups, one consisting of 62 patients with normal coronary arteries of grade 0 or mild coronary aneurysms of grade I (low-risk group), and the other consisting of 16 patients associated with significant aneurysms of grade II or III (high-risk group). This is because the prognosis of grade I aneurysms

TABLE 3. Comparison of Clinical and Laboratory Findings
on Admission Between the Two Groups with Aspirin Therapy

Items	Low-risk group (n=62)	High-risk group (n=16)	p Value
Sex (male:female)	36:26	7:9	NS
Age of onset (yr)	2 3/12±1 8/12	1 5/12±1 1/12	NS
C-reactive protein (+)	3.2±1.4	4.9±1.5	<0.001
White blood cell count	14,300±4,800	15,800±5,000	NS
Hematocrit (%)	34.3±2.9	33.8±2.9	NS
Platelet count (×10^4)	36.0±11.8	31.7±10.5	NS
GOT (IU/1)	34±38	31±30	NS
Serum albumin (g/100 ml)	3.6±0.5	3.4±0.4	NS
IgG (mg/100 ml)	790±250	670±270	NS

Values are mean ± standard deviation.
GOT = glutamic oxaloacetic transaminase; IgG = immunoglobulin
G; NS = not significant. (From Nakano H et al.: Scoring
method for identifying patients with Kawasaki disease at
high risk of coronary artery aneurysm. Am J Cardiol 58:740,
1986. By permission of Technical Publishing Company.)

is not serious compared to that of grade II or III aneurysms,
and in clinical practice, it is frequently difficult to
accurately identify slight ectasia of the coronary artery
by echocardiography (Feigin and Barron, 1986). We believe
that significant coronary aneurysms with a diameter of over
4.0 mm can be easily detected with echocardiography even in
small infants.

Second, patient profiles and laboratory data obtained
at the time of admission between 4 and 7 days after onset
of the illness were compared between the two groups of high-
risk and low-risk patients. Items selected were sex, age at
onset of Kawasaki disease, C-reactive protein (CRP), white
blood cell count, hematocrit, platelet count, glutamic oxaloacetic transaminase, serum albumin and immunoglobulin G
(IgG). Simple comparison showed no significant differences
of variables between the two groups except for CRP, as indicated in Table 3, and therefore multivariate analysis was
performed in order to determine whether the two groups could
be separated using the method of quantification II (Hayashi,

1959).

After each item has been categorized into 2 or 4 grades, the partial correlation coefficient contributing to the separation of high-risk and low-risk was obtained by discrimination analysis; the coefficient was higher for CRP (0.61), age (0.50), IgG (0.35) and platelet count (0.34), in that order. Then, discrimination was again studied using 3 high-ranking variables except for IgG because of the presence of a significant correlation with age (r=0.46). From these results, a scoring system was devised by proportionally simplifying the weighting of each category (Table 4). A patient was predicted to have a significant coronary aneurysm when his or her total score for 3 variables was negative, while a patient was predicted not to develop any significant coronary lesion when the total score was 0 or positive.

TABLE 4. Scoring Method for Prediction of Development of Coronary Artery Aneurysm

Items	Category	Weight of category	Score
Age of onset	under 1 yr	-0.51	- 1
	1 - 2 yr	+0.01	0
	over 2 yr	+0.36	+ 1
CRP	0 - 1+	+0.96	+ 2
	2+ - 4+	+0.41	+ 1
	5+	-0.01	0
	6+	-1.94	- 3
Platelet count	under 30×10^4	-0.47	- 1
	over 30×10^4	+0.26	+ 1

Low-risk group is composed of patients whose total score is 0 or positive, while high-risk group is composed of patients whose total score is negative. (From Nakano H et al.: Scoring method for identifying patients with Kawasaki disease at high risk of coronary artery aneurysms. Am J Cardiol 58: 742, 1986. By permission of Technical Publishing Company.)

RETROSPECTIVE EVALUATION OF TREATMENT USING THE DEVISED
SCORING METHOD

Using the scoring method devised, the effect of aspirin
and immunoglobulin on the occurrence of coronary artery dis-

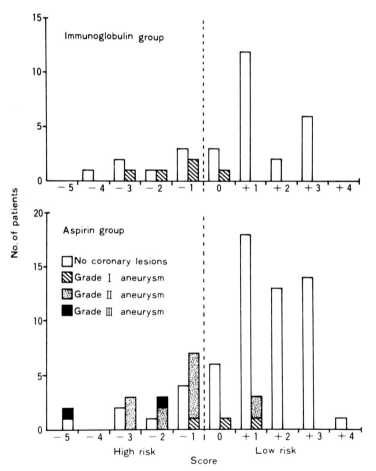

Figure 1. Coronary artery lesions and use of the scoring
system in patients who received immunoglobulin or aspirin.
(From Nakano H et al.: Scoring method for identifying
patients with Kawasaki disease at high risk of coronary
artery aneurysm. Am J Cardiol 58:741, 1986. By permission
of Technical Publishing Company.)

ease was retrospectively studied (Fig. 1). Of the 78 patients who received aspirin alone and were studied in order to obtain a score, 16 patients had significant coronary aneurysms; 12 of the 14 patients with grade II aneurysms and the 2 patients with grade III aneurysms were in the high-risk group. As indicated in Fig. 1, false positive results were seen in 7 of the 62 low-risk patients (11.3%) and false negative results in 2 of the 16 high-risk patients (12.5%) using these criteria.

Immunoglobulin was used in combination with aspirin in a total of 35 patients in our hospital until October 1985 (Fig. 1). The total amount of immunoglobulin administered was 400 to 2,000 mg/kg according to the recommendations of an incorporated joint study (Furusho et al., 1984). Fortunately, we had no patients who developed significant coronary artery aneurysms of grade II or III regardless of immunoglobulin dosage. Five patients had slight coronary grade I dilatation, but 4 of these patients were in the high-risk group.

PROSPECTIVE STUDY OF IMMUNOGLOBULIN THERAPY USING THE DEVISED SCORING METHOD

A prospective randomized controlled trial for immunoglobulin therapy was conducted in patients with Kawasaki disease, using the devised scoring system, from November 1985 onward. Patients who were admitted between 4 and 7 days after onset of illness were divided into high-risk or low-

TABLE 5. Clinical and Laboratory Findings in the Prospective Controlled Trial of Immunoglobulin Therapy for Kawasaki Disease

Group	n	Age	Sex (m:f)	Days at admission	CRP (mg/dl)	Platelet ($\times 10^4$)	Score
Low-ASA	9	1y 7m±1y4m	5:4	4.2±0.7	7.8±2.8	37.7±7.5	+1.7±1.0
Low-IG	11	2y 1m±1y3m	8:3	4.4±1.1	6.1±2.5	39.4±7.9	+2.1±0.9
High-ASA	4	1y10m±1y4m	2:2	5.3±0.5	15.1±2.2	44.7±14.8	-2.5±1.9
High-IG	5	2y 7m±1y5m	2:3	4.6±0.5	17.3±4.0	32.2±11.1	-2.6±0.5
Total	29	2y 0m±1y3m	17:12	4.5±0.9	9.8±5.3	38.4±9.6	+0.5±2.3

Values are mean ± standard deviation.
CRP = C-reactive protein; ASA = aspirin; IG = immunoglobulin.

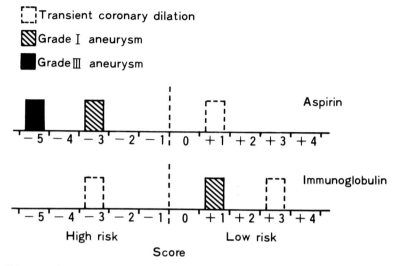

Figure 2. Coronary artery lesions and use of the scoring system in the prospective controlled study of immuno-globulin therapy.

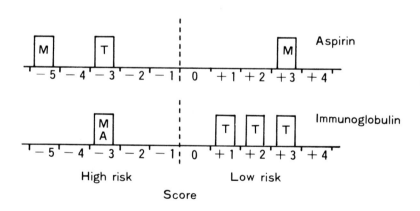

Figure 3. Valvular complication and use of the scoring system in the prospective controlled study of immuno-globulin therapy.
M = mitral regurgitation; T = tricuspid regurgitation; A = aortic regurgitation.

risk groups according to the scoring method, and we administered aspirin alone or immunoglobulin, 200 mg/kg, for 3 days, in combination with aspirin to one patient in each group according to an order determined randomly beforehand (Table 5). As seen in Fig. 2, giant aneurysms of grade III were recognized in one patient of the high-risk group who received aspirin alone (High-ASA), and mild aneurysms of grade I were seen in one High-ASA patient and one patient in the low-risk group who received immunoglobulin, respectively. Transient coronary ectasia was demonstrated in 3 patients regardless of group. Although no firm conclusions could be reached because of the small number of patients, the present scoring method appears to provide useful information for the prediction of coronary artery involvement in Kawasaki disease.

Transient regurgitant signals from the cardiac valve were demonstrated in 7 patients by pulsed Doppler echocardiography, but no significant relationships were seen between immunoglobulin therapy or severity of the disease and valvular complications (Fig. 3). Most cases of valvular regurgitation following Kawasaki disease are recognized for a short time during the acute febrile period and are suggested to be the result of carditis (Nakano et al., 1985; Nakano et al., 1986). On the other hand, there were significant differences in the length of the febrile period and the number of days after onset of illness at which CRP becomes negative between the high-risk and low-risk groups, but immunoglobulin administration was unable to shorten these periods (Table 6). These observations imply that immunoglobulin therapy may substantially prevent the occurrence of coronary artery aneurysms, but may not critically affect the clinical course of the systemic inflammatory process associated with Kawasaki disease. We hypothesize that immunoglobulin acts locally at the site of the coronary artery wall and inhibits the interaction between platelets and coronary arteritis. Although the precise mechanism of action of immunoglobulin still needs to be fully investigated, the present results suggest that platelets play an important role in the development of coronary artery lesion in this disease (Burns et al., 1984).

SUMMARY

The prediction of the severity of Kawasaki disease in terms of coronary artery disease is important for the evalu-

TABLE 6. Comparison of Clinical Course in Each Group

Group	Febrile period	No. of days at negative CRP
Low-ASA	7.6 ± 1.9	16.2 ± 4.7
Low-IG	7.2 ± 2.3	16.6 ± 6.3
High-ASA	12.8 ± 9.0	16.7 ± 9.5
High-IG	13.8 ± 10.4	24.0 ± 14.5
Low-risk	7.4 ± 2.1 ⎤ p<.001	16.5 ± 5.5 ⎤ p<.001
High-risk	13.3 ± 9.2 ⎦	23.6 ± 13.1 ⎦
Aspirin	9.2 ± 5.4 ⎤ NS	18.3 ± 8.4 ⎤ NS
Immunoglobulin	9.3 ± 6.5 ⎦	18.9 ± 9.7 ⎦

Values are number of days of illness as means ± standard
deviation. Low-risk group includes Low-ASA and Low-IG
groups, while High-risk group includes High-ASA and High-
IG groups. Similarly, Aspirin group includes Low-ASA and
High-ASA groups, while Immunoglobulin group includes Low-
IG and High-IG groups.
CRP = C-reactive protein; ASA = aspirin; IG = immunoglobulin.

ation of prognosis as well as for making decisions on an
appropriate form of treatment. Coronary artery lesions develop as early as 8 days after onset of illness and immunoglobulin is known to be ineffective in aneurysms which have
already developed. Therefore, we advocate the selection of
suitable candidates for immunoglobulin therapy as early as
possible after disease onset. Our scoring system is composed
of only 3 items which are confined to the results of routine
laboratory examinations, and it is desired to be available
for use by any hospital offering primary care for patients
with Kawasaki disease. However, such a simple procedure may
be associated with a reduced level of reliability for evaluation in clinical practice. Early and simple, but reliable,
predictors of coronary risk in Kawasaki disease should
therefore be further studied in order to reduce the morbidity
and mortality through appropriate treatment and care.

REFERENCES

Burns JC, Glode MP, Clarke SH, Wiggins J Jr, Hathaway WE
    (1984). Coagulopathy and platelet activation in Kawasaki

syndrome: identification of patients at high risk for development of coronary artery aneurysms. J Pediatr 105:206–211.

Feigin RD, Barron KS (1986). Treatment of Kawasaki syndrome. New Engl J Med 315:388–390.

Furusho K, Sato K, Soeda T, Matsumoto H, Okabe T, Hirota T, Kawada S (1983). High-dose intravenous gammaglobulin for Kawasaki disease. Lancet 2:1359.

Furusho K, Kamiya T, Nakano H, Kiyosawa N, Shinomiya K, Hayashidera T, Tamura T, Hirose O, Manabe Y, Yokoyama T, Kawarano M, Baba K, Baba K, Mori C (1984). High-dose intravenous gammaglobulin for Kawasaki disease. Lancet 2: 1055–1058.

Hayashi C (1959). Fundamental concept of the theory of quantification and prediction. Ann Inst Stat Math 7:43–48.

Kato H, Koike S, Yokoyama T (1979). Kawasaki disease: effect of treatment on coronary artery involvement. Pediatrics 63:175–179.

Kijima Y, Kamiya T, Suzuki A, Hirose O, Manabe H (1982). A trial procedure to prevent aneurysm formation of the coronary arteries by steroid pulse therapy in Kawasaki disease. Jpn Circ J 46:1239–1242.

Nakano H, Nojima K, Saito A, Ueda K (1985). High incidence of aortic regurgitation following Kawasaki disease. J Pediatr 107:59–63.

Nakano H, Ueda K, Saito A, Nojima K (1985) Repeated quantitative angiograms in coronary arterial aneurysm in Kawasaki disease. Am J Cardiol 56:846–851.

Nakano H, Ueda K, Saito A, Tsuchitani Y (1986). Doppler detection of tricuspid regurgitation following Kawasaki disease. Pediatr Radiol 16:123–125.

Nakano H, Saito A, Ueda K, Nojima K (1986). Clinical characteristics of myocardial infarction following Kawasaki disease: report of 11 cases. J Pediatr 108:198–203.

Nakano H, Ueda K, Saito A, Tsuchitani Y, Kawamori J, Miyake T, Yoshida (1986). Scoring method for identifying patients with Kawasaki disease at high risk of coronary artery aneurysms. Am J Cardiol 58:749–753.

Newburger JW, Takahashi M, Burns JC, Beiser AS, Chung KJ, Duffy E, Glode MP, Mason WH, Reddy V, Sanders SP, Shulman ST, Wiggins JW, Hicks RV, Fulton DR, Lewis AB, Leung DYM, Colton T, Rosen FS, Melish ME (1986). The treatment of Kawasaki syndrome with intravenous gamma globulin. New Engl J Med 315:341–347.

Kawasaki Disease, pages 299–304
© 1987 Alan R. Liss, Inc.

PREDICTORS OF CORONARY RISK IN KAWASAKI DISEASE

L. N. Benson, M.D., and R. D. Rowe, M.D.

Department of Pediatrics, Division of Cardiology,
The Hospital for Sick Children, Toronto, Canada
M5G 1X8

The elucidation of the etiologic factors, treatment
modalities and prognostic factors for cardiovascular
involvement in Kawasaki Disease are elusive today as when
the disease was first described in 1967 (Kawasaki et al,
1967), although much has been learned in the past twenty
years (Sekiguchi et al, 1986).

Kawasaki Disease is an acute disorder affecting infants
and young children, 75% under 4 years of age. The Japan
Mucocutaneous Lymph Node Syndrome Research Committee has
provided clinically useful guidelines in diagnosis (1978).
However, it is the cardiovascular manifestations which
present the most serious complications and may lead to death
(Sekiguchi et al, 1986). Clearly the prognosis for Kawasaki
Disease depends on the degree of this coronary artery involvement, and despite the use of aspirin, flurbiprofen,
dipyridamole or steroids to prevent these aneurysms, the
incidence remains about 20% (Kamiya et al, 1981).

In 1983, Furusho proposed administration of large doses
of immunoglobulin for prevention of coronary aneurysms and
subsequent reports supporting the efficacy of this therapy
has surfaced in both the Japanese and North American literature (Furusho et al, 1983; Newburger et al, 1986). However,
80% of affected children do not develop aneurysms (Sekiguchi
et al, 1986). Predictors of the high risk population for
development of coronary aneurysms would be most useful for
the clinician in managing individual patients, in assessing
the efficacy of therapies, the elimination of potential side-
effects of therapies in low risk patients and reducing

costs (Feigin et al, 1986). Since the substrate for aneurysm formation occurs in the first ten days of the illness when perivascular inflammation gives way to a panvasculitis, it is critical that high-risk patients be differentiated early in their clinical course. A number of factors have been assessed to predict the presence of coronary artery involvement. Asai in 1976 proposed a scoring system to help the clinician decide if coronary angiography was indicated (Asai et al, 1983), and a modification of this scoring system has been applied to a cohort of patients by Heilbut and her colleagues at The Hospital for Sick Children in Toronto (Heilbut et al, 1982), as well as assessing the influence of fever duration (Koren et al, 1986), from the same institution - all appear to have some value in detecting the presence of coronary involvement.

In the Asai score (Asai et al, 1983) or its modification (Heilbut et al, 1982), points were given for various observed general clinical features and routine laboratory findings (table 1) with a 6 point threshold indicating the presence of an aneurysm. However, the highest risk factors, given 2 points, include observations made over 16 or 30 days - making either scores more retrospective rather than predictive. Nevertheless, a nationwide Japanese survey in which the Asai score and coronary angiography were compared in 426 patients (Sekiguchi et al, 1986) yielded a sensitivity of 88%, specificity of 54%, a predictive value of a positive test 35% and predictive value of a negative test 94%. Similiar magnitude figures were found in the Toronto experience (table 2). The study by Koren emphasizes the influence of prolonged inflammation as a coronary risk as represented by fever beyond 14 days - a suggestion initially made by Asai that the most severely affected patients tended to have coronary involvement.

Other risk factors found in the Japanese experience are male gender, and age at disease onset of one year or less. However, age appeared not to be significant in the Toronto experience with 55% of affected children between 1 and 4 years and only 26% under one year (Turner-Gomes et al, 1986). Thus, none of the scoring systems can be used until the fever ceases, limiting their clinical usefulness.

Recently, investigators (Iwasa et al, 1986; Nakano et al, 1986) have attempted to relate variables measured early from fever onset which would predict coronary artery disease.

Table 1.   Scoring Method to Evaluate Kawasaki Disease (Sekiguchi et al, 1986)

Factors	● 2 points ●	1 point	0 point
Sex		Male	Female
Age of onset		under 1 year	over 1 year
● Duration of fever	over 16 days	14–15 days	under 13 days
Double-peaked fever	observed		not observed
Skin eruption		observed	not observed
Under 10 g/dl hemoglobin or under 3.5 million erythrocytes		observed	not observed
Highest leukocyte count during illness	over 30,000/mm^{-3}	over 26,000 and under 30,000/mm^{-3}	under 26,000/mm^{-3}
Highest erythrocyte sedimentation rate during illness	over 101 mm/hr	60–100 mm/hr	under 60 mm/hr
● Day of illness until normalization of C-reactive protein level or erythrocyte sedimentation rate	after 30th day		prior to 29th day
Double-peaked C-reactive protein level or double-peaked erythrocyte sedimentation rate	observed		not observed
Cardiomegaly		observed	not observed
Arrhythmia		observed	not observed
Q:R ratio increase in leads II, III, and aV$_f$	observed		not observed
Myocardial infarction	observed		not observed
Recurrence of the disease		observed	not observed

Table 2. Prediction of Presence of Coronary
Lesion in Kawasaki Disease

	Sensitivity	Specificity	Pred. Value Pos. Test	Pred. Value Neg. Test
ASAI(N=426) (Sekiguchi, 1986)	88%	54 %	35%	94%
Mod. Score (N=64) (Heilbut, 1982)	100%	76%	35%	100%
Fever (N=54) (Koren, 1986)	100%	65%	50%	100%
Iwasa (1985a)	83%	75%	50%	94%
Nakano (1986)	87%	87%	63%	96%

Iwasa related age, sex, red blood cell count, hematocrit and serum albumin concentration. The developed score has a sensitivity of 83% specificity of 75%, predictive value of a positive test (score less than 0) 50% and negative test (score greater than 0) of 94% (table 2). Clinical trials applying this score have been useful in selecting high-risk patient groups for immunoglobulin therapy (Iwasa et al, 1986b). A similiar approach evaluating early predictors of high risk was addressed in a discriminative analysis study on patients at 5 days of illness (Nakano et al, 1986). Looking initially at 9 clinical variables, and dividing the patient groups into low-risk (normal or ectatic coronary lesions) or high-risk (aneurysmal lesions), 3 discriminative functions were identified. The age of onset, C-reactive protein (radioimmunodiffusion) and platelet count were graded and scored, with scores of 0 or greater assigned to the low risk group versus those with negative scores, the high risk group. The sensitivity and specificity was 87% with a predicitive value for a positive test of 63% and predictive value of a negative test 96% (table 2). Patients with lower numerical scores tended to have more severe disease. The system has a low false negative and false positive rate (12.9% and 12.5% respectively). These are considerable improvements from previous systems with the distinct advantage of being applied early in the disease. Clearly, they lack predictive value of identifing patients who will develop aneurysm (table 2), but may define those at low risk. However, further clinical traits of both scores are warranted.

With all this said and done Kawasaki Syndrome, its etiology and protean manifestations, therapy and prognosis can be characterized still in 1986 as "a riddle wrapped in a mystery inside an enigma". -W. Churchill 1939.

REFERENCES

Asai T (1983). Evaluation method for degree of seriousness in Kawasaki Disease. Nippon Shonika Gakkai Zasshi (Act Pediatr Jpn; overseas ed.) 25:170.

Feigin R, Barron KS (1986). Treatment of Kawasaki Syndrome: N Engl J Med 315:388-390.

Furusho K, Sato K, Soeda T, Matsumoto H, Okabe T, Hirota T, Kawada S (1983). High-dose intravenous gammaglobulin for Kawasaki Disease. Lancet 2:1359.

Heilbut MD, Rose V, Duncan WJ et al (1982). Kawasaki Disease (KD) Assessment of risk factors for cardiovascular sequelae (abstract). Pediatr Res 16:100A.

Iwasa M, Sugiyama K, Kawase A, Yoshino M, Nakano M, Katoh T, Wada Y (1986a). Prevention of coronary artery involvement in Kawasaki Disease by early intravenous high-dose gamma globulin. In Doyle EF, Engle MA, Gersony WM, Rashkind WJ and Talner NS (eds): Pediatric Cardiology: Proceedings of the Second World Congress, New York:Springer-Verlag, pp 1083-1085.

Iwasa M, Sugiyama K, Ando T, Nomura H, Katoh T, Wada Y (1986b). Selection of high risk children for immunoglobulin therapy in Kawasaki disease. Presented at the Second International Kawasaki Disease Symposium, Dec., 1986, Kauai, Hawaii.

Japan MCLS Research Committee (1978). Diagnostic guideline of infantile acute febrile muco-cutaneous lymphnode syndrome, 3rd revised edition, Dept. of Epidemiology, Institute of Public Health, Tokyo.

Kamiya T, Suzuki A, Kijima Y, Hirose O (1981). Coronary arterial lesion in children with Kawasaki Disease (abstract). Circulation 64: suppl. IV:IV - 278.

Kawasaki T, Kouasaki F (1967). Febrile oculo-orocutaneo-acrodesquamatous syndrome with or without acute non-supperative cervical lymphadenitis in infancy and childhood: clinical observations of 50 cases. Allergy (Jpn J Allergy) 16:178. (In Japanese with English Abstract).

Koren G, Lavi S, Rose V, Rowe R (1986). Kawasaki Disease: Review of risk factors for coronary aneurysms. J Pediatr 108:388-392.

Nakano H, Ueda K, Saito A, Tsuchitani Y, Kawamori J, Miyake, Yoshida T (1986). Scoring method for identifying patients with Kawasaki Disease at high risk of coronary artery aneurysm. Am J Cardiol 58:739-742.

Newburger JW, Takahashi M, Burns JC et al (1986). The treatment of Kawasaki Syndrome with intravenous gammaglobulin. N Engl J Med 315:341-347.

Sekiguchi M, Takao A, Endo M, Asai T, Kawasaki T (1986). On the mucocutaneous lymph node syndrome or Kawasaki Disease. In, Progress in Cardiology 97-144.

Suzuki M, Kaneda Y, Tsuda M, Ri Y, Fukuda Y, Furukawa K, Ishige H, Sugimota A (1983). On the experience of using massive immunoglobulin in Kawasaki Disease (in Japanese). Pediatr Jpn 24:391-395.

Turner-Gomes S, Rose V, Brezina A, Smallhorn J, Rowe R (1986). High persistence rate of estabsished coronary artery lesions secondary to Kawasaki Disease among a panethnic Canadian population. J Pediatr 108:928-932.

Kawasaki Disease, pages 305–309
© 1987 Alan R. Liss, Inc.

LATE ONSET VALVULAR DYSFUNCTION IN KAWASAKI DISEASE

Samuel S. Gidding

Division of Pediatrics, The Children's Memorial
Hospital, Chicago, Illinois 60614

The long-term follow-up of patients with Kawasaki Disease
has been primarily focused upon coronary artery aneurysms and
their sequelae (Melish, 1982). Because of recent experience
with a patient who more than one year following acute Kawasaki
disease developed severe mitral and aortic insufficiency, an investigation of late-onset cardiac valvular dysfunction as a manifestation of Kawasaki disease was undertaken (Gidding et al, 1986).
Twenty-three major pediatric cardiac centers across the continental United States were contacted to assess their experience with
new cardiac valvular dysfunction in patients with resolution
of the acute manifestations of Kawasaki disease.

The following definition for late-onset valvular dysfunction
was developed: onset of cardiac valvular insufficiency at least
one month after resolution of the acute manifestations of Kawasaki
disease, including resolution of any valvular insufficiency that was
associated with acute disease. Other potential etiologies of
acquired valvular dysfunction, including infectious endocarditis
and rheumatic fever, had to be excluded.

At least one staff cardiologist from each of 23 centers across
the United States was contacted by telephone. These centers
collectively have identified 3500 to 4000 patients with Kawasaki
disease. Late-onset valvular insufficiency which fit our clinical
definition was identified in seven cases. Thus, the incidence of
late-onset valvular insufficiency was very low, approximately
1 in 500 cases or 0.2%. This number can only be considered an
estimate of the incidence of late-onset valvular insufficiency
in the United States for several reasons: 1) the duration of late
follow-up varied greatly among institutions; 2) many patients

without coronary aneurysms have been discharged or lost to follow-up; 3) it has not been routine practice to perform Doppler assessment of cardiac valves during follow-up echocardiographic examinations; and 4) the sample size is biased by referral patterns in various parts of the country.

There were nine insufficient cardiac valves in the seven identified patients (Table 1). Four patients had isolated mitral insufficiency, two patients had involvement of both mitral and aortic valves, and the seventh patient, in whom the diagnosis of Kawasaki disease was strongly suspected but not completely established, had isolated aortic insufficiency.

CASE REPORTS

Two cases with isolated mitral insufficiency are described below. The first presented with Kawasaki disease at age three months and developed aneurysms of both main coronary arteries. At five months of age, myocardial infarction was suspected by electrocardiogram and angiography revealed occlusion of the right coronary artery and aneurysms of the left coronary artery. At two years of age a new murmur of mitral insufficiency was detected. An acute ischemic event was not identified at this time. This patient has subsequently gone on to have a second myocardial infarction involving the antero-septal and inferior walls. The mitral insufficiency remains mild to moderate and therapy in this patient has been directed towards treatment of the myocardial infarction.

The second case initially presented at 14 months of age. Mitral insufficiency developed three months after resolution of acute Kawasaki disease. This patient had significant aneurysms of both right and left coronary systems, but no cardiac dysfunction or myocardial ischemia by electrocardiographic criteria. Coronary aneurysms subsequently resolved. However, five years after onset of disease, the patient still has mild mitral insufficiency.

The remaining two cases of late-onset mitral insufficiency had onset of mitral insufficiency related to acute myocardial infarction. One of these latter two patients has expired secondary to the myocardial infarction and is the only death in this series. Although myocardial ischemia can be implicated in all four cases of isolated mitral insufficiency, in at least two cases chronic valvulitis cannot be excluded as a possible etiology because mitral insufficiency developed independent of acute ischemic episodes.

TABLE 1

Clinical Data on Patients with Late Onset Valvular Insufficiency

Case	Valves Involved	Suspected Pathogenesis	Coronary Aneurysms	Clinical Features
1	Mitral	Papillary muscle ischemia or valvulitis	Yes	Myocardial infarction, onset of insufficiency not related to acute ischemia
2	Mitral	Papillary muscle ischemia or valvulitis	Yes	Aneurysms resolving when insufficiency noted
3	Mitral	Papillary muscle Ischemia	Yes	Myocardial infarction
4	Mitral	Papillary muscle ischemia	Yes	Myocardial in farction, expired
5	Mitral/ aortic	Valvulitis	Yes	Required valve replacement, abdominal aortic aneurysm
6	Mitral/ aortic	Probable valvulitis	No	
7	Aortic	Aortic root dilatation	No	Atypical presentation of acute illness

The two cases of combined mitral and aortic insufficiency include one which has been previously reported (Gidding et al, 1986). In that child, mitral and aortic valvular insufficiency were first detected 17 months after resolution of acute symptoms and also after apparent resolution of mild coronary artery aneurysms, as determined by echocardiogram. This patient developed severe congestive heart failure over the next two to three months, necessitating mitral and aortic valve replacement. Histologic examination of the excised cardiac valves revealed the presence of a dense inflammatory infiltrate. The normally avascular dense stroma of both aortic and mitral valves was coursed by well-formed capillaries. The inflammatory infiltrate was composed of predominately mononuclear cells, although some polymorphonuclear leucocytes were also seen. The electronic microscopic studies showed that the inflammatory infiltrate was composed of lymphoid cells, plasma cells, monocytes, and macrophages, with focal areas containing polymnorphonuclear leucocytes. Activated plump fibroblasts were freely admixed with inflammatory cells. Though this patient had a very stormy postoperative course, she is currently doing well two years following valve replacement. It is of interest that she also has an abdominal aortic aneurysm. The second patient presented at four months of age with typical features of Kawasaki disease. Two and a half years later, new cardiac murmurs of mitral and aortic insufficiency were noted. There was no evidence of acute inflammatory disease or recurrent Kawasaki disease. She had not been known previously to have coronary artery aneurysms, although her intial echocardiographic studies were performed in a laboratory which does not see a large volume of Kawasaki patients. At this time she has not developed clinical evidence for congestive heart failure.

The patient with isolated aortic insufficiency developed a prolonged febrile illness suggestive of Kawasaki disease at three years of age. The acute illness was characterized by two months of spiking fevers to 101-102° F, arthralgias, mild pharyngitis, rash involving the palms and soles as well as the trunk, mild cervical adenopathy, mild conjunctivitis, and subsequent peeling of the hands and trunk. Unusual features of this illness included a somewhat longer duration of fever than is usually seen, lack of temperatures above 102°, and the prominence of arthralgias as a symptomatiac complaint. Extensive evaluation did not identify a viral or bacteriologic etiology for this illness. Coronary aneurysms were not detected. Approximately two years later, the patient returned and at this time had a new murmur of aortic insufficiency of moderate severity. Two-dimensional echocardiography and angiography showed a mildly dilated aortic root with an irregular appearance. Coronary arteries appeared normal. The aortic valve was tricuspid but thickened. Rheumatic fever and endocarditis were excluded as possible etiologies. This patient may represent a case of late-onset valvular insufficiency secondary to aortic root dilatation.

CONCLUSIONS AND RECOMMENDATIONS

From this survey of 23 major pediatric cardiac centers in the continental United States, we conclude the following: 1) late-onset valvular insufficiency is a rare but definite sequela of Kawasaki disease; 2) mitral and aortic valves are most commonly affected; and 3) pathogenesis of late-onset valvular insufficiency may be related to chronic valvulitis, myocardial infarction, papillary muscle dysfunction, or to aortic root dilatation.

We recommend that all patients with Kawasaki disease, including those without coronary aneurysms, have careful cardiac auscultation every six months for three years after resolution of the acute disease. The time interval of three years is chosen because this time interval would have allowed identification of all patients in this series. Patients undergoing echocardiographic evaluation for coronary artery aneurysms should also have Doppler assessment for mitral and aortic insufficiency. Patients who are at high risk (i.e., those with myocardial infarction, evidence of left valvular dysfunction, or with aortic aneurysms) should be followed more closely.

ACKNOWLEDGEMENT

I would like to thank Nestor Alincastre, M.D., Fred Bierman, M.D., Frank Crussi, M.D., Jerry Jacobs, M.D., Jane Newberger, M.D., and Masato Takahashi, M.D., for contributing clinical information and material for this report. I would also like to thank Stanford T. Shulman, M.D. and C. Elise Duffy, M.D., for their careful review of the paper, and Shann Bulger for her preparation of the manuscript.

REFERENCES

1. Melish ME: Kawasaki Syndrome (the mucocutaneous lymph node syndrome). Ann Rev Med 1982;33:569-585.

2. Gidding SS, Shulman ST, Ilbawi M, Crussi F, Duffy CE: Mucocutaneous lymph node syndrome (Kawasaki disease): Delayed aortic and mitral insufficiency secondary to active valvulitis. J Amer Col Cardiol 1986;7:894-897.

Kawasaki Disease, pages 311–323
© 1987 Alan R. Liss, Inc.

MITRAL REGURGITATION IN KAWASAKI DISEASE

Atsuyoshi Takao, Koichiro Niwa, Chisato Kondo,
Toshio Nakanishi, Gengi Satomi, Makoto Nakazawa,
Masahiro Endo*
Department of Pediatric Cardiology and *Cardio-
vascular Surgery, The Heart Institute of Japan,
Tokyo Women's Medical College, Tokyo 162, Japan

SUMMARY

The clinical characteristics and prognosis of 16 cases
of mitral regurgitation (MR) secondary to Kawasaki disease
(KD) were studied, and its pathogenesis was discussed. The
observation period ranged from 3 years and 17 months to 15
years. Six of the 16 patients died, and 10 are alive. MR
has disappeared spontaneously in 2 of these survivors.
Thirteen of the 16 patients were male and 3 were female,
there being a predominance in male, which is a striking
contrast to rheumatic mitral regurgitation which is predominant in females. The age at the time of diagnosis ranged
from 3 months to 7 years. The appearance time of MR showed
two different patterns, one with early onset within a few
weeks to one month after affliction with KD and the other
with MR developing months or years later during the course
of the follow-up. The cardiothoracic ratio was greater in
those who had a progressively downhill course, and whose
$\Sigma RV1\text{-}6$ decreased with time course. This was considered to
be due to the decrease of the remaining functioning myocardial mass. The outcome of the patients with a severe degree
of coronary arterial stenosis and occlusion observed on the
coronary angiogram was poor. The prognosis of the patients
with severe left coronary arterial stenosis was especially
poor. MR due to KD is regarded as a new clinical entity,
and its pathogenesis is thought to be due to ischemia,
papillary muscle dysfunction, coronary angitis, myocardial
failure and valvulitis. Incidence of MR will increase when
examined by Doppler echocardiography especially in the acute
stage. Our experience as well as that of others indicates
the presence of valvulitis, myocarditis or left ventricular
dilatation leading to MR in the acute stage.

In 1973, we first reported three cases of coronary arterial lesions found on coronary angiography associated with mitral regurgitation (MR) in Kawasaki disease (KD) (Hamada et al., 1973). Since then we have experienced 16 cases of MR secondary to KD.

Rheumatic fever, myocarditis, congenital heart abnormalities, myocardial diseases, and metabolic disorders are known to cause MR in children (Freedom, 1978). However, following our first report, MR has recently been found to develop after KD. We investigated the pathogenesis of MR secondary to KD in 16 cases, and its clinical profiles.

SUBJECTS

At the Heart Institute, 186 patients were diagnosed as having KD and had cardiac catheterization and angiography between 1972 and 1986. Sixteen cases (13 males and 3 females, ranging in age from 3 months to 7 years) were diagnosed as having MR by left ventriculogram. They were divided into those who died (6), and those who are alive (10), including 2 in whom MR disappeared. The observation period ranged from 3 years and 17 months to 15 years from the onset of MR.

METHODS

The clinical outcome, chest Xrays, electrocardiograms coronary angiograms, and the possible pathogenesis of MR were studied. An autopsy was performed in those 10 patients who died.

The total summation of amplitude of RV1-6 on the electrocardiograms was expressed as $\Sigma RV1-6$. To quantitate the numbers of precordial leads showing QS or rS pattern, each one lead of the V4R-7 that showed a QS or rS pattern was counted as one point for scoring. The sum was calculated and its correlation to prognosis was examined.

The degree of stenosis expressed as % at the site of severest stenosis in the left main trunk of the coronary artery (LTM), the left anterior descending artery (LAD), the left circumflex artery (LCX) and the right coronary artery (RCA) was determined, and the relationship between the sum of these values and prognosis was examined. When the severest stenosis was in the LMT, the degree of stenosis was counted as double of the expressed %.

RESULTS

Out of 186 cases, 83 (45%) including 65 males and 18 females showed abnormal coronary angiographic findings such as stenosis, obstruction, aneurysm formation or narrowing (Fig. 1). MR secondary to KD occurred in only 1 of the 103 patients (1%) who had a normal coronary angio- gram and 15 of the 83 patients (18%) who had abnormal findings. The male to female ratio among the 16 with persis- tent MR was 13:3. Fourteen of these 16 patients had stenosis or occlusive lesions. The site of the abnormality of the coronary angiogram was bilateral in 60 of the 83 patients (72%), on the left side in 16 patients (19%) and on the right side in 7 patients (9%). This tendency of prevalence, bilateral, left and right in order, was also seen in the 15 patients who had secondary MR (Fig. 2).

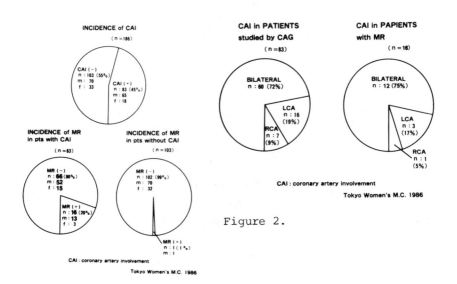

Figure 2.

Figure 1.

At the onset of KD, the 15 patients who developed
secondary MR had typical symptoms, but the history of one
patient was atypical for the committee criteria. The age
at the onset of KD was between 3 months and 6 years, there
being no difference between the survivors and those who
died. Three patients had relapse and two of them died.
The mode of the therapy given consisted of the administration of steroids in 7 patients, aspirin in 4 patients,
and only antibiotics in 4 patients. The definite onset of
the disease in one of the patients who died was uncertain,
but autopsy revealed an occluded coronary arterial lesion
typical for KD. (Fig. 3-1, 3-2).

Figure 3-1.   **Clinical Course of K.D. with MR in Deceased Cases (after onset of K.D.)**

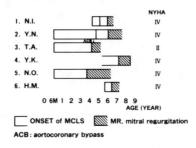

Figure 3-2.   **Clinical Course of K.D. with MR in Surviving Cases (after onset of K.D.)**

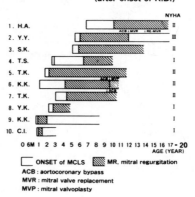

Twelve cases in which the chronological description of AMI was clear were studied. AMI occurred from one month to 5 years after the onset of KD with the mean being 2 years and 2 months, and there was no difference between survivors and those who died. The symptoms at the time of AMI consisted of chest pain in 2 cases, chest pain and vomiting in 2, palpitation in 2, vomiting in 1, high pitched crying in 1, and vague complaint in 4 cases (Fig. 3-1, 3-2).

MR occurred from within 1 month to 5 years after the onset of KD. MR persisted in 14 cases, but disappeared in 2 cases. In 10 of the 14 patients (71%) with persisting MR, MR occurred after 4 years of age. Both patients in whom MR disappeared had developed MR before they were 1 year old (3 months, 5 months), and MR disappeared within a year after the onset of KD. MR appeared concomitantly with AMI in 10 of the 12 patients, within 1 month after AMI in 1 patient and within 10 months after AMI in 1 patient. The clinical outcome of the patients with MR secondary to KD revealed death in 6 patients (38%; 5 males and 1 female), survival of 8 patients (72%; 7 males, 1 female), and disappearance of MR in 2 patients (1 male and 1 female). Five of the 6 deaths occurred within 2 years of the onset of MR. One of the 6 deaths was a sudden death due to the occlusion of a bypass 6 months after aorto-right coronary artery bypass grafting. The other 5 patients died of severe congestive heart failure. One of the survivors had aorto-coronary bypass grafting (ACB) and mitral valve replacement (MVR) twice. One had ACB and mitral valve plasty (MVP) and one had ACB only. According to the NYHA functional classification, 2 patients remained in stage I, 6 patients in stage II and 1 patient in stage III. Disappearance of MR occurred within 1 year after the occurrence of MR in two cases, and MR did not recur thereafter. Both cases now have NYHA stage I (Fig. 3-1, 3-2).

The relationship between the cardiothoracic ratio (CTR) on the chest Xrays and clinical outcome was examined. In 5 of the 6 deaths, MR became the factor aggravating the congestive heart failure with CTR exceeding 70%, resulting in death. The patient who died after ACB occlusion had decreased CTR following ACB, but death occurred suddenly due to the occlusion of the ACB (Fig. 4-1). CTR was unchanged or decreased after surgery or spontaneously in the 8 survivors (Fig. 4-2). CTR was normalized in cases in which MR had disappeared.

Changes of Cardiothoracic Ratio in
DECEASED cases (after onset of K.D.)

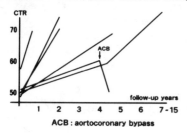

Changes of Cardiothoracic Ratio in
SURVIVING Cases (after onset of K.D.)

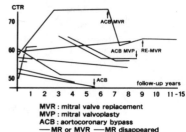

Figure 4-1.

Figure 4-2.

The change in electrocardiogram was examined in terms of prognosis. The two patients who showed left bundle branch block pattern took a fatal course. One of the 3 patients who developed atrial fibrillation died, and the other two survived. The ΣRV1-6 value, QS-rS score, and infarction range on the electrocardiogram could be examined in 5 of the fatal patients, 6 of the survivors and 2 in whom MR had disappeared. The ΣRV1-6 decreased gradually after the occurrence of KD in the fatal cases, and death occurred after the value decreasing to less than 50 mm in 4 cases excluding those who had ACB. Among the survivors, the ΣRV1-6 increased to greater than 100 mm or was unchanged (Fig. 5). The QS and rS score increased rapidly to over 5 points in the patients who died. One patient temporarily had QS-rS score of 0, but again developed QS and rS patterns leading to death. The survivors had little change in QS-rS scores, being under 3 points (Fig. 6).

All the patients who had anterior wall infarction with additional infarction of the septal, lateral or inferior wall died. In particular, all four patients with antero-septal infarction or anteroinferior myocardial infarction died. On the other hand, all five patients with inferior myocardial infarction alone or inferiolateral infarction survived (Fig. 7).

The patients who survived had either no stenosis or occlusion of the right coronary artery (RCA) alone or of the anterior descending artery alone. On the other hand, all

Figure 5.

Changes of $\Sigma RV_{1 \sim 6}$ on ECG (after onset of K.D.)

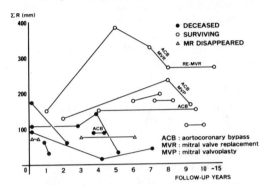

Figure 6.

Changes of Numbers of Precordial Leads with Qs or rS Pattern (after onset of K.D.)

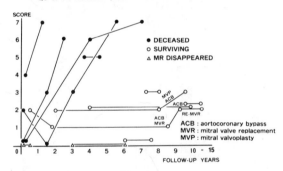

Figure 7.

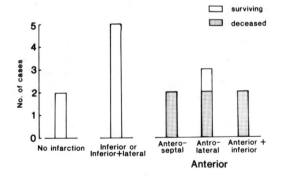

Site of myocardial infarction diagnosed from EKG in KD with MR

the patients with left main coronary trunk occlusion died
(Fig. 8). Then the total summation score of the coronary
artery stenosis or occlusion as described in methods section was examined in relation to prognosis. Ten of the 13
patients with 50% or more occlusion of RCA and with 75% or
more occlusion of LCA had secondary MR. Six of the 8 patients with LCA occlusion of 125% or more died. Two of the
12 patients with 100% occlusion of RCA died. All the
patients with secondary MR who died had a total count of
stenosis value of over 200%. With the exception of one
patient, all the patients who survived (7 patients) had a
total sum of less than 190%. All 4 patients who had
complete occlusion of the left main trunk died. On the
other hand, all four patients with complete occlusion of
only the RCA survived. There was one patient with 25%
stenosis of the left anterior descending artery (LAD). In
1 patient with mild LMT dilatation but not stenosis, MR
disappeared, and the coronary arterial aneurysm disappeared
on the echocardiogram several months after the coronary
angiogram (Table 1, Fig. 9).

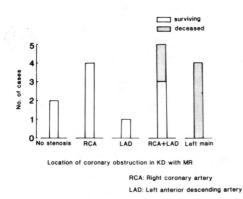

Location of coronary obstruction in KD with MR

RCA: Right coronary artery

LAD: Left anterior descending artery

Figure 8.

Stenosis or Obstruction of CA on CAG
LMCA, LAD, LCX, RCA & Degree of
MR on LVgram

	LCA	RCA	Total	MR
deceased				
N . I .	200%	75%	275	3
Y . N .	200%	0%	200	2 ~3
M . K .	180%	90%	270	1 ~2
T . A .	165%	75%	240	1
N . O .	125%	100%	225	2
H . M .	100%	100%	200	3 ~4
surviving				
Y . Y .	90%	95%	185	3
K . K .	90%	99%	189	1 ~3
S . K .	0%	99%	99	1
H . A .	165%	99%	255	2 ~3
T . S .	90%	99%	189	0 ~1
T . K .	25%	0%	25	1
T . K .	75%	100%	175	1
Y . K .	0%	100%	100	1 ~2
MR disappeared				
K . K .	0	0	0	1 ~2 ·0
C . I .	0	0	0	1 ~2 ·0

Table 1.

Figure 9.

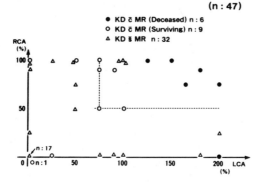

MR vs. Degree of Stenosis of Coronary Arteries in K.D.
(n : 47)

● KD c̄ MR (Deceased) n : 6
○ KD c̄ MR (Surviving) n : 9
△ KD s̄ MR n : 32

DISCUSSION

KD was first reported by Kawasaki as a new clinical entity in 1967 (Kawasaki et al., 1967). The cause of KD is still unknown, but KD is now a well-recognized disease entity which is characterized by cardiovascular involvement such as coronary angitis, myocarditis, and pericarditis which may lead to ischemic complications or sequelae (Takao et al., 1980).

We performed coronary angiography in 186 cases of KD at our institute. The incidence of coronary arterial involvement was 45%, which is much higher than the approximately 10% reported by others. This may be due to the fact that our institute specializes in cardiovascular diseases.

The two patients who had no coronary arterial stenosis with only slight cardiomegaly on the chest Xray and no QS or rS pattern on the electrocardiogram had mild MR, which disappeared, and they have NYHA stage I. The score for QS or rS pattern increased with time in the patients who had ischemic coronary angiographic findings and who died; the cause of death was congestive heart failure aggravated by the extensive myocardial infarction and MR. The CTR on the chest roentgenogram increased markedly and ΣRV1-6 decreased progressively. The survivors among the patients who had abnormal coronary arterial findings had relatively mild stenosis, and the score for QS or rS hardly increased. The increase in CTR with time was not prominent and there was no decrease in ΣRV1-6. This may be due to the compensatory behavior of the remaining functional myocardium. MR occurs following stenosis or occlusion in either the right or left coronary artery alone, but more readily occurs when the stenosis is moderate or marked in both arteries. However, the fact that the patients who developed complete occlusion of the right coronary artery showed less tendency to fatal outcome indicates that the prognosis is correlated to the degree of stenosis of the left coronary artery.

One of the patients who had MR of grade 1 on the left ventriculogram had a low ejection fraction of 0.26 at the time. However, the coronary angiographic findings in this case showed only a mild degree of stenosis of 25% in the LAD. This case may represent a dilated cardiomyopathy subsequent to myocarditis due to KD (Nakanishi et al., 1985).

Stenosis was detected on the coronary angiograms of 14 of the 16 patients who had secondary MR, and 6 of them died. On the other hand, the patient who had no abnormalities on the coronary angiogram, and the case with the dilated coronary lesion alone soon disappearing without any residual stenosis of the coronary artery showed MR appearing in the acute stage, and it disappeared in convalescent stage. This suggests that the mechanism of MR formation in the two differed. Generally, MR is considered to occur pathologically based on abnormalities of mitral valve leaflets, papillary muscle and chordae, and valvular or annular enlargement (Perloff et al., 1972). Clinically it is caused by rheumatic fever, myocarditis, congenital malformation, complications with other heart diseases, cardiomyopathies, and metablic disorders in childhood. However, as described and illustrated here on 16 cases, MR subsequent to the affliction with KD is a new clinical entity of acquired mitral regurgitation. The coronary arterial lesions in the patients with late onset MR secondary to KD reported in this series are extensive, and the ischemia in the myocardium and papillary muscles is prominent (Takao et al., 1982). Therefore, the cause of such MR after KD is considered to be due to dysfunction of the papillary muscle resulting from myocardial ischemia. In 1982, Uemura et al made histological studies on patients with MR subsequent to KD who died of valvulitis in acute stage, and regarded MR caused by endocarditis. Our two cases without abnormalities in the coronary arterial findings may have had valvulitis, but since we found no clinical evidence of myocarditis on the electrocardiogram,

it is not clear whether they can be regarded as pure valvulitis. Several reports of aortic valve regurgitation after
KD caused by valvulitis have been reported (Honda et al.,
1979)(Shiraishi et al., 1983). Most recently a case of KD
with delayed aortic and mitral insufficiency secondary to
active valvulitis has been reported (Gidding et al., 1986).
KD exhibits endocarditis, myocarditis, pericarditis, and
pancarditis like rheumatic fever (Markowitz et al., 1972),
but the incidence of endocarditis is not as high as that of
rheumatic fever in KD. The difference between endocarditis
in KD and that associated with rheumatic fever must be studied further regarding etiology of KD.

Although in the study of this series, only the MR proven
by left ventriculography was investigated, detection rate of
MR will increase if we use Doppler echocardiography especially in acute stage. Such is the trend that we also observed
MR in a series of cases examined recently in acute stage
which disappeared with clinical improvement. In this
regard, our experience as well as that of others indicates
the presence of valvulitis, myocarditis or left ventricular
dilatation leading to MR in acute stage (Fig. 10, 11).

Figure 10. **MR on Doppler echocardiography
in patients with MCLS
in acute phase (within 4 wks)
: 29 %**

Figure 11.

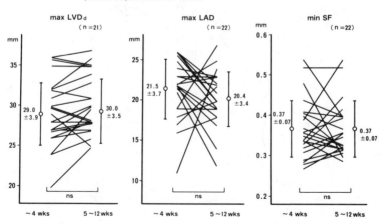

Dimensional changes between acute and convalescent
phases in patients with MCLS

max LVDd
(n =21)

max LAD
(n =22)

min SF
(n =22)

REFERENCES

Freedom RM (1978). Congenital valvular regurgitation. In Keith JD; Rowe RD, Vlad P (eds): "Heart Disease in Infancy and Childhood (3rd edition)," New York: Macmillan Publishing Co., pp 828-833.

Gidding SS, Shulman ST, Ilbawi M, Crussi F, Duffy CE (1986). Mucocutaneous lymph node syndrome (Kawasaki disease): Delayed aortic and mitral insufficiency secondary to active valvulitis. J Amer Coll Cardiol 7:894-897.

Hamada I, Takao A, Nakazawa M (1973). Two cases of MCLS associated with angiographically proven coronary artery aneurysm. In "Research Conference of the Society for Japanese Pediatric Cardiology, July 22, 1973".

Hamada I, Takao A, Mimori S, Nakazawa M, Takamizawa K, Imai M, Iinuma H, Koizumi Y, Shida H (1973). Cardiovascular complications of mucocutaneous lymphnode syndrome. Mainly discussed about mitral insufficiency and coronary arterial aneurysm. Rinsho Shoni Igaku (Clinical Pediatrics) 21:163-182.

Honda S, Matsumoto H, Mizoguchi Y, Hamasaki Y, Sunagawa H (1979). Aortic regurgitation following acute febrile mucocutaneous lymphnode symdrome (MCLS) in an infant. Jpn. Circ J 43:363-468.

Kawasaki T. Kosaki F (1967). Febrile oculo oro cutaneo acro desquamatous syndrome with or without acute non-suppurative cervical lymphadenitis in infancy and childhood. Clinical observations of 50 cases. Japanese Journal of Allergy 16:178-222.

Markowitz M, Gordis L (1972). "Rheumatic Fever." Philadelphia: W.B. Saunders Co., pp 62-70.

Nakanishi T. Takao A. Nakazawa M. Endo M. Niwa K, Takahashi Y (1985). Clinical, hemodynamic and angiographic features of coronary obstructive disease in the mucocutaneous lymphnode syndrome. Am J Cardiol 55:662-668.

Perloff JK, Roberts WC (1972). Functional anatomy of mitral regurgitation. Circulation 46:227-239.

Shiraishi T. Jinnai H, Hiramoto K, Ozaki H (1983). A case of aortic regurgitation following MCLS valvulitis. An autopsy case. Acta Paed Jap 87:739-845.

Takao A, Kawamura T. Nishihara S. Niwa K, Endo M (1980). Kawasaki's disease:clinical aspects of the cardiovascular lesions. In Godman M (ed): "Pediatric Cardiology, vol. 4," Edinburgh: Churchhill Livingstone, 635-648.

Takao A, Niwa K, Takahashi Y, Satomi G, Nakazawa M, Endo M
(1982). Mitral regurgitation as sequela of Kawasaki
disease: Prognosis and treatment. Chiryo 64:1701-1790.
Uemura S. Negoro H, Minami Y, Nakagawa K, Uehara T,
Miyashiro E, Koike M, Ohno T (1982). A case of mitral
regurgitation following MCLS valvulitis. An autopsy
case. Acta Paed Jap 86:38-43.

Kawasaki Disease, pages 325–339
© 1987 Alan R. Liss, Inc.

PROGNOSTIC SIGNIFICANCE OF CORONARY ARTERY ANEURYSM AND
ECTASIA IN THE CORONARY ARTERY SURGERY STUDY (CASS)
REGISTRY

Thomas Robertson, M.D. and Lloyd Fisher, Ph.D.

Cardiac Diseases Branch, National Heart, Lung Blood
Institute (T.R.), and CASS Coordinating Center,
University of Washington (L.F.)

Following acute Kawasaki Syndrome (KS) in childhood,
coronary artery aneurysms may persist into adulthood and
lead to acute myocardial infarction or sudden death.
Coronary arteriographic and pathologic examinations have
revealed large aneurysms, on the order of 1cm in diameter
or larger. Therapeutic recommendations have included
long-term anticoagulation and coronary artery bypass
grafting. Smaller aneurysms or ectasia also follow in the
wake of KS and the prognosis is unclear. Nevertheless, a
substantial number of children who experience clinical or
subclinical KS and develop coronary artery aneurysms can be
anticipated to reach adulthood in the coming years.

Aneurysms and ectasia occur in patients with coronary
heart disease. Although the pathophysiology is different,
it may be instructive to consider long-term prognosis in
such aneurysms as a possible model of future expectations
for patients who survive into adulthood with the stigmata
of KS.

The National Heart, Lung and Blood Institute Coronary
Artery Surgery Study (CASS) maintained a large registry
with a number of individuals with arteriographically
determined dilatation of the coronary arteries (Principal
Investigators of CASS and their Associates, 1981). These
data are examined in this report. A prior CASS paper on
such patients has been published (Swaye et al., 1983); this
report includes additional updated follow-up information
and analyses.

MATERIALS AND METHODS

The Coronary Artery Surgery Study (CASS) enrolled 24,959 patients with suspected or proven coronary artery disease between August 1975 and July 1979. These consecutive patients, subject to obtaining informed consent, had clinical, laboratory and angiographic data collected in a standardized fashion near the time of coronary angiography. Fifteen clinics in the United States and Canada participated in this study (Appendix 1).

The coronary arteriographic data were recorded on a previously published form (Principal Investigators of CASS and their Associates, 1981). The arterial tree was divided into 27 defined segments (Ringqvist et al., 1983). The morphology of each segment could be coded as discrete aneurysmal disease, or as diffuse aneurysmal disease (among other options). This was defined as coronary dilatation that exceeded the diameter of normal adjacent segments or the diameter of the patient's largest coronary vessel by 1 1/2 times. Figure 1 shows an aneurysmal CASS arteriogram.

Coronary stenoses were read as the maximal percent luminal diameter narrowing for each segment. An obstruction of 50% or more in the left main coronary artery was considered clinically significant, while obstructions of 70% or more were considered clinically significant in the other arterial segments. Disease was classified as 0, 1, 2 or 3 vessel disease depending upon the presence or absence of clinically significant disease in the major segments of the right, left and circumflex artery systems. Details of the computation are published (Ringqvist et al., 1983). The zero vessel disease patients were subdivided into totally normal (no observed narrowings, minimal (some but less than 50% stenosis) and moderate some (nonleft main) lesions of between 50% and 69% narrowing. The CASS used a left ventricular score (Principal Investigators of CASS and their Associates, 1981) to assess left ventricular function. The right anterior oblique ventriculogram was divided into five segments: anterobasal, anterolateral, apical, diaphragmatic and posterobasal. Left ventricular wall motion abnormalities were subjectively assessed and scored numerically as follows: 1, normal; 2, moderate hypokinesis; 3, severe hypokinesis; 4, akinesis; 5, dyskinesis; and 6, ventricular aneurysm. The score (conceptually ranging from 5 to 30) is the sum of the

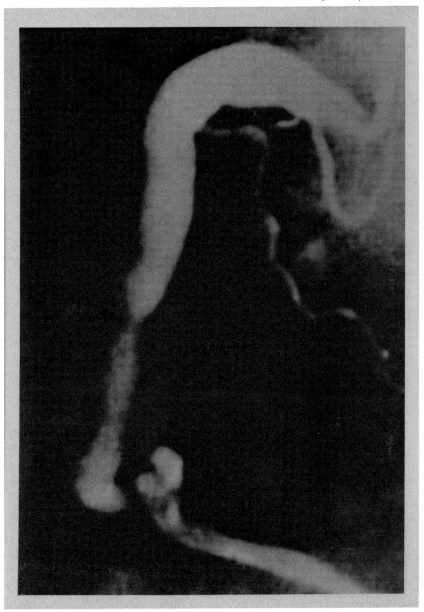

Figure 1a. Right coronary arteriograms of coronary aneurysmal cases. (Courtesy of Paul Swaye, M.D. and Circulation.)

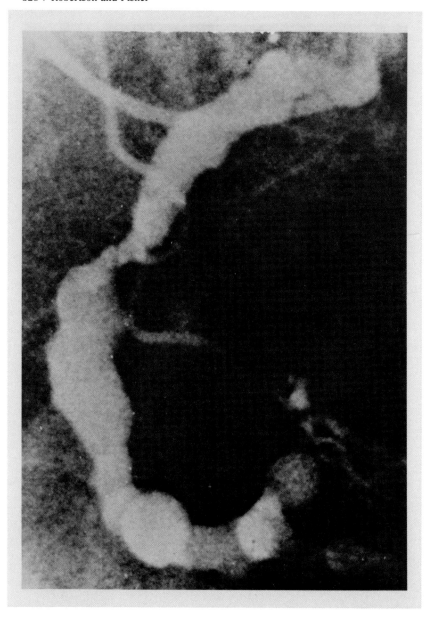

Figure 1b. Right coronary arteriograms of coronary aneurysmal cases. (Courtesy of Paul Swaye, M.D. and Circulation.)

scores for the five segments. Thus, a normally contracting left ventricle has a score of five.

Many of the patients enrolled in the CASS registry had anginal chest pain. Such pain was graded from 1-mild to 4-severe using the Canadian Heart Association classification (Campeau, 1976).

The interpretation of the CASS data is complicated by coronary artery bypass surgery with its possible impact. The patients were divided into groups treated early with medicine or surgery. This was done as follows: the number of days after enrollment within which 95% of the first year bypass surgeries occurred was determined for each clinic. Patients with surgery within this period, or within 90 days of angiography, were considered surgical cases. This survival follow-up time began at the time of surgery. The remaining cases were the medically treated cases. Their follow-up began at the site specific average time to surgery for the surgical cases.

STATISTICAL METHODS

Comparisons on discrete characteristics between patients with and without coronary aneurysm were made using the Chi-square test. The comparison of survival experience between groups was visually made using the life table method, and the log rank statistic was used to assess statistical significance (Kalbfleisch and Prentice, 1980). To see if an identified variable (in this case presence or absence of a coronary aneurysm) had additional prognostic power above and beyond an additional set of variables the following was done. The Cox proportional hazard regression model was used (Kalbfleisch and Prentice, 1980). A step-up stepwise model was constructed using the additional set of variables. The variables in this model plus the identified variable were all used as predictive variables in a further Cox survival run. The Chi-square statistic was used for the p-value for the identified variable. The statistical significance of the identified variable univariately was found using the score statistic Chi-square with no predictive variables in the model.

TABLE 1. Comparison of the Patient Characteristics Among Those With and Without Coronary Aneurysm. Entries are Number and Percent of the Column Heading.

Characteristic	Subdivision		Coronary Aneurysm		No Coronary Aneurysm		P-value Comparing Those With and Without Coronary Aneurysm
--			1,055	100%	22,231	100%	--
Sex	Male		938	89%	16,568	75%	<0.0001
	Female		117	11%	5,663	26%	
Age	<25		0	0%	74	0.3%	
	26-35		18	2%	857	4%	0.0003
	>36		1,037	98%	21,300	96%	
Vessels Diseased	Zero	Normal	16	2%	4,456	20%	
		Minimal	41	4%	1,330	6%	
		Moderate	49	5%	877	4%	
	One		217	21%	4,601	21%	<0.0001
	Two		292	28%	4,912	22%	
	Three		440	42%	6,007	27%	
>50% Stenosis of the Left Main Coronary Artery	No		953	90%	20,604	93%	0.0022
	Yes		102	10%	1,589	7%	

Left Ventricular Score					
5	323	32%	10,487	49%	<0.0001
6-9	332	33%	5,510	26%	
10-14	234	23%	3,783	18%	
≥15	119	12%	1805	8%	
Canadian Heart Association Anginal Classification					
N/A	214	20%	6,144	28%	<0.0001
I	58	6%	1,039	5%	
II	246	23%	4,947	22%	
III	286	27%	5,718	26%	
IV	152	14%	2,640	12%	
Unrelated to Exertion	99	9%	1,739	8%	
Congestive Heart Failure					
Never	925	88%	20,008	90%	
Impairment None Now	21	2%	311	1%	
Mild	41	4%	781	4%	0.13
Moderate	49	5%	821	4%	
Severe	19	2%	307	1%	
Drugs Used					
Beta Blockers	513	49%	10,235	46%	0.10
Nitroglycerin	666	63%	13,910	63%	0.72
Long-Acting Nitrates	591	56%	10,928	49%	<0.0001
Aspirin	43	4%	826	4%	0.55
Anticoagulants	90	9%	1,727	8%	0.37
Race					
White	1026	97%	21,556	97%	0.64
Black	25	2%	540	2%	
Other	4	0.4%	135	0.6%	

RESULTS

The individuals with coronary aneurysm do not look like a representative subgroup of the CASS registry. Nine characteristics are compared between those with and without coronary aneurysm (Table 1). The presence of coronary aneurysm is associated with more coronary artery disease and impaired ventricular function. Those with a coronary aneurysm had more vessels diseased, more narrowing of the left main coronary artery, more angina, poorer left ventricular score and use more long-acting nitrates (all $p<0.003$); anticoagulation use at the time of study was the same in both groups. Those with coronary aneurysm were more often male (89% versus 75%) and were older. This is not surprising in light of the other data since increasing age and male sex were associated with more coronary artery disease in the CASS registry.

The extent of the coronary dilatation is given in Table 2 in terms of the number of arterial segments involved. The majority, 55%, of the patients had only one segment involved. There were more segments with the disease characterized as diffuse, rather than discrete. The precise segments involved are shown in Table 3; note that the entries are restricted to those with at least one aneurysmal segment. Coronary aneurysm was especially common in the right coronary artery.

An unadjusted survival comparison (Figure 2) shows that those patients with coronary aneurysm had a worse prognosis than those without coronary aneurysm ($p<0.0001$). However, since the presence of aneurysm was associated with more coronary artery disease and poorer ventricular function it is of interest to see if there is an added risk to coronary aneurysm. Cox survival models were used. First a stepup stepwise Cox regression was run selecting variables with statistically independent ($p\leq0.05$) predictive power from among 48 possible predictor variables. A variable indicating presence or absence of coronary aneurysm was then added to see if it had additional predictive power. This was done separately for three subsets of patients: 1) those with early surgery; 2) patients with zero vessel disease; and 3) patients with 1, 2 or 3 vessel disease and treated early with medicine. In all three subsets of patients the presence or absence of aneurysm did not add to the model with significance level ≤0.05; this is shown in Table 4.

TABLE 2. Distribution of the Number of Aneurysmal Segments per Patient Among Patients with Coronary Aneurysms. (Number and Column Percent)

Number	Discrete Aneurysmal Segments		Diffuse Aneurysmal Segments		Total Aneurysmal Segments	
0	655	62%	350	33%	---	---
1	293	28%	345	33%	576	55%
2	57	5%	137	13%	191	18%
3	20	2%	83	8%	112	11%
4	10	1%	49	5%	58	6%
5	11	1%	39	4%	54	5%
6	4	0.4%	27	3%	31	3%
7	3	0.3%	15	1%	19	2%
8	2	0.2%	5	0.5%	8	0.8%
9	0	0%	2	0.2%	2	0.2%
10	0	0%	2	0.2%	3	0.3%
11	0	0%	0	0%	0	0%
12	0	0%	1	0.1%	1	0.1%

TABLE 3. Distribution of Aneurysmal Disease by Arterial
Segment Among Patients with Aneurysm. (Number and Percent)

Segment	No Aneurysm		Discrete Aneurysm		Diffuse Aneurysm	
Proximal RCA	784	74%	43	4%	228	22%
Mid RCA	793	75%	56	5%	206	20%
Distal RCA	869	82%	53	5%	133	13%
Right Posterior Decending Artery	982	93%	34	3%	39	4%
Right Postero-lateral Segment	969	92%	26	3%	60	6%
1st Branch	993	94%	28	3%	34	3%
2nd Branch	979	93%	24	2%	52	5%
3rd Branch	964	91%	19	2%	72	7%
Acute Marginal	1040	99%	8	1%	7	1%
Left Main Coronary Artery	1020	97%	8	1%	27	3%
Proximal LAD	890	84%	50	5%	115	11%
Mid LAD	930	88%	59	6%	66	6%
Distal LAD	1008	96%	31	3%	16	2%
1st Diagonal	996	94%	25	2%	34	3%
2nd Diagonal	1026	97%	15	1%	14	1%
1st Septal	1040	99%	14	1%	1	0.1%
Prox Cx	943	89%	35	3%	77	7%
Distal Cx	953	90%	33	3%	69	7%
First Ob Marg	1014	96%	25	2%	16	2%
2nd Ob Marg	999	95%	13	1%	43	4%
3rd Ob Marg	965	92%	9	1%	81	8%
Left Atrial Ventricular Artery	994	94%	7	1%	54	5%
1st LPL	1014	96%	3	0.3%	38	4%
2nd LPL	1012	96%	2	0.2%	41	4%
3rd LPL	1006	95%	2	0.2%	47	5%
Left Posterior Descending Artery	1008	96%	1	0.1%	46	4%

Abbreviations: RCA = right coronary artery; LAD = left
anterior descending; Cx = circumflex; Prox = proximal;
Ob Marg = obtuse marginal; LPL = left posteriolateral

Figure 2: Patients with and without coronary aneurysm

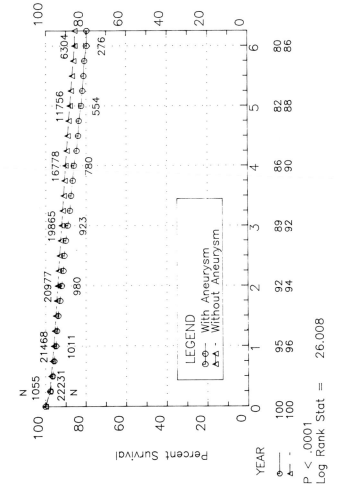

Figure 2. Unadjusted survival experience of the CASS patients with and without coronary aneurysm.

TABLE 4. Results of Cox Survival Analyses to Assess Additional Risk Due to the Presence of Aneurysm.

Patient Group	Univariate p-value for Aneurysm	Final p-value for Aneurysm
Early Surgically Treated Cases	0.012	0.087
Medically Treated Zero Vessel Disease Cases	0.544	0.281
1, 2, and 3 Vessel Disease, Early Medical Treatment	0.256	0.574

In addition, separate life table comparisons were performed for different subsets by vessels diseased and ventricular function. The results confirmed that coronary aneurysm did not increase the risk.

Figure 3 presents the survival experience by the number of diseased vessels among those patients with coronary aneurysms. The six year survival of patients with zero vessel disease is 95%.

DISCUSSION

One important question in interpreting these data is the accuracy of the readings of coronary aneurysm. The CASS had an ongoing quality control program in which randomly selected films were reviewed on an ongoing basis (Swaye, et al., 1983). independently reviewed 54 randomly selected CASS films read as aneurysmal coronary artery disease. They report 70.2% agreement, 9.4% of the findings as equivocal and disagreement in the remaining 20.4% of the films.

The impact of aneurysmal coronary disease in CASS is greatly confounded because of the association with advanced coronary artery stenotic disease. An additional prognostic impact of the aneurysm on coronary disease cannot be demonstrated. This is perhaps clearest in the zero vessel

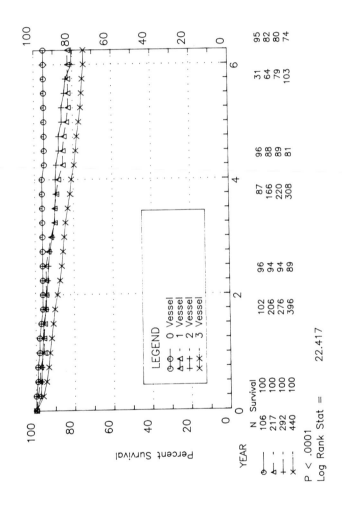

Figure 3: Coronary aneurysm patients by number of vessels diseased

Figure 3. Survival experience by number of arteries with clinically significant atherosclerotic heart disease among patients with coronary aneurysm.

disease patients; the five year 95% survival is near the
U.S. population experience for a similar age cohort.

The inference of the CASS results to Kawasaki's
syndrome is unclear and tenuous. The pathophysiologic
mechanisms of disease are likely very different. The
selection of CASS patients for angiography was linked to
many factors, most usually presumed ischemic pain.
Nevertheless, the good news is that under some circumstances aneurysmal coronary artery disease carries little
if any penalty for survival over at least a 6 year time
period. More long-term follow-up of Kawasaki syndrome
patients is needed to establish the prognostic significance
in these patients with observed coronary aneurysms. The
CASS data give reason for guarded optimism.

REFERENCES

Campeau L: Grading of Angina Pectoris. Circulation
    54:522, 1976.
Kalbfleisch JD, Prentice RL: The Statistical Analysis of
    Failure Time Data. New York, John Wiley and Sons,
    1980.
Principal Investigators of CASS and their Associates:
    National Heart, Lung, and Blood Institute Coronary
    Artery Surgery Study. Circulation 63 (Suppl II):II-1,
    1981.
Ringqvist I, Fisher LD, Mock M, Davis KB, Wedel H, Chaitman
    BR, Passamani E, Russel RO, Alderman EL, Kouchoukas NT,
    Kaiser GC, Ryan TJ, Killip T, Fray D: Prognostic Value
    of Angiographic Indices of Coronary Artery Disease from
    the Coronary Artery Surgery Study (CASS). J Clin
    Invest 71:1854, 1983.
Swaye PS, Fisher LD, Litwin P, Vignole PA, Judkins MP, Kemp
    HG, Mudd JG, Gosselin AJ: Aneurysmal Coronary Artery
    Disease. Circulation 67:134, 1983.

APPENDIX 1

Cooperating Clinical Sites

University of Alabama in Birmingham: William J. Rogers,
M.D.*, Richard O. Russell, Jr., M.D., Albert Oberman, M.D.,
and Nicholas T. Kouchoukos, M.D. Albany Medical College:

Eric D. Foster, M.D.*, Julio A. Sosa, M.D.*, Joseph T.
Doyle, M.D., Martin F. McKneally, M.D., Joseph B. McIlduff,
M.D., Harry Odabashian, M.D., and Thomas M. Older, M.D.
Boston University: Thomas Ryan, M.D.*, David Faxon, M.D.,
Laura Wexler, M.D., Robert L. Berger, M.D., Donald Weiner,
M.D. and Carolyn H. McCabe, B.S. Loma Linda University:
Joan Coggin, M.D.* Marshfield Medical Foundation, Inc. and
Marshfield Clinic: William Myers, M.D.*, Richard D.
Sautter, M.D.*, John N. Browell, M.D., Dieter M. Voss,
M.D., and Robert D. Carlson, M.D. Massachusetts General
Hospital: J. Warren Harthorne, M.D.*, W. Gerald Austen,
M.D.*, Robert Dinsmore, M.D., Frederick Levine, M.D., and
John McDermott, M.D. Mayo Clinic and Mayo Foundation:
Robert L. Frye, M.D.*, Bernard Gersh M.D., David R. Holmes,
M.D., Michael B. Mock, M.D., Hartzell Schaff, M.D., and
Ronald E. Vlietstra, M.D. Miami Heart Institute: Arthur
J. Gosselin, M.D.*, Parry B. Larsen, M.D., and Paul Swaye,
M.D. Montreal Heart Institute: Martial G. Bourassa M.D.*,
Claude Goulet, M.D., and Jacques Lesperance, M.D. New York
University: Ephraim Glassman, M.D.* and Michael Schloss,
M.D. St. Louis University: George Kaiser, M.D.*, J.
Gerard Mudd, M.D.*, Robert D. Wiens, M.D., Hendrick B.
Barner, M.D., John E. Codd, M.D., Denis H. Tyras, M.D., and
Vallee L. Willman, M.D., Bernard R. Chaitman, M.D., St.
Luke's Hospital Center: Harvey G. Kemp, Jr., M.D.*, and
Airlie Cameron, M.D. Stanford University: Edwin Alderman,
M.D.*, Francis H. Koch, M.D., Paul R. Cipriano, M.D., James
F. Silverman, M.D. and Edward B. Stinson, M.D., Medical
College of Wisconsin: Felix Tristani, M.D.*, Harold L.
Brooks, M.D.*, and Robert J. Flemma, M.D. Yale University:
Lawrence S. Cohen, M.D.*, Rene Langou, M.D., Alexander S.
Geha, M.D., Graeme L. Hammond, M.D., and Richard K. Shaw,
M.D.
Central Electrocardiographic Laboratory, University of
    Alabama:
    L. Thomas Sheffield, M.D.*, David Roitman, M.D., and
    Carol Troxell, B.S.
Coordinating Center, University of Washington:
    Kathryn Davis, Ph.D.*, Mary Jo Gillespie, M.S., Lloyd
    Fisher, Ph.D., J. Ward Kennedy, M.D., Richard
    Kronmal, Ph.D., and Kevin Cain, Ph.D.
Chairman of the Steering Committee:
    Thomas Killip, M.D., Beth Israel Medical Center
National Heart, Lung and Blood Institute:
    Eugene R. Passamani, M.D., Thomas Robertson, M.D.,
    and Peter Frommer, M.D.
    * Principal Investigator

Kawasaki Disease, pages 341-346
© 1987 Alan R. Liss, Inc.

CORONARY FINDINGS POST KAWASAKI DISEASE IN CHILDREN WHO
DIED OF OTHER CAUSES

Shiro Naoe, Kei Takahashi, Hirotake Masuda,and
Noboru Tanaka

Research Laboratory of Pathology, Ohashi Hospital,
Toho University, 2-17-6 Ohashi Meguroku, Tokyo,
Japan 153

INTRODUCTION

It is well known that Kawasaki disease produces coronary artery aneurysms or luminal stenosis as its sequelae.
Over 85 autopsy cases of Kawasaki disease were collected
from our own hospital and other institutions throughout Japan. Among them, there are some cases in which sudden death
occurred a few years after an apparent complete recovery from
the disease as indicated in Fig.-1. In most of these cases,

Cases of Coronary findings post KD in children who died of other causes

Case	Age	Sex	Cause of Death	Duration from onset of K.D. to death
1	1y7m	F	Traffic accident	60d
2	2y	F	Influenza meningitis	9m
3	2y6m	F	Chronic myeloid leukemia	2y
4	3y	M	Neuroblastoma	2y
5	15y	M	Sepsis, Staphylococcal pneumonia	14y

Fig-1

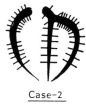
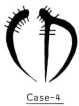
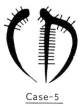

Case-2   Case-4   Case-5

sequelae were the immediate cause of death. On the other

hand, there are other cases in which children in good health and without any clinical signs, died of unrelated causes.

We felt that it might be beneficial to examine coronary artery involvement in these cases in which patients with a history of Kawasaki disease died of unrelated causes.

MATERIAL AND PROCEDURE

In this study, pathological examinations were performed in 5 such cases. These investigations concentrated mainly on the coronary arteries and in these cases they were examined in considerable detail. We studied the distribution of these lesions using the sectioning as indicated in Fig-1.

RESULTS

In every one of these five cases, intimal thickening, destruction of the internal elastic lamina and thinning of the media were observed, but an inflammatory cell infiltrate, thrombosis, recanalization of the affected artery, appearance of foam cells and calcification were observed in none.

In Case 1, the patient died 60 days after an apparent complete recovery from the disease. Partial thickening of the intima appears symmetrical and edematous with an elastic stain, it looks like the so-called intimal cushion structure but without any branching nearby. From this observation we consider it to be arterial involvement, not an intimal cushion.

In case 2, the patient died of influenza meningitis 9 months after complete recovery from Kawasaki disease. The intima shows edematous and cellular fibrous thickening. As indicated in Photo-1, these changes are seen throughout the coronary arteries bilaterally.

In case 3, the patient died of chronic myeloid leukemia. There is also fibrous thickening of the intima.

On the other hand, case 4, in which death occurred 2 years after recovery, shows its intima divided into two concentric circles. It appears fibrous on the adventitia side, but on the lumen side, there are scattered spindle cells which are considered to be myointimal. (Photo-2)

In case 5, in which the patient died 14 years after recovery, fibrous intimal thickening is observed and is accompanied by a new formation of the internal elastic lamina.

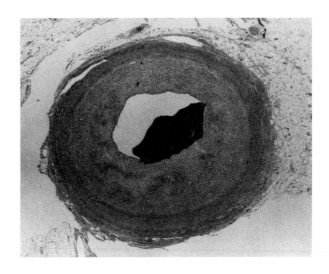

Photo −1

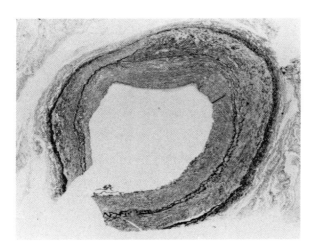

Photo −2

Also irregular production of external elastic fiber is marked.

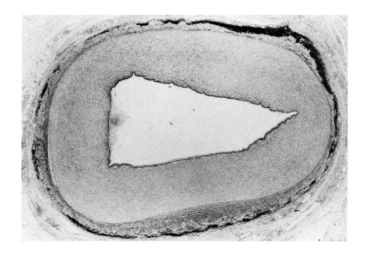

Photo-3

In Fig-2, coronary arteries of children of approximately the same age, without a history of Kawasaki disease, are shown as a control.

In case 5 and 2, enlargement of the arterial diameter

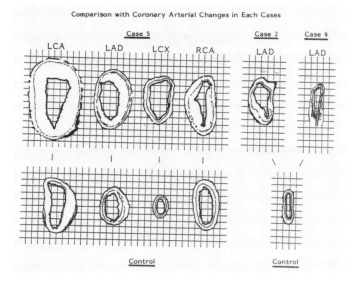

Comparison with Coronary Arterial Changes in Each Cases

Fig-2

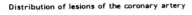

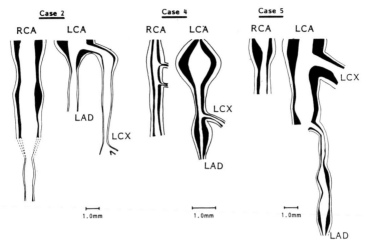

Fig-3

is seen, but the lumen remains relatively patent.

If we consider the distribution of lesions in each of these cases, we find the following (Fig-3);

In case 2, dilatation of vessels and intimal thickening are found at the branching points of the left and right coronary arteries, but not in the distal portions of the coronary arteries.

In case 4, the left coronary artery has slight dilatation at two sites and there, intimal thickening appears. However, these changes are not found in the right coronary artery.

In case 5, in which 14 years had passed since the patient suffered from Kawasaki disease, intimal thickening extends to the periphery, and dilatation of vessel is observed.

In every one of the five cases in this study, arterial involvement, primarily changes of intima and internal elastic lamina, is observed. The segmental involvement and distribution of the lesions are not inconsistent with late stage lesions of Kawasaki disease, but in almost every case of sudden death with a previous history of the disease, coronary artery aneurysms, stenotic lumen, a thrombosis and recanalization of the affected vessel appeared. In these five cases there was no such involvement.

Based on these observations, we have considered it possible that patients with a history of Kawasaki disease may have some coronary artery lesions not serious enough to become an immediate cause of death, but which might lead to juvenile arteriosclerosis in the future. When arterial involvement is very slight, however, as in case 1, there might be complete resolution, such as that of the intimal cushion in childhood.

Finally, there are cases in which the lumen remains relatively patent in spite of the existence of arterial lesions. It should be pointed out that these are sometimes not noticed by coronary angiography.

At the present time it is not understood at all how these affected vessels morphologically change in adaptation to blood volume, speed of the blood stream and blood pressure as they grow.

REFERENCES

Masuda H, Shozawa T, Naoe S, Tanaka N(1986). The intercostal artery in Kawasaki disease. Arch Pathol Lab Med 110: 1336-1142

Naoe S, Atobe T, Masuda H, Tanaka N (1983). Kawasaki disease-particularly on arterial changes. Pathol Clinic Med 1: 1156-1166.

Naoe S, Masuda H (1981). Kawasaki disease as a risk factor of juvenile arteriosclerosis. J Jpn Arterioscler,Soc 9: 27-35.

Tanaka N, Naoe S, Masuda H, Ueno T (1986). Pathological study of sequelae of Kawasaki disease (MCLS) with special reference to heart and coronary arterial lesions. Acta Pathol Jpn 36:1513-1527.

Kawasaki Disease, pages 347–355
© 1987 Alan R. Liss, Inc.

ISCHEMIC HEART DISEASE IN KAWASAKI DISEASE

Tetsuro Kamiya, M.D. and Atsuko Suzuki, M.D.

Department of Pediatrics, National Cardiovascular Center
5-7-1, Fujishirodai, Suita, Osaka, 565 Japan

Under the title of Ischemic Heart Disease in Kawasaki
Disease (K.D.), five selected subjects will be
discussed.

1. Aggravation of stenotic lesion of the coronary artery

In K.D., it is well known that the coronary artery may
be involved in an acute phase, and dilated lesions (aneurysm
and dilatation) may persist thereafter. We reported, in
1982, the incidence of coronary artery lesions observed by
2D echo. By echocardiographic observation daily in
60 cases with K.D., (1) the initial change was increased
density at and around the coronary arterial wall. It appeared on 5.4 ± 1.1 days of illness in 100% of the examined
cases. Dilatation was first documented on echocardiogram
on 9.5 ± 2.7 days of illness in 47.5%. Aneurysm was first
detected on 11.4 ± 1.9 days of illness in 28.8%. Pericardial effusion was first observed on 9.0 ± 2.0 days of illness in 51.8%.
Once a dilated lesion has developed, two major
changes may follow. One is decrease in size of dilated
lesion, and the other is new appearance and aggravation of
stenotic lesion. (1) (2) The latter, new appearance and
aggravation of stenotic lesion, is one of the most important problems in K.D., because it is the major cause of
myocardial ischemia and death. As mentioned later, it is
rather difficult to detect correctly the presence of
stenotic lesion with the routine noninvasive methods. Even
coronary angiography may miss this stenotic lesion. To
visualize stenotic lesions clearly on angio, selective

coronary arteriography with appropriate tilting in multiple views is indispensable, because stenotic lesion is produced just at the inlet and outlet of aneurysm. In our study in 262 cases with angiographic evidence of coronary artery lesion (CAL), 37% of the cases combined stenotic lesion (occlusion, segmental stenosis and/or localized stenosis) with dilated lesion.

To confirm the actual state of this progressive stenotic lesion, in our hospital, follow-up angios including selective coronary arteriography (CAG) were performed in the cases with angiographic evidence of CAL. As source of materials, as shown in Fig. 1, 2D echo was done in 3,536 cases with a history of K.D. in our hospital, and in 1,100 cases among them, CAG was performed. in the cases with documentation of CAL on the first CAG (CAG1), the second CAG (CAG2) was scheduled after one year, and in the cases with evidence of CAL on CAG2, the third CAG (CAG3) was scheduled after 3 years. In 76 cases, follow-up study with three CAGs was done up to date. In these cases, age at the onset

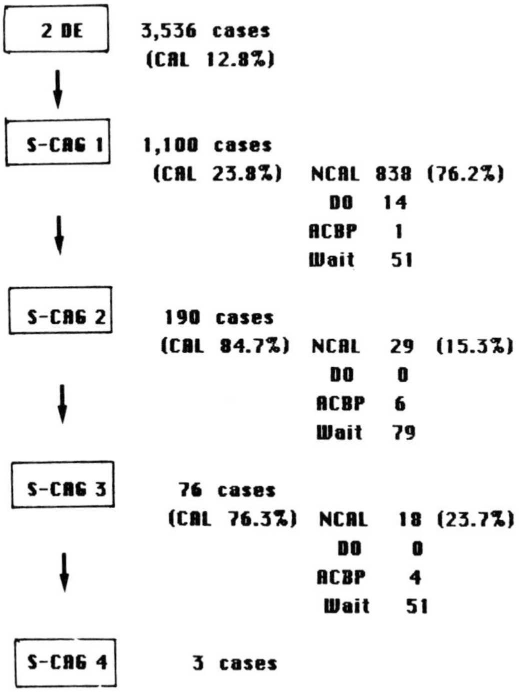

2 DE	3,536 cases (CAL 12.8%)	
↓		
S-CAG 1	1,100 cases (CAL 23.8%)	NCAL 838 (76.2%) DO 14 ACBP 1 Wait 51
↓		
S-CAG 2	190 cases (CAL 84.7%)	NCAL 29 (15.3%) DO 0 ACBP 6 Wait 79
↓		
S-CAG 3	76 cases (CAL 76.3%)	NCAL 18 (23.7%) DO 0 ACBP 4 Wait 51
↓		
S-CAG 4	3 cases	

Fig. 1. Source of Materials

of K.D. was 2y4m ± 2y1m (mean ± standard deviation), and interval from the onset to CAG1 was 1y8m ± 2y8m. Interval from CAG1 to CAG2 was 1y3m ± 1y1m, and that from CAG2 to CAG3 was 3y8m ± 1y1m. Twenty two cases out of these 76 cases dropped out during this study. Seven cases among them had AC bypass surgery after CAG1 or CAG2. Among 40 cases with documentation of stenotic lesion on any of three angios, 72.5% of the cases showed new appearance or aggravation of stenotic lesion (AGGR), as shown in Fig. 2 and 3. On the contrary, 22.5% of the cases disclosed improvement of stenotic lesion. Cases with no apparent change on angio

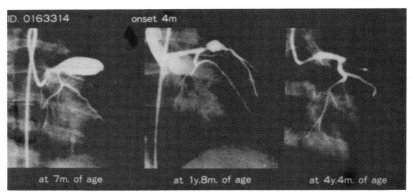

Fig. 2. Follow-up Angios

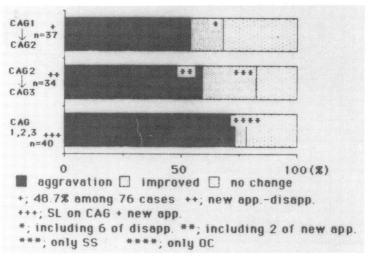

Fig. 3. Follow-up of SL with Three CAGs in 76 Cases

were only 5%, and all of them were those with occlusion of
the coronary artery. Statistical analysis using logistic
regression model showed close relationship between the size
of aneurysm and the possibility of AGGR. In conclusion,
the most clinically significant problem of coronary artery
lesion in K.D., stenotic lesion, tends to be aggravated
when it appears, even several years after the onset of
K.D.

2. Medical treatment to prevent the aggravation of
   stenotic lesion

   Among 177 cases, in which CAG1 and CAG2 were done, the
effect of the drugs to prevent AGGR was analyzed. Six
kinds of drugs (Warfarin, Aspirin, Flurbiprofen,
Dipyridamole, Ticlopidine and Nifedipine) were chosen and,
in 34, 34, 36, 20, 30 and 23 cases with evidence of CAL on
CAG1 respectively, each drug had been administered for
one year and then, CAG2 was performed. Of these
177 cases, 15 cases were omitted from this study mainly
because of the alteration of the drug during this one year.
The findings of stenotic lesion on CAG1 and CAG2 were compared in each cases, and the judgement was made as follows;
AGGR, improvement and no change. The results of this study
are shown in Fig. 4. Incidence of AGGR in the group
treated with Flurbiprofen was the lowest (7%), and it was

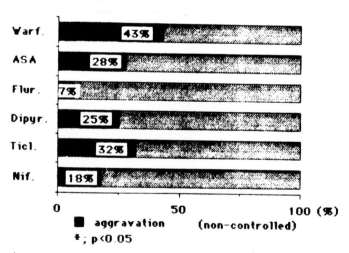

Fig. 4. Incidence of Aggravation of SL (CAGL vs CAG2)

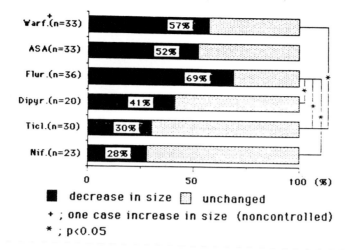

Fig. 5   Incidence of Decrease in Size of Medium and Large
         Aneurysms (CAG1 vs CAG2)

significantly lower than that in the group with Warfarin
(43%).

Regarding decrease in size of dilated lesion, the
change of medium- and large-sized aneurysms is shown in
Fig. 5. Incidence of decrease in size in the group treated
with Flubiprofen (69%) was significantly higher than those
in the groups with Dipyridamole (41%), Ticlopidine (30%)
and Nifedipine (28%). Incidence in the group with Warfarin
(57%) was also significantly higher than that in the group
with Ticlopidine. Among all the cases, only one case in
the group treated with Warfarin revealed increase of the
size of aneurysm during the follow-up.

Based on this study, it can be said that there seems
to be two types of the effect of drugs; one is, as observed
in Flurbiprofen, prevention of AGGR *with* decrease in size
of dilated lesion, and the other type is, as in Nifedipine,
prevention of AGGR *without* decrease in size (Fig. 6). Both
types may have each problem, advantage and disadvantage.
In the former type (type A in Fig. 6), metabolic disorder
may occur in the abnormally thickened arterial wall at
dilated lesion, although blood stream in dilated lesion is
improved. In the latter group (type B in Fig. 6), eddy
stream in dilated lesion may cause thrombus formation or
derangement of intima, although metabolism in the arterial
wall at dilated lesion is not disturbed.

It may be
needless to say
that the study
of the effect
of drugs for
aneurysm is
important. Our
study is a
tentative one,
and the study
was done under
non-controlled
and non-
randomized con-
dition. But,
as far as our
knowledge, our
study is only one for this purpose. Now we have been
studying the effect of drugs under controlled and
randomized condition, and the result will be presented in
near future.

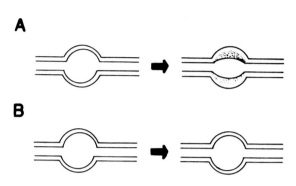

Fig. 6. Types of the Effect of Drugs

3. Clinical detection of myocardial ischemia

It is rather difficult to detect myocardial ischemia
clinically. When stenotic lesion is aggravated significantly, myocardial ischemia may occur. In our study among
33 cases with significant stenosis of coronary artery
(occlusion, segmental stenosis and localized stenosis more
than 75%), the sensitivity was 0.12 for 2D echo (dyskinesis
of wall motion), 0.09 for ECG at rest, 0.39 for ECG with
Dipyridamole load, 0.21 for ECG with Master's doubled two
step test, 0.27 for Holter ECG, 0.52 for treadmill test.
These methods with echo and ECG are not sensitive enough to
detect myocardial ischemia in the cases with CAL in K.D.,
although specificity of these methods are good enough.
Only one noninvasive way which is useful at present is
thallium myocardial imaging with a load by exercise or
Dipyridamole. The sensitivity of myocardial imaging to
detect myocardial ischemia was 0.82. It can be said that
myocardial imaging with a load is the best and indispensable way at present to detect myocardial ischemia non-
invasively.

4. Myocardial infarction

Myocardial infarction is the major cause of death in
K.D. In our experience, even small infarction in the area
of right coronary artery may be a cause of sudden death. A
5 year old boy, in whom severe localized stenosis was demonstrated only in the right coronary artery (segment 2)
with aneurysms of both coronary arteries on angio, died
suddenly and unexpectedly 5 days after angio. Postmortem
angiography of the coronary artery revealed the same
findings, indicating no possibility of acute thrombus
formation in the aneurysms. Small myocardial infarction
(a scar with a diameter of 5mm) was found at the
posterior wall (Fig. 7). This may be a case showing that
even a small old scar can evoke total arrhythmia.

5. Adult
   case

In
Japan, 7
adult
cases
with a
history
of K.D.
were
reported
(Fig. 8).
Age of
the cases
distri-
buted
from 17
to 41
years old.

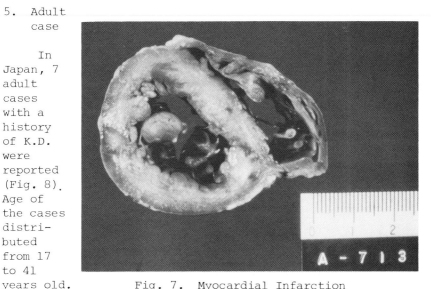

Fig. 7. Myocardial Infarction

The onset of
K.D. in these cases was 14 years old or less. Outcome was
severe in all the proven cases except for one without any
description of it. AC bypass was performed in 4 cases,
PTCA was done in one case and one case died suddenly
during anticoagulant therapy. Adult cases may be increased in the future with possible severe stenotic lesion
and myocardial ischemia.

Because of the possibility that the normal coronary
artery on echo or even angio does not mean the normal

Case	Age,Sex	Onset	Involved Artery	Outcome
1	26Y, M	14Y	LM, RCA	ACBP
2	17Y, M	4Y	LAD,LCX	ACBP
3	20Y, F	5Y?	LAD, RCA	died
4	37Y, M	6Y	LM, LAD, RCA	unknown
5	19Y, F	0Y	LM, RCA	ACBP
6	41Y, M	8Y	RCA	PTCA
7	19Y, F	0Y	RCA,LAD, LCX	ACBP

Fig. 8. Reported Adult Cases

arterial structure histologically, an autopsied case was presented. In our case, who died suddenly 4 years after the onset of K.D. at the age of 8 years, even though postmortem angio showed normal right coronary artery (fig.9), the histological examination of that artery showed destruction of elastic laminae and marked thickening of intima (Fig. 10). As there is no definitive way to

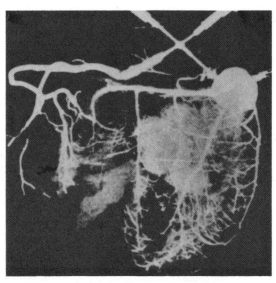

Fig. 9. Postmortem Angiography

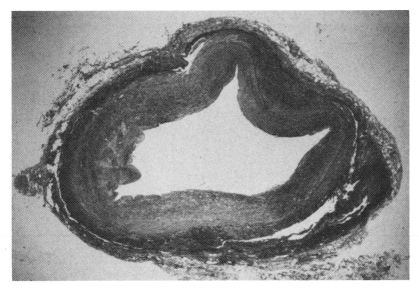

Fig. 10. Histological Findings of the Right Coronary Artery

visualize the coronary arterial wall itself, careful
follow-up must be necessary at least in the cases with
"regression" of aneurysm.

REFERENCES

1) T. Kamiya, A. Suzuki, Y. Kijima, O. Hirose and O.
   Takahashi (1982). Coronary arterial lesion in Kawasaki
   Disease – Occurrence and Prognosis - . Recent Advances
   in Cardiovascular Disease, 3: 19-27 (in Japanese)
2) T. Kamiya, A. Suzuki, Y. Kijima and O. Hirose (1981).
   Coronary arterial lesion in children with Kawasaki
   disease. Circulation, 64: IV-278

Kawasaki Disease, pages 357-365
© 1987 Alan R. Liss, Inc.

INCOMPLETE KAWASAKI DISEASE WITH CORONARY ARTERY
INVOLVEMENT

Anne H. Rowley, Frank Gonzalez-Crussi, Samuel S.
Gidding, C. Elise Duffy, and Stanford T. Shulman

Departments of Pediatrics and Pathology,
Northwestern University Medical School, Children's
Memorial Hospital, Chicago, IL   60614

INTRODUCTION
    The diagnostic criteria for Kawasaki Disease are
extremely useful in establishing the diagnosis and
particularly useful in preventing overdiagnoses. However,
strict adherence to such criteria may result in incomplete
forms of illness being unrecognized. Accurate early
diagnosis of all cases of Kawasaki Disease is especially
important because intravenous gammaglobulin administered
early in the course of illness significantly prevents the
development of coronary artery abnormalities, and sequelae
such as myocardial infarction and sudden death may be
prevented by antithrombotic therapy.

    Over a recent two-year period at Children's Memorial
Hospital in Chicago, we saw four patients with Kawasaki
Disease who developed characteristic coronary artery
abnormalities following illnesses which did not fulfill
diagnostic criteria. An additional patient lacked any
history of acute manifestations of Kawasaki Disease but had
severe Kawasaki-like arterial changes at autopsy. During
this two-year period, we saw 22 other children with Kawasaki
Disease who developed coronary artery abnormalities.
Therefore, 5 of 27 or 18.5% of patients with Kawasaki-like
coronary abnormalities had acute illnesses which did not
fulfill classic diagnostic criteria.

CLINICAL PRESENTATIONS
    The first patient presented at 7 months of age with a 5
day history of high fever and irritability. On examination

he had posterior cervical adenopathy and red, fissured lips.
There was no history or findings of conjunctival injection,
rash, or swelling or erythema of the hands or feet. The
white blood cell count was elevated with a left shift, and
the sedimentation rate and platelet count were also
elevated. Several days after presentation, desquamation of
the fingers and toes developed. Echocardiogram showed a
fusiform aneurysm of the left main coronary artery which
extended into the proximal left anterior descending and left
circumflex coronary arteries. There was also a saccular
aneurysm of the proximal right coronary artery. These have
slightly decreased in size over time.

The second patient presented at 4 months of age with
seven days of high fever unresponsive to antibiotics and a
one day history of a bulging fontanelle. She had a diffuse
erythematous rash for the first few days of her illness. A
lumbar puncture was consistent with aseptic meningitis. When
seen by us she had no rash, conjunctival injection, oral
mucous membrane changes, erythema or swelling of the hands or
feet, or lymphadenopathy. The white blood cell count and
sedimentation rate were elevated. The platelet count was
initially normal but became elevated after one week.
Extensive evaluation for prolonged fever did not reveal an
etiology. Because of the persistent fever and elevated
platelet count, an echocardiogram was performed which showed
a small pericardial effusion and aneurysms of the left
anterior descending, left circumflex, and proximal right
coronary arteries. Two days after aspirin was begun, the
infant's fever, which had persisted for 14 days,
disappeared. One year later she had a persistent saccular
aneurysm at the origin of the right coronary artery and
diffuse dilatation of the left main coronary artery.

The third patient presented at 6 months of age after a
two week illness characterized by fever for 7 days,
erythematous lips, and swelling of the hands and feet. She
had no conjunctival injection, lymphadenopathy, or rash.
When peeling of the fingers was noted, she was sent to us for
evaluation. Echocardiogram revealed fusiform dilatation of
the left anterior descending coronary artery and a saccular
aneurysm of the right coronary artery. Subsequently the
right coronary aneurysm has resolved, and the dilatation of
the left anterior descending has improved.

The fourth patient presented at 12 months of age, 3 weeks after an illness manifested by two days of fever and five days of conjunctival injection. He had no rash, mucous membrane or extremity changes, or lymphadenopathy. He developed desquamation of the lateral sides of both feet and one hand two weeks later. Because Kawasaki Disease was suspected, he underwent echocardiography which showed dilatation of the right coronary artery system and a large aneurysm of the left anterior descending coronary artery.

The fifth patient was a 2 year old male who presented with a one day history of labored breathing and vomiting. On examination he had findings of severe congestive heart failure. Extensive evaluation revealed no explanation for the illness. He died of intractible congestive heart failure and multi-organ system failure. There was no history of an antecedent febrile illness or diagnostic findings of Kawasaki Disease, but he had had significant peeling of the fingers and hands several months prior to admission. At autopsy, there was marked intimal proliferation of the major coronary arteries with reduction of the lumen to a slit-like space (Figure), typical of the pathology found in aneurysms which have regressed in patients with Kawasaki Disease.

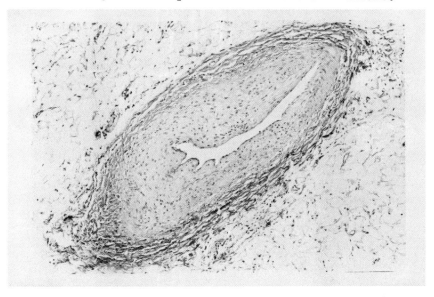

Figure: Coronary Artery Showing Intimal Fibrous Proliferation without Inflammatory Infiltrate in Case 5 (250x)

The most consistent clinical findings in this group of patients with incomplete or atypical Kawasaki Disease were prolonged fever and subsequent desquamation.

DISCUSSION

There are many reports in the English-language literature of coronary artery aneurysms in childhood associated with a febrile illness, excluding cases associated with bacterial endocarditis and pericarditis or congenital arteriovenous fistulas, the most common other causes of coronary aneurysms in children (Neufeld and Schneeweiss, 1983). These cases usually had an illness with features suggestive of Kawasaki Disease, and had serious or fatal late sequelae. There are at least nine reports from 1871 to 1969 of children who had myocardial infarction or sudden death shortly after a febrile illness suggestive of Kawasaki Disease but not meeting diagnostic criteria (Burns and Manion, 1969; Crocker et al, 1957; Gee, 1871; Martelle, 1955; Rae, 1937; Ramsay and Crumrine, 1931; Scott and Miller, 1946; Sherkat et al, 1967). In addition, there are at least seven cases reported from 1951 to 1986 of children with myocardial infarction or sudden death several years after an illness which probably represented Kawasaki Disease but was not recognized as such at the time (Bharati et al, 1975; Gorgels et al, 1986; Kempton, 1951; Kohr, 1986; McMartin et al, 1974; Pounder, 1985). There are more than 20 similar cases from 1939 to 1976 reported as infantile periarteritis nodosa, an entity now recognized as pathologically indistinguishable from Kawasaki Disease (Benyo and Perrin, 1968; Chamberlain and Perry, 1971; Glanz et al, 1976; Liddicoat et al, 1974,; Munro-Faure, 1959; Pickard et al, 1947; Roberts and Fetterman, 1963; Scott and Rotondo, 1944; Sinclair and Nitsch, 1949; Stimson, 1939; Tang and Segal, 1971). There are also at least 14 reports from 1948 to 1983 of young adults with coronary artery aneurysms but no evidence of atherosclerosis or other risk factors for coronary disease, some of whom had a history of an illness suggestive of Kawasaki Disease as children (Ahronheim, 1977; Ashton and Munro, 1948; Cafferky et al, 1969; Dawson and Ellison, 1972; Ellis and Kurth, 1968; Ebert et al, 1971; Flugelman et al, 1983; Ghahramani et al, 1972; Kitamura et al, 1983; Mattern et al, 1972; Oliveira et al, 1984; Seabra-Gomes et al, 1974; Stephens et al, 1982; van den Brock and Segal, 1973). Since the illnesses in these cases usually did not fulfill diagnostic criteria, it is likely that some of these represented incomplete or atypical presentations of the

illness, although there may have been additional features
diagnostic of Kawasaki Disease which were not recognized at
the time.

Of great concern are reports of children without known
prior illness who presented with myocardial infarction or
sudden death due to coronary artery aneurysms. Seabra-Gomes
et al(1974) reported a 4 year old who was healthy until he
presented in heart failure secondary to a myocardial infarction after an appendectomy. Wilson et al(1975) reported a 15
year old who died suddenly after exercise, and had no prior
illness. Trillo et al(1980) reported a 6 year old who died
suddenly during play with no history of a prior illness. It
is possible that these children had classic Kawasaki Disease
which had been missed, but it is perhaps more likely that
they had an illness with few or no clinical manifestations.

There are several reports of patients similar to ours
with incomplete or atypical Kawasaki Disease who developed
coronary artery disease. Fukushige et al(1980) reported an
8 month old and a 6 month old with only fever and rash who
both developed coronary disease and fatal myocardial infarction. Canter et al(1981) reported a 28 month old with only
fever, rash and fissured lips who developed bilateral coronary aneurysms and myocardial infarction. Reller et al(1984)
reported a 7 year old with fever, conjunctival injection,
oral mucous membrane changes, and lymphadenopathy. Despite
an elevated ASO titer and throat culture positive for
group A streptococcus, he did not improve with penicillin
and developed bilateral coronary artery aneurysms. Fujiwara
et al(1986) reported 6 children with fewer than 4 diagnostic
criteria who died of myocardial infarction secondary to
thrombosis of coronary aneurysms. Salo et al(1986) reported
one patient with 3 diagnostic criteria who developed a left
coronary aneurysm. Burns et al(1986) reported a 3 month old
with 4 diagnostic criteria who developed coronary aneurysms
and died, and a 6 week old who had only 3 days of fever but
all other diagnostic criteria and developed coronary
aneurysms.

In summary, strict application of Kawasaki Disease diagnostic criteria may result in failure to recognize atypical
patients, some of whom will develop significant coronary
artery abnormalities with long-term sequelae that are theore-
tically preventable. It is likely that with the increasing
incidence of Kawasaki Disease there will be an increasing

number of children with subclinical and incomplete presentations of the illness. Over a two-year period, 5/27 or 18.5% of our patients with Kawasaki-like coronary abnormalities had acute illnesses which did not fulfill classic diagnostic criteria. The most consistent clinical findings in this group were prolonged fever and subsequent desquamation. Children with a prolonged unexplained febrile illness with features suggestive of Kawasaki Disease should undergo echocardiography, particularly if subsequent peripheral desquamation is noted. Obviously, reliable early identification of all patients with subclinical or incomplete Kawasaki Disease will depend upon detection of the etiologic agent or agents of the illness and development of a specific diagnostic test.

REFERENCES

1. Ahronheim JH (1977). Isolated Coronary Periarteritis: Report of a Case of Unexpected Death in a Young Pregnant Woman. Am J Cardiol 40:287-90.
2. Ashton N, Munro M (1948). Coronary Artery Aneurysm with Occlusion Due to a Calcified Thrombus. Br Heart J 10:165-6.
3. Benyo RB, Perrin EV (1968). Periarteritis Nodosa in Infancy. Amer J Dis Child 116:539-44.
4. Bharati S, Fisher EA, Yaniz RA, et al (1975). Infarct of the Myocardium with Aneurysm in a 13-year old girl. Chest 67:369-73.
5. Burns CJ, Manion WC (1969). Sudden Unexpected Death of a Two-year-old Child from Thrombosis of Both Coronary Arteries with Aneurysmal Dilatation of the Vessels. Med Annals DC 38:381-22.
6. Burns JC, Wiggins JW, Toews WH, et al (1986). Clinical Spectrum of Kawasaki disease in infants younger than 6 months of age. J Pediatr 109:759-63.
7. Cafferky EA, Crawford DW, Turner AF, et al (1969). Congenital Aneurysm of the Coronary Artery with Myocardial Infarction. Am J Med Sci 257:320-7.
8. Canter CE, Bower RJ, Strauss AW (1981). Atypical Kawasaki Disease with Aortic Aneurysm. Pediatrics 68:885-8.
9. Chamberlain JL, Perry LW (1971). Infantile periarteritis nodosa with coronary and brachial aneurysms: A case diagnosed during life. J Pediatr 78:1039-42.
10. Crocker DW, Sobin S, Thomas WC (1957). Aneurysms of the Coronary Arteries. Amer J Path 33:819-37.

11. Dawson JE, Ellison RG (1972). Isolated Aneurysm of the Anterior Descending Coronary Artery. Am J Cardiol 29:868-71.
12. Ebert PA, Peter RH, Gunnells JC, Sabiston DC (1971). Resecting and Grafting of Coronary Artery Aneurysm. Circulation 43:593-8.
13. Ellis R, Kurth RJ (1968). Calcified Coronary Artery Aneurysms. JAMA 203:105-7.
14. Flugelman MY, Hasin Y, Bassan MM, et al (1983). Acute Myocardial Infarction 14 Years After an Acute Episode of Kawasaki Disease. Amer J Cardiol 52:427-8.
15. Fukushige J, Nihill MR, McNamara DG (1980). Spectrum of Cardiovascular Lesions in Mucocutaneous Lymph Node Syndrome: Analysis of Eight Cases. Am J Cardiol 45:98-107.
16. Fujiwara H, Fujiwara T, Kao TC, et al (1986). Pathology of Kawasaki Disease in the Healed Stage. Acta Pathol Jpn 36:857-67.
17. Gee SJ (1871). Cases of morbid anatomy: Aneurysms of coronary arteries in a boy. St. Barth Hosp Rep 7:148.
18. Ghahramani A, Iyengar R, Cunha D, et al (1972). Myocardial Infarction Due to Congenital Coronary Arterial Aneurysm. Am J Cardiol 29:863-67.
19. Glanz S, Bittner SJ, Berman MA, et al (1976). Regression of Coronary-Artery Aneurysms in Infantile Periarteritis Nodosa. N Engl J Med 294:939-40.
20. Gorgels APM, Braat SHGJ, Becker AE, et al (1986). Multiple Aneurysms of the Coronary Arteries as the Cause of Sudden Death in Childhood. Amer J Cardiol 57:1193-4.
21. Kempton JJ (1951). Calcified Aneurysms of the Coronary Arteries. Proc RSM 44:733-4.
22. Kitamura S, Kawachi K, Harima R, et al (1983). Surgery for Coronary Heart Disease Due to Mucocutaneous Lymph Node Syndrome (Kawasaki Disease). Amer J Cardiol 51:444-8.
23. Kohr, RM (1986). Progressive asymptomatic coronary artery disease as a late fatal sequela of Kawasaki disease. J Pediatr 108:256-9.
24. Liddicoat JE, Bekassy SM, O'Donnell MJ, DeBakey ME (1974). Coronary artery aneurysms in a 9-year old child. Surgery 76:845-7.
25. Martelle RR (1955). Coronary Thrombosis in a Five-Month-old Infant. J Pediatr 46:322-6.
26. Mattern AL, Baker WP, McHale JJ, Lee DE (1972). Congenital Coronary Aneurysms with Angina Pectoris and Myocardial Infarction Treated with Saphenous Vein Bypass Graft. Am J Cardiol 30:906-9.

27. McMartin DE, Stone AJ, Franch RH (1974). Multiple Coronary-Artery Aneurysms in a Child with Angina Pectoris. N Engl J Med 290:669-70.
28. Munro-Faure H (1959). Necrotizing Arteritis of the Coronary Vessels in Infancy. Pediatrics 23:914-26.
29. Neufeld HN, Schneeweiss A (1983). Coronary Artery Disease in Infants and Children. Philadelphia, Lea & Febiger.
30. Oliveira DBG, Foale RA, Bensaid J (1984). Coronary artery aneurysms and Kawasaki's disease in an adult. Br Heart J 51:91-3.
31. Pickard CM, Owen JG, Dammin GJ (1947). Aneurysms of the Coronary Arteries Due to Polyarteritis Nodosa Occurring in an Infant. J Lab Clin Med 32:1513-14.
32. Pounder DJ (1985). Coronary Artery Aneurysms Presenting as Sudden Death 14 Years After Kawasaki Disease in Infancy. Arch Pathol Lab Med 109:874-6.
33. Rae MV (1937). Coronary Aneurysms with Thrombosis in Rheumatic Carditis. Arch Path 24:369-76.
34. Ramsay RE, Crumrine RM (1931). Coronary Thrombosis. Arch Dis Child 42:107-10.
35. Reller M, DeCristofaro J, Schwartz DC (1984). Coronary Aneurysms in a Patient with Atypical Kawasaki Syndrome and a Streptococcal Infection. Pediatr Cardiol 5:205-8.
36. Roberts FB, Fetterman GH (1963). Polyarteritis Nodosa in infancy. J Pediatr 63:519-29.
37. Salo E, Pelkonen P, Pettay O (1986). Outbreak of Kawasaki Syndrome in Finland. Acta Pediatr Scand 75:75-80.
38. Scott EP, Miller AJ (1946). Coronary Thrombosis. J Pediatr 28:478-80.
39. Scott EP, Rotondo CC (1944). Periarteritis Nodosa. J Pediatr 25:306-10.
40. Seabra-Gomes R, Somerville J, Ross DN, et al (1974). Congenital coronary artery aneurysms. Br Heart J 36:329-35.
41. Sherkat A, Kavanagh-Gray D, Edworthy J (1967). Localized Aneurysms of the Coronary Arteries. Radiology 84:24-6.
42. Sinclair W, Nitsch E (1949). Polyarteritis Nodosa of the Coronary Arteries. Am Heart J 38:898-904.
43. Stephens DD, Parsillo JE, Dinsmore RE, et al (1982). Circumflex Coronary Artery Aneurysm Visualized by Real-Time Cross-Sectional Echocardiography. Chest 81:513-15.

44. Stimson, PM (1939). Clinical Conference at Willard Parker Hospital, New York. Arch Pediatr 56:319-24.
45. Tang PHL, Segal AJ (1971). Polyarteritis Nodosa of Infancy. JAMA 217:1666-70.
46. Trillo AA, Scharyj M, Prichard RW (1980). Coronary artery aneurysm and myocardial infarction resulting in sudden death of a 6 year-old child. Am J Forensic Med Path 1:349-54.
47. van den Brock H, Segal BL (1973). Coronary Aneurysms in a Young Woman: Angiographic Documentation of the Natural Course. Chest 64:132-4.
48. Wilson CS, Weaver WF, Zeaman ED, Forker AD (1975). Bilateral Nonfistulous Congenital Coronary Arterial Aneurysms. Am J Cardiol 35:319-23.

Kawasaki Disease, pages 367–378
© 1987 Alan R. Liss, Inc.

ATYPICAL KAWASAKI DISEASE

Tomoyoshi Sonobe, Tomisaku Kawasaki

Department of Pediatrics, Japanese Red Cross
Medical Center, Tokyo, Japan 150

INTRODUCTION

Kawasaki disease is increasing in numbers in Japan.
According to the 1985 nation wide survey, as of the end of
1984, about 60,000 cases were registered (Yanagawa, 1986).
The 3rd major nation wide epidemic was seen thereafter in
Japan from the winter of 1985 to the spring of 1986. As the
number has increased, the number of atypical cases which did
not meet the criteria of the Kawasaki Disease Research Committee has increased concomitantly. Here we present fatal
and nonfatal atypical Kawasaki disease cases with coronary
artery involvement and discuss   the clinical aspects in
our 5 years' experience.

MATERIALS AND METHODS

The definition of atypical Kawasaki disease is as follows: The patients should have 3 or 4 of 6 principal symptoms listed in the 3rd revised diagnostic guideline (1979)
prepared by the Japan Kawasaki Disease Research Committee
and have no clinical and laboratory evidence of any other
disease known to mimic Kawasaki disease.

From 1981 to 1985 at the Japanese Red Cross Medical
Center we have seen 45 atypical Kawasaki disease cases.
Forty-three patients received Aspirin (50mg/kg/day) and two
patients received Flurbiprofen (nonsteroidal anti-inflammatory drug, 4mg/kg/day) therapy. The incidence, age distribution, sex ratio, 6 principal symptoms, duration of fever,

major laboratory data (maximum WBC, ESR, C-reactive protein
and thrombocyte count) and the incidence of coronary artery
involvement were compared with those of definitive Kawasaki
disease cases. The incidence of other significant symptoms
and findings of Kawasaki disease was also studied in atypical cases.

The assesment of coronary artery involvement was made
by two dimensional echocardiography (2DE) which was performed more than once a week after admission till the 30th
day of illness. When abnormalities were found by 2DE at
the 30th day of illness, additional 2DE was performed again
at the 60th day of illness. Coronary artery involvement was
classified as normal, having dilatation, or having aneurysm,
mainly according to the inner wall diameter of proximal portions of coronary arteries and partly to the shape of dilated coronary arteries and diameter of aorta. Normal was
defined when the diameter was less than 2mm for children
less than 2 years of age and less than 2.5mm for children
over 2 years of age. Dilatation was less than 4mm of dilating lesion and aneurysm was when the diameter exceeded 4mm.

A fatal atypical case experienced in 1976 is presented
as well as two cases from these 45 atypical cases.

CASE REPORTS

Case 1. This 5-month-old girl was admitted to our hospital on the 11th day of illness with persisting high fever
of 11 days duration, rash and congestion of bilateral conjunctivae (March, 1976). However physical examination on
admission revealed no signs of typical Kawasaki disease except for fever. Laboratory data showed marked leukocytosis
with shift to the left and strong positive acute phase reactants. She received Aspirin, Warfarin and Prednisolone
with the tentative diagnosis of Kawasaki disease after negative blood culture. Faint desquamation of the finger tips
was noted after persisting fever of 19 days duration. On
the 40th day of illness, ECG revealed deep Q waves in leads
II, III and $_aV_F$. With the diagnosis of inferior myocardial
infarction, she received intravenous Urokinase therapy.
Post myocardial infarction course was uneventful and she was
discharged on the 87th day of illness. Six days after discharge
from the hospital she died suddenly with a shrill cry on
feeding.

Autopsy revealed bilateral huge coronary aneyrysms with thrombotic occlusion. Histopathological findings were compatible with typical arteritis seen in Kawasaki disease.

Case 2. A 4-year-old girl was admitted to our hospital for the evaluation of fever of 8 days duration, marked cervical lymphadenopathy with wry neck, red lips and knee pain (Nov., 1984). Her past history was uneventful. Aspirin therapy (50mg/kg/day) was started on the day of admission. Fever lasted for 14 days and then mild desquamation was noted from the tips of fingers. Rash and congestion of bilateral conjunctivae were not noted throughout the course. The diameter of coronary arteries detected by 2DE increased gradually up to 7mm in the left and 6mm in the right coronary artery by the 14th day of illness. Aneurysm formation was also seen in the peripheral portion of the right coronary artery. This case should be classified as a definitive case by the definition of the 4th revised diagnostic guideline because of the presence of 4 symptoms and dilating coronary artery lesion.

Case 3. A 10-month-old boy was admitted for the evaluation of prolonged fever of 7 days duration, mild congestion of bilateral conjunctivae and febrile convulsion (July, 1983). There were no symptoms of Kawasaki disease other than fever on admission. Laboratory examinations revealed leukocytosis, positive acute phase reactants and pleocytosis of mononuclear cells in CSF ($64/mm^3$). He was treated with the diagnosis of aseptic meningitis. Desquamation from finger tips was noticed on the 16th day of illness. Aneurysms of bilateral coronary arteries were detected by the first 2DE performed on the same day. Presence of coronary artery involvement with 3 principal symptoms led us to make the diagnosis of atypical Kawasaki disease. Ticlopidine (antiplatelet drug) therapy was started. He became afebrile on the 24th day of illness. The diameter of dilated coronary arteries decreased gradually and complete regression of coronary aneurysms was confirmed by selective coronary angiography 1 year after the onset.

RESULTS

The total number of definitive Kawasaki disease cases to our hospital during this period was 630. The ratio of atypical cases to definitive cases was 7.1:100. Male to female ratio in atypical cases was 1.14:1. Age distribution ranged from 2 months to 9 years of age and 56% of the cases were less than 2 years of age. Mean age was 26 ± 20 months (Mean ± SD). Thirty-six of 45 cases (80%) had 4 of 6 principal symptoms and 9 cases (20%) had 3 principal symptoms.

The incidence of 6 principal symptoms among atypical cases were as follows: 1. Fever persisting 5 days or more: 73%, 2. Bilateral conjunctival congestion: 78%, 3. Changes of lips and oral cavity: 76%, 4. Acute nonpurulent cervical lymphadenopathy: 36%, 5. Polymorphous exanthema: 40%, 6. Changes of peripheral extremities: 80%. Duration of fever was 7.0 ± 4.6 days (Mean ± SD).

Major laboratory data of 30 cases who were admitted before the 8th day of illness were analyzed. Maximum WBC was 12,900 ± 4,500/mm^3 (Mean ± SD). Maximum ESR was 60 ± 24/h (Mean ± SD). Maximum C-reactive protein was 3.0 ± 1.7 (+) (Mean ± SD). Maximum thrombocyte count was 54 ± 13 x 10^4/mm^3 (Mean ± SD). Table 1 and 2 show the comparison of clinical symptoms and laboratory data in the atypical cases and 300 definitive cases who were treated with Aspirin at our hospital. Hydrops of gall bladder (1/30), pleocytosis of CSF (6/11), increase of serum transaminase (15/30), hypoalbuminemia (6/30) and urine abnormalities (5/30) were present in these 30 atypical cases. Skin changes at the site of BCG were seen in 16 of 24 atypical cases (67%) who received the inoculation within 2 years before the onset of the disease.

The incidence of coronary artery involvement during the acute phase (analysis of 39 cases who were admitted before the 15th day of illness), on the 30th day of illness (45 cases) and on the 60th day of illness (45 cases) were 21% (dilatation: 8%, aneurysm: 13%), 11% (dilatation: 4%, aneurysm: 7%) and 8% (dilatation: 4%, aneurysm: 4%), respectively. The incidence of coronary artery involvement during the acute phase of the disease (up to the 30th day of illness) was 14% (5/36) in the group with 4 principal symptoms and 33% (3/9) in the group with 3 principal symptoms and 18% (8/45) in all, respectively. Figure 1 shows the comparison of the incidence of coronary artery involvement in atypical and definitive cases at our hospital.

Incidences of 6 Principal Symptoms in Atypical Kawasaki Disease

Principal Symptoms	Atypical Cases n=45	Definitive Cases n=300
① Fever (≥5 days)	73 %	98 %
② Conjunctival congestion	78 %	100 %
③ Changes of lips and oral cavity	76 %	99 %
④ Cervical lymphadenopathy	36 %	72 %
⑤ Polymorphous exanthema	40 %	97 %
⑥ Changes of peripheral extremities	80 %	100 %

Table 1. Incidence of 6 Principal Symptoms in Atypical Kawasaki Disease.

Duration of Fever and Laboratory Data of Atypical Cases

	Atypical Cases n=30	Definitive Cases n=300
Duration of Fever	7.0±4.6*	9.9±4.8
WBC (max.) (/mm³)	12,900±4,500 (5,600~24,200)	15,100±4,000 (7,000~29,200)
ESR (max.) (/h)	60±24 (35~116)	69±27 (15~142)
CRP (max.) (+)	3.0±1.7 (0~6+)	4.3±1.5 (0~6+)
Platelet (max.) (×10⁴/mm³)	54±13 (30~90)	66±15 (29~105)

★Analysis of 45 cases

Table 2. Duration of Fever and Laboratory Data of Atypical Cases.

Incidence of Coronary Artery Involvement(CAI)

CAI ☐(N) : Normal, ▨(D) : Dilatation, ■(A) : Aneurysm(≥4mm by 2DE)

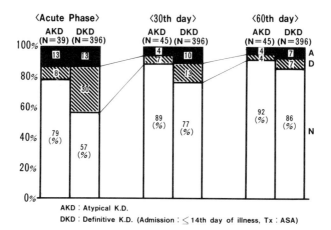

AKD : Atypical K.D.
DKD : Definitive K.D. (Admission : ≤14th day of illness, Tx : ASA)

Figure 1. Incidence of Coronary Artery Involvement in Atypical and Definitive Cases.

Definition of Kawasaki Disease
(Changes of Diagnostic Guideline)

Diagnostic Guideline	Year	Definition
① First	1970	① plus 3 or 4 of symptom ②~⑤
② First revised	1972	same as above
③ Second revised	1974	5 or 6 of symptom ①~⑥
④ Third revised	1978	same as above
⑤ Fourth revised	1984	ⓐ same as above ⓑ 4 of symptom ①~⑥ plus coronary involvement

Symptoms ① fever ≥5 days ② conjunctival congestion ③ changes of lips and oral cavity
④ rash ⑤ changes of extremities ⑥ cervical lymphadenopathy

Table 3. Definition of Kawasaki Disease (Changes of Diagnostic Guideline).

DISCUSSION

Every disease has atypical cases or "formes fruste," and Kawasaki disease is no exception. In order to discuss atypical cases, we must review the changes in the definition of the disease which has been revised several times in Japan as shown in Table 3 (Kusakawa, 1986). The disease was first described in 1967 by T. Kawasaki (Kawasaki, 1967) under the name of acute febrile mucocutaneous lymph node syndrome (MC-LS). In order to survey the epidemiology, clinical aspects and etiology, the MCLS Research Committee was organized under the sponsorship of the Japanese Ministry of Health and Welfare and the Committee made the first diagnostic guideline in 1970. The criteria at that time were that the patient should have 4 or 5 of 5 principal symptoms (1. Fever persisting 5 days or more, 2. Bilateral conjunctival congestion, 3. Changes of lips and oral cavity, 4. Polymorphous exanthema, 5. Changes of peripheral extremities) but always including number 1. An important modification was made in the 2nd revised diagnostic guideline in 1974. Cervical lymphadenopathy was added to the 5 principal symptoms and the diagnosis of the disease was made when the patient had at least 5 of 6 principal symptoms. There were no significant changes in the 3rd revised diagnostic guideline. The latest 4th revised guideline (Table 4) had an important provision that patients with four principal symptoms can be diagnosed as Kawasaki disease when coronary aneurysm is recognized by 2DE or coronary angiography. Since 2DE examination and angiography are not always available, in this article we have selected the 3rd revised diagnostic guideline to establish our definition of atypical case as mentioned previously.

The ratio of definitive to atypical cases was 100:7.1 in our series. This ratio was nearly the same as that of Ohta's series (136:11) (Ohta et al., 1983). There was no significant difference between definitive to atypical cases regarding age distribution and sex ratio (Yanagawa, 1986). Five of 36 cases with 4 principal symptoms had coronary artery involvement. These 5 cases were classified as definitive cases if they were defined according to the latest 4th revised diagnostic guideline. The increment of the definitive cases due to the additional provision was 0.8% (5:630).

By the comparison of the incidences of principal symptoms between atypical and definitive cases, there was signif-

DIAGNOSTIC GUIDELINE
of
Kawasaki Disease
(MCLS: Infantile Acute Febrile Mucocutaneous Lymph Node Syndrome)

(4th Revised Edition, September 1984)

This is a disease of unknown etiology affecting most frequently infants and young children under 5 years of age. The symptoms can be classified into two categories, principal symptoms and other significant symptoms or findings.

A. PRINCIPAL SYMPTOMS

1. Fever persisting 5 days or more
2. Changes of peripheral extremities:
   [Initial stage]: Reddening of palms and soles, Indurative edema
   [Convalescent stage]: Membranous desquamation from fingertips
3. Polymorphous exanthema
4. Bilateral conjunctival congestion
5. Changes of lips and oral cavity: Reddening of lips, Strawberry tongue, Diffuse injection of oral and pharyngeal mucosa
6. Acute nonpurulent cervical lymphadenopathy

At least five items of 1–6 should be satisfied for diagnosis of Kawasaki disease. However, patients with four items of the principal symptoms can be diagnosed as Kawasaki disease when coronary aneurysm is recognized by two dimensional echocardiography or coronary angiography.

B. OTHER SIGNIFICANT SYMPTOMS OR FINDINGS

The following symptoms and findings should be clinically considered:

1. Cardiovascular: Auscultation (heart murmur, gallop rhythm, distant heart sounds), ECG changes (prolonged PR·QT intervals, abnormal Q wave, low voltage, ST·T changes, arrhythmias), Chest X-ray findings (cardiomegaly), 2-D echo findings (pericardial effusion, coronary aneurysms), Aneurysm of peripheral arteries other than coronary (axillary etc.), Angina pectoris or Myocardial infarction
2. GI tract: Diarrhea, Vomiting, Abdominal pain, Hydrops of gall bladder, Paralytic ileus, Mild jaundice, Slight increase of serum transaminase
3. Blood: Leukocytosis with shift to the left, Thrombocytosis, Increased ESR, Positive CRP, Hypoalbuminemia, Increased α_2-globulin, Slight decrease in erythrocyte and hemoglobin levels
4. Urine: Proteinuria, Increase of leukocytes in urine sediment
5. Skin: Redness and crust at the site of BCG inoculation, Small pustules, Transverse furrows of the finger nails
6. Respiratory: Cough, Rhinorrhea, Abnormal shadow on chest X-ray
7. Joint: Pain, Swelling
8. Neurological: Pleocytosis of mononuclear cells in CSF, Convulsion, Unconsciousness, Facial palsy, Paralysis of the extremities

REMARKS: 1. For item 2 under principal sympotoms, the convalescent stage is considered important.
2. Male : Female ratio: 1.3 ~ 1.5 : 1, patients under 5 years of age: 80 ~ 85%, fatality rate: 0.3 ~ 0.5%
3. Recurrence rate: 2 ~ 3%, proportion of sibling cases: 1 ~ 2%

Prepared by The Japan Kawasaki Disease Research Committee, c/o Department of Pediatrics, Japan Red Cross Medical Center, 4-1-22 Hiroo, Shibuya-ku, Tokyo, 150 Japan. (Telephone: 03-400-1311)

Table 4. The 4th Revised Diagnostic Guideline of Kawasaki Disease.

icant decrease of the incidence of cervical lymphadenopathy
(36% vs 72%) and exanthema (40% vs 96%) among atypical
cases. Ohta reported that the incidence of cervical lymphadenopathy was 36% in his 11 atypical cases (Ohta et al.,
1983). The assessment of cervical lymphadenopathy is somewhat difficult or uncertain compared to the remaining principal symptoms. The incidence of atypical and definitive
cases may change by the criterion of cervical lymphadenopathy. In the United States, usually, the size of cervical
lymphadenopathy must exceed 1.5cm (Newburger et al., 1986),
while the Japanese criterion does not define the size.

The duration of fever of atypical cases was shorter
than that of definitive cases because there were 1 afebrile
case and 11 cases whose duration of fever was less than 5
days. The duration of fever of the cases with coronary artery involvement was usually longer in both atypical and
definitive cases. Leukocytosis, increased ESR, positive C-
reactive protein and thrombocytosis,which were common in the
acute phase of the disease,were also seen in atypical cases.
Although abnormalities of these laboratory data were milder
in atypical cases, there were no significant differences between the two groups.

Hydrops of gall bladder, pleocytosis of CSF, increase
of serum transaminase, hypoalbuminemia and urine abnormalities were also present in our series. Redness and crust at
the site of BCG inoculation was one of the conspicuous symptoms of Kawasaki disease as was hydrops of gall bladder.
These skin changes were seen in 54% of the definitive cases
who received BCG within 2 years before the onset of the disease (Takayama et al., 1982). Sixteen of 24 cases (67%) in
our atypical series showed the same skin changes. These abnormalities were listed in the 4th revised diagnostic guideline as other significant symptoms or findings. Since there
is no infallible diagnostic test for Kawasaki disease, these
significant symptoms and findings are useful for making a
diagnosis, especially in atypical cases.

The most serious complication of Kawasaki disease is
cardiovascular, especially coronary artery involvement (Kato
et al., 1982). Ohta (Ohta et al., 1983) and Tada (Tada et
al.,1983) reported that the coronary artery involvement in
atypical cases were seen in 18% (2/11) and 40% (6/15) of the
cases, respectively. In our atypical cases the incidence of
coronary artery involvement was smaller than that of defini-

tive cases, especially in the acute phase of the disease.
However it is worth remembering the incidence of aneurysm
(inner wall diameter of coronary artery exceeding 4mm) was
the same as that of definitive cases in the acute phase of
the disease.

Although there were no patients with other cardiovascular involvement in our series, there were reports of mitral
regurgitation (Ishizaka et al., 1983), aortic aneurysm and
peripheral artery involvement (Canter et al., 1981) in atypical cases. Huge aneurysms (diameter of coronary artery exceeding 8mm) which tend to be occluded easily (Nakano et
al., 1985, Ichinose et al., 1985, Sonobe et al., 1985) were
not present in our atypical series. However huge aneurysm
cases with or without myocardial infarction were reported by
several authors (Ishizaka et al., 1983, Nakano et al., 1983,
Reller et al., 1984, Harima et al., 1985).

Besides our fatal case, fatal cases have been reported
(Fukushige et al., 1980, Fujiwara et al., 1985). Pathological findings of fatal atypical cases were identical with
those of fatal definitive cases like ours (Fujiwara et al.,
1985). Landing and Larson (Landing and Larson, 1977) stated
that pathological findings of fatal definitive Kawasaki disease cases were not distinguishable from those of infantile
periarteritis nodosa (IPN). Therefore the difference between Kawasaki disease and IPN became more obscure. However
we must remember that Kawasaki disease is a clinical entity,
while IPN is a pathological entity. We believe that the
discovery of the etiology of Kawasaki disease can provide us
the differential clue whether the two diseases are identical
or not.

In conclusion, all the evidence mentioned above suggests
that atypical Kawasaki disease as defined here is essentially identical to definitive Kawasaki disease. Therefore the
same treatment and management of definitive cases including
anticoagulant therapy and 2DE examinations are required for
the atypical Kawasaki disease cases.

REFERENCES

Canter CD, Bower RJ, Strauss AW (1981). Atypical Kawasaki
    disease with aortic aneurysm. Pediatrics 68:885-888.
Fujiwara H, Fujiwara T, Hamashima Y (1985). Pathology of

Kawasaki disease in the healed stage: Relationship among Kawasaki disease with clinically typical and un-typical cases, and IPN. Prog Med 5:13-18 (in Japanese with English abstract).

Fukushige J, Nihill MR, McNamara DG (1980). Spectrum of cardiovascular lesions in mucocutaneous lymph node syndrome: Analysis of eight cases. Am J Cardiol 45:98-107.

Harima Y, Kojima S, Yoshimoto T, Tanaka J, Nishimura K, Mimura Y, Sakai T (1985). A case of atypical Kawasaki disease with huge aneurysms and uveitis. Prog Med 5: 165-169 (in Japanese).

Ichinose E (1985). Prognosis of coronary aneurysm in Kawasaki disease. Acta Paediatr Jpn 89:1595-1603 (in Japanese).

Ishizaka Y, Miyake T, Seto S, Hirao T, Setoya T, Saito A, Ueda K, Nakano H (1983). A cases of atypical MCLS. Jpn J Pediatr 36:1267-1272 (in Japanese).

Kato H, Ichinose E, Yoshioka F, Takechi T, Matsunaga S, Suzuki K, Rikitake N (1982). Fate of coronary aneurysms in Kawasaki disease: Serial coronary angiography and long-term follow-up study. Am J Cardiol 49:1758-1766.

Kawasaki T (1967). Acute febrile mucocutaneous lymph node syndrome: Clinical observation of 50 cases. Jpn J Allerg 16:178-222 (in Japanese).

Kusakawa S (1986). Diagnostic guideline of Kawasaki disease and its chronological change. In The Study Committee on Cause of Kawasaki Disease, Japan Heart Foundation (eds): "Kawasaki Disease -Epidemiological Data Book-," Tokyo: Soft Science Publications, pp 188-191 (in Japanese with English abstract).

Kusuhara A, Saito K, Ogino H, Kouno S, Matsumura T (1983). Clinical analysis of definitive and atypical Kawasaki disease. Proceedings of the Kinki Area Kawasaki Disease Research 4:44-46 (in Japanese).

Landing BH, Larson EJ (1977). Are infantile periarteritis nodosa with coronary artery involvement and fatal mucocutaneous lymph node syndrome the same? : Comparison of 20 patients from North America with patients from Hawaii and Japan. Pediatr 59:651-662.

Nakano H, Ueda K, Saito A, Nojima K (1985). Repeated quantitative angiograms in coronary arterial aneurysms in Kawasaki disease. Am J Cardiol 56:846-851.

Nakano M, Somiya K, Hirata Y, Iguma M (1983). A case of atypical Kawasaki disease with huge aneurysms. Proceedings of the Kinki Area Kawasaki Disease Research 4:37-39 (in Japanese).

Newburger JW, Takahashi M, Burns JC, Beiser AS, Chung KJ,
Duffy CE, Glodes MP, Mason WH, Reddy V, Sanders SP,
Shulman ST, Wiggins JW, Hicks RV, Fulton DR, Lewis AB,
Leung DYM, Colton T, Rosen FS, Melish ME (1986). The
treatment of Kawasaki Syndrome with intravenous gamma
globulin. N Engl J Med 315:341-347.
Ohta K, Miyake T, Seto S, T Hirano (1983). Diagnosis and
management of Kawasaki disease. Proceedings of the Kinki
Area Kawasaki Disease Research 4:55-56 (in Japanese).
Reller M, DeCristofaro J, Schwartz DC (1984). Coronary
aneurysms in a patient with atypical Kawasaki syndrome and
a streptococcal infection. Pediatr Cardiol 5:205-208.
Sonobe T, Goto A, Mekaru M, Ishiwara T, Kataoka T, Kawasaki
T, Furukawa T (1985). The prognosis of coronary lesions
due to Kawasaki disease. Proceedings of the Kinki Area
Kawasaki Disease Research 8:41-44 (in Japanese with Eng-
lish abstract).
Tada A, Issiki G, Makino S, Yoshikawa S, Sakai Y (1983).
Study on so-called atypical cases of MCLS. Proceedings
of the Kinki Area Kawasaki Disease Research 4:40-43 (in
Japanese).
Takayama J, Yanase Y, Kawasaki T (1982). Study on the skin
changes at the site of BCG inoculation in MCLS. Acta
Paediatr Jpn 88:567-572 (in Japanese).
Yanagawa H (1986). Results of nationwide surveys on Kawasa-
ki disease. In The Study Committee on Cause of Kawasaki
Disease, Japan Heart Foundation (eds): "Kawasaki Disease
-Epidemiological Data Book-," Tokyo: Soft Science
Publications, pp 198-200 (in Japanese with English
abstract).
Yanagawa H, Nakamura Y (1986). Nationwide epidemic of Kawa-
saki disease in Japan during winter of 1985-1986. Lancet
2:1138-1139.

Kawasaki Disease, pages 379-382
© 1987 Alan R. Liss, Inc.

NON-INVASIVE IMAGING OF THE HEART AND CORONARY ARTERIES IN
CHILDREN WITH KAWASAKI DISEASE

Kyung J. Chung, M.D., F.A.C.C. and
David J. Sahn, M.D., F.A.C.C.

Department of Pediatrics, University of
California at San Diego, School of Medicine,
La Jolla, CA

Kawasaki disease (mucocutaneous lymph node syndrome) is
an acute febrile exanthematous illness with multiple organ
involvement. This disease appears to be benign and self-
limited in most cases. However, extensive cardiac involvement may cause sudden death due to myocardial infarction
from occlusive coronary aneurysm or conduction abnormality.
Since the prognosis of Kawasaki disease mainly depends on
the extent of cardiac and coronary arterial involvement, it
is extremely important to establish non-invasive techniques
to investigate these areas for immediate management and
long-term follow-up.

Many investigators have discussed the possibility of
predicting coronary artery disease, myocardial injury, and
left ventricular dysfunction in children with Kawasaki
disease with various non-invasive techniques. Echocardiogram (M-mode, two-dimensional, and Doppler) has been used
for detecting anatomical and functional cardiac abnormalities. Recently, several reports indicated that coronary
artery aneurysms can be imaged with two-dimensional echocardiograms (2-D echo).

We have evaluated 62 infants and children with Kawasaki
disease with 2-D echo and compared the result with cine-
angiographic study. We were able to detect coronary
aneurysms or dilatation in the proximal coronary arteries
in all patients, except in one child with an isolated
distal coronary aneurysm, corroborated by angiography.
Capannari et al also reported that the sensitivity of 2-D
echo was 100% for detecting proximal coronary aneurysms
because there were no patients in their study who had

isolated distal coronary aneurysms. Since coronary
aneurysms in Kawasaki disease are mainly in the proximal
portions and isolated distal aneurysms are rare and usually
hemodynamically insignificant, 2-D echo has great advantage
over angiography since it is non-invasive and has no known
complications.

To obtain optimum quality echo images for coronary
artery disease, one must have high resolution echo
equipment and transducers. Also, the examiner should be
experienced in obtaining high quality images. Often
sedation may be necessary to examine a young child. We
find Chloral Hydrate (80-100 mg/kg) orally, provides
excellent sedation without causing respiratory difficulty
or hemodynamic compromise. The current dilemma with 2-D
echo is that there is no specific criteria for normal
coronary arteries in different aged children. We usually
assume that the coronary artery is normal when its diameter
is less than 3mm and the inner surface is smooth throughout
the course of the coronary artery. In a questionable case,
the patient himself often serves as control. The patient's
own subsequent examinations of the coronary arteries would
determine whether the initial study was normal or not. To
obtain optimum images of the coronary artery, one starts
with precordial short axis view. Once the aortic root is
visualized at the level of the great arteries, the transducer is angled slightly superiorly. At this level, the
ostium of left main coronary artery (LCA) is seen. To
trace the coronary artery further distally, the transducer
is rotated 20° to 30° clockwise or counterclockwise for
optimum visualization. To trace the left anterior
descending branch (LAD), one continues to visualize the LAD
segment from main LCA, following anterially near the plane
of the pulmonic valve, and continuing inferiorly along the
anterior interventricular groove toward the ventricular
apex. The LAD may be best seen by modified long axis view.
To detect the right coronary artery (RCA), one uses
techniques similar to those used for LCA detection, but
moves the transducer inferiorly to find the tricuspid
annulus. At this point, one can see proximal third of RCA.
Beyond this portion of RCA, there are no good anatomical
landmarks distinguishable by 2-D echo. Parts of distal RCA
may be seen on subxiphoid view.

During the first two weeks of illness, which is
considered the acute febrile period, M-mode echo abnormalities as described below were present in 45% of the

patients studied. These abnormalities include: pericardial effusion (21%), decreased ventricular septal motion (28%) and decreased left ventricular function (10%). All children who subsequently developed coronary artery disease had one or more findings of M-mode echo abnormalities suggesting that these abnormalities were the early markers for possible coronary artery disease in Kawasaki disease. It is also interesting to note that M-mode echo showed a much higher incidence of abnormalities than did 2-D echo. This suggests that many patients with Kawasaki disease have subclinical cardiac involvement without major changes, since M-mode echo is extremely sensitive to changes in the myocardium. This also supports the pathological findings of Yutani et al. They found that some degree of inflammation of the biopsied myocardium is present in all patients with this disease.

During the acute febrile period in our patients, ECG showed first or second degree heart block and ST-T wave changes in 36% of the patients studied. These findings were normalized within six months after the onset of the disease in all children except in two infants. These two patients continued to show abnormal q-waves on ECG and 2-D echo showed multiple coronary aneurysms with left ventricular dysfunction. Abnormally deep q-waves in children after Kawasaki disease appears to be a serious finding and almost always reflects myocardial damage.

In conclusion, screening by ECG, M-mode, and 2-D echo appears to be sufficient to rule out cardiac and coronary arterial involvement in children with Kawasaki disease. Angiocardiograms should be reserved for those who require detailed anatomy of the coronary arteries for surgical planning with a high suspicion of coronary involvement which has not been visualized by 2-D echo.

REFERENCES

1. Kawasaki, T (1967). Acute febrile mucocutaneous ayndrome with lymphoid involvement with specific disquamation of the fingers and toes in children. Clinical observation of 50 cases. Jpn J Allergy 16:178-222.

2. Melish, ME (1982). Kawasaki syndrome (mucocutaneous lymph node syndrome). Pediatric Annals 11:2-11.

3. Chung KJ, Brandt L, Fulton DR et al (1982). Cardiac and coronary arterial involvement in infants and children from New England with mucocutaneous lymph node syndrome (Kawasaki disease). Amer J Cardiol 50:136-142.

4. Capannari TE, Daniels SR, Meyer RM et al (1986). Sensitivity, specifity and predictive valve of two-dimensional echocardiography in detecting coronary artery aneurysms in patients with Kawasaki disease. J Amer Coll Cardiol 7:355-360.

5. Yutani C, Go S, Kamiya T et al (1981). Cardiac biopsy of Kawasaki disease. Arch Pathol Lab Med 105:470-473.

6. Fujiwara H, Chen C, Fujiwara T et al (1980). Clinicopathologic study of abnormal Q-wave in Kawasaki disease (mucocutaneous lymph node syndrome). Amer J Cardiol 45:797-804.

7. Hakanishi T, Takao A, Kondoh C et al (1986). Q-wave in myocardial infarction after Kawasaki disease (Abst.). Circulation 74:II-206.

Kawasaki Disease, pages 383–394
© 1987 Alan R. Liss, Inc.

PATHOGENETIC MECHANISMS OF ARTERITIS IN KAWASAKI DISEASE - A CRITICAL ANALYSIS

Göran K. Hansson

Department of Clinical Chemistry, Gothenburg University, Sahlgren's Hospital, S-413 45 Gothenburg, Sweden

INTRODUCTION

Kawasaki disease is often accompanied by servere cardiovascular lesions, which may be fatal for the patient (Fujiwara et al., 1980; Japan MCLS, 1980). These lesions are basically characterized by (i) an inflammatory arteritis of the coronary arteries, (ii) an aneurysmic dilation of segments of the affected artery, and (iii) the development of a thrombosis on the surface of the vessel. None of these features is unique to Kawasaki disease; they are observed also in other vasculitides, and to some extent even in atherosclerosis. The exceptional situation in Kawasaki disease is that these phenomena occur as part of what appears to be an acute infectious illness in a young child. The fact that the vascular lesions are known from other fields of pathology merits an analysis of the condition from the point of view of basic vascular biology.

In this chapter, I will describe some of the cellular and molecular events that may underlie the vascular lesions of Kawasaki disease. I will limit the analysis to three important phenomena: endothelial injury, adhesion of platelets and leukocytes, and disturbances of vascular smooth muscle function.

ENDOTHELIAL INJURY

The vascular endothelium consists of a monolayer of flat cells, which form the interface between the blood and the vessel wall. With this location, the endothelium is the major regulator of vascular permeability, and any perturbation of the monolayer is likely to have drastic effects on the permeability of plasma components into the underlying vascular tissue (Reidy, 1985).

There is a multitude of factors that have been reported to cause endothelial injury, but unfortunately, the criteria for establishing a cytotoxic effect on the endothelium have been rather loose. The best defined system is obviously the cell culture, usually employing bovine aortic or human umbilical vein endothelium. With the use of endpoints such as trypan blue uptake or release of ^{51}Cr, both of which reflect plasma membrane damage, several endothelial cytotoxic factors have been identified (Hansson and Schwartz, 1983a). The best documentation is probably for bacterial endotoxins (Harlan et al., 1983; Reidy and Schwartz, 1983; Hansson et al., 1985), which may be relevant for the pathogenesis of Kawasaki disease, as is pointed out elsewhere in this volume. The effects of endotoxins from gram-negative bacteria on the endothelium are, however, very variable between species, and possibly also between different vascular regions (Harlan et al., 1983). In fact, human endothelium is much less sensitive to endotoxin than are bovine endothelial cells.

In vivo, it has been more difficult to identify agents that cause endothelial injury. The problem is partly due to the fact that there is a continuous, low level of spontaneous cell death and turnover in the arterial endothelium of the unmanipulated individual (Hansson and Schwartz, 1983b). This cell death is clustered in focal areas, which also exhibit a higher frequency of cell replication (Hansson et al., 1985). This implies that there are foci of increased endothelial turnover on the artery, which can be visualized by immunocytochemical techniques (Hansson and Schwartz, 1983b; Hansson et al., 1985).

This spontaneous occurrence of foci of cell injury creates a tremendous sampling problem in attempts at assessing endothelial injury by a conventional morphologic technique such as transmission electron microscopy of cross-sections, since an analysis of such a focus will show a much higher frequency of dead cells, than an analysis of a surrounding area (Hansson et al., 1985). For in vivo studies, techniques which visualize endothelial cells en face and permit the sampling of large numbers of cells, are therefore recommended. The two best characterized methods are the direct indentification of dead cells by immunocytochemistry (Hansson and Schwartz, 1983b), and the indirect method of identifying cells in S-phase of the cell cycle by ^{3}H-thymidine autoradiography

(Schwartz and Benditt, 1973). Their majordrawbacks are that both methods are rather laborious, and that they can only be used for experimental animals. For studies of human endothelial cells, one therefore has to rely on cell culture experiments.

Studies of experimental models of atherosclerosis show that the earliest event that occurs, e.g. after the initiation of cholesterol feeding in the rabbit, is injury to the endothelium (Bondjers et al., 1977). This is a true cell injury, characterized by deteriorating intermediate metabolism, plasma membrane defects, and finally overt cell death (Hansson and Bondjers, 1980; Hansson and Bondjers, 1986).

At later stages of hypercholesterolemia, endothelial injury occurs predominantly in the shoulder region of the atherosclerotic lesion, which is the growth region of the lesion (Bondjers et al., 1977; Hansson and Bondjers, 1980). Endothelial injury therefore appears to be central to both initiation and progression of the disease - although we know very little about the molecular mechanisms involved in the destruction of endothelial cells in atherosclerosis.

This contrasts with the situation for Kawasaki disease, where an important cytotoxic mechanism has been identified by Leung et al. (1986). As is described in detail in another chapter of this volume, they have shown that sera from patients with Kawasaki disease contain complement-activating antibodies that recognize an endothelial surface antigen. Antibody binding to the endothelium will therefore result in complement-mediated lysis of the cell. The endothelial antigen is, however, not constitutively expressed by the endothelium; its synthesis is induced by gamma interferon, which is a secretion product of activated T lymphocytes. This antibody-dependent endothelial cytolysis therefore requires the presence of activated T cells in the vicinity of the endothelium, or alternatively, high systemic gamma-interferon levels. In any event, it highlights the importance of interactions between the immune system and the vessel wall for the development of arterial lesions in Kawasaki disease.

One fascinating aspect of Kawasaki disease is that vascular lesions appear selectively in the coronary arteries (Fujiwara et al., 1980; Japan MCLS, 1980). This is difficult to explain from our current knowledge of the regional variations in the vasculature. We do know, however, that spontaneous endothelial injury is non-randomly distributed over the aortic surface in the rat, with foci of increased cell death and replication (Hansson et al., 1985). It has furthermore been proposed that hemodynamic pertubations such as turbulence and the appearance of low-shear and/or high-shear regions, promotes the development of endothelial injury (Fry, 1968; Nerem and Cornhill, 1980; Davies et al., 1986). Finally, it is obvious from epidemiology that certain risk factors are more important in one region of the vasculature than in another; for instance, hypercholesterolemia is an important risk factor for coronary atherosclerosis, but less important for atherosclerosis of the leg arteries, where smoking is totally dominant (Hopkins and Williams, 1981). None of these observations explain the selectivity for the coronaries in the case of Kawasaki disease. They clearly illuminate, however, the importance of realizing that the endothelium is not an entirely homogenous cell layer throughout the vasculature, but subject to variations in structure, metabolism, and other features as part of a regional specialization.

INTERACTIONS BETWEEN BLOOD CELLS AND VESSEL WALL

It has been proposed by Ross and others, that endothelial injury leads to an exposure of the subendothelial collagen, which induces platelet sticking, aggregation, and release of platelet constituents (Ross et al., 1977; Ross, 1986). Among these, the platelet-derived growth factor (PDGF), is both a chemoattractant and a growth promoter for smooth muscle cells (Ross et al., 1986). The model has essentially been verified for arterial injury models in which a balloon catheter is used to remove the endothelium (and part of the subendothelial intima); this damage is followed by a repair response characterized by platelet aggregation, smooth muscle migration into the intima, and finally, a drastic proliferation of intimal smooth muscle cells (Ross et al., 1977).

It is, however, less clear whether PDGF is involved in the response to more subtle - and pathophysiologically more relevant - types of vascular injury. Reidy and Schwartz (1981) have shown that removal of endothelial cells per se does not lead to platelet aggregation, or to the formation of an intimal tickening. Instead, the critical event appears to be a damage to the subendothelial structural components. Even a massive toxic assault on the endothelium, which occurs in endotoxinemia, does not cause any significant platelet sticking (Hansson et al., 1985).

The intimal lesion of the Kawasaki arteritis appears to be an exception in at least two respects: it is covered by a significant thrombus, and it is associated with an increase rather than a decrease in vascular diameter (Fujiwara et al., 1980; Japan MCLS, 1980). This clearly indicates that we must look for additional factors that contribute to the Kawasaki arteritis, in addition to those which initiate the repair process of the intima.

It is important to realize that the endothelium has a tremendous capacity to repair defects in the monolayer. After spontaneous endothelial cell death both in vivo and in vitro, the subendothelium is exposed only during a few minutes before the defect is covered by migrating neighbour cells (Hansson and Schwartz, 1983b). Instead, the dead cell remains in the monolayer for a long time while the reorganization of the monolayer takes place, and this is both an advantage and a disadvantage for the vessel. We have calculated the residence time of a dying endothelial cell in the rat aorta, and found it to be up to 24 hours (Hansson and Schwartz, 1983). During this period, the dying cell can be the target for pathophysiologic reactions which may initiate a disease process in the artery. The continuity of the endothelial monolayer is therefore maintained at the expense of rapid removal of defective cells, and the price paid for this is the presence of dying cells in the monolayer.

The platelets which form the surface thrombus of Kawasaki arteritis have at least two different structures to stick to: the subendothelial collagen, which may after all be exposed in this particular lesion, and the injured endothelial cell. The remnants of an endothelial cell that has been lysed, e.g. by the mechanism elucidated by Leung et al. (1986), will expose cytoskeletal structures to the circulating blood. Among these structures are intermediate filaments, which carry Fc receptors for IgG (Hansson et al., 1984). Immune complexes may therefore bind to these filaments, and unbound Fc ends of the complexes could be recognized by surface Fc receptor-carrying cells such as platelets. Monocytes and granulocytes, which both carry Fc receptors, might also be recruited by such a mechanism.

If this proposed mechanism is correct, one would expect the sticking of platelets and leukocytes to be reduced in the presence of an excess of free immunoglobulins, which would compete with immune complexes for binding to cytoskeletal Fc receptors. In this context, it is fascinating to notice that infusion of gammaglobulin significantly reduces cardiovascular complications in

Kawasaki disease (Newburger et al., 1986). It would be interesting to learn whether Fc fragments are also effective in this respect. Alternatively, the administration of gamma-globulin might transfer regulatory antibodies to the patients.

Finally, lymphocytes are also found in the vascular lesions of Kawasaki patients (Fujiwara et al., 1980), as well as in atherosclerosis and other vascular diseases (Jonasson et al., 1986). One mechanism for recruitment of lymphocytes to the vessel wall has been identified by Masuyama et al. (1986). They found that $CD4$-positive T-helper cells bind to endothelial cells that express class II MHC antigens (Ia antigens), and in culture, this binding was dependent on pretreatment of endothelium with gamma interferon, which is a product of activated T cells. Gamma interferon can also render the endothelium the capacity to present foreign antigens to T cells, by inducing the expression of class II antigens (Pober et al., 1983). This could be important for the development of autoimmune responses to the vasculature in Kawasaki disease.

Lymphocyte activation may thus be important for both recruitment of T cells to the vessel wall, antigen presenting capacity of vascular cells, and induction of specific endothelial antigens to which antibodies may develop in Kawaski disease. The conditions which activate T lymphocytes may therefore turn out to be crucial for our understanding of the pathogenesis of this arteritis.

SMOOTH MUSCLE FUNCTION IN ARTERITIS

Vascular smooth muscle cells exhibit prominent responses to several products of both monocytes and lymphocytes, and the phenotypic changes that smooth muscle cells undertake during these responses may be important in the pathogenesis of arteritis, in Kawasaki disease as well as in other conditions.

The best established of these interactions is the response of smooth muscle cells to PDGF, which is transported in the alpha granules of platelets and released during platelet activation (Ross et al., 1986). As mentioned above, medial smooth muscle cells respond chemotactically to a PDGF gradient and migrate up into the intima in response to PDGF released from degranulating platelets on the vascular surface (Ross, 1986; Ross et al., 1986). Once in the intima, these smooth muscle cells start proliferating, and thereby form an intimal thickening (Ross et al., 1977). The growth-promoting effect of PDGF has been characterized in great detail; PDGF is a commitment factor, which stimulates the entrance of G_0 cells into the cell cycle (Ross et al., 1986). On the molecular level, the growth factor acts by inducing the phosphorylation of tyrosin residues in its receptor (Heldin and Westermark, 1984). This, in turn, starts a series of metabolic reactions in the membrane and cytoplasm of the target cell, which result in DNA synthesis as well as reorganization of structural cellular components (Ross el al., 1986).

The platelet is, however, only one of many cells which can express the PDGF genes (Ross et al., 1986). Monocytes and macrophages are, in fact, important PDGF producers (Shimakado et al., 1985), and in the arteritic lesion, they may be as important as sources of PDGF, as the platelet. In addition, PDGF is also secreted by endothelial cells, at least under cell culture conditions (DiColieto and Bowen-Pope, 1983). The role of the endothelial-derived PDGF is, however, uncertain in the pathophysiology of arteritis.

Other secretory products of macrophages may be more deleterious to smooth muscle cells. The activated macrophage is a rich source of proteases and of oxygen radicals (Nathan et al., 1980; Niwa and Schmiya, 1984), which may both injure the vascular cell and thus contribute to the tissue destruction that is seen in arteritis. Finally, the macrophage produces a procoagulant activity (Schwartz and Edgington, 1981), and this could be important for the formation of the mural thrombus in Kawasaki arterititis.

It has recently been clarified that smooth muscle cells, as well as endothelial cells, are affected by T-cell lymphokines. In vitro, smooth muscle cells respond to gamma interferon by expression of class II MHC antigens, implying that they can acquire the molecular apparatus required for antigen presentation (Jonasson et al., unpublished observations).

In animal studies, the MRL mouse has been shown to develop arteritis in addition to other inflammatory lesions on an auto-immune basis (Moyer and Reinish, 1984). Arterial smooth muscle cells of these mice express class II MHC antigens and apparently present autoantigens to autologous T cells, which induce the destructions of the smooth muscle cells by cell-mediated immune responses (Moyer and Reinish, 1984). Moreover, we have recently observed that a number of intimal smooth muscle cells express class II MHC antigens during the normal arterial response to injury (Jonasson et al., unpublished observations). The expression of these antigens occurs concomitantly with the infiltration of lymphocytes into the vessel wall and is blocked by inhibitors of T-cell activation, implying that the expression of these antigens by smooth muscle cells is under T-cell control (Hansson et al., unpublished observations).

Finally, in man, smooth muscle cells of atherosclerotic plaques express the class II antigens, HLA-DR and HLA-DQ, in high frequency, and again, there is a significant infiltration of T cells into the tissue (Jonasson et al., 1985). In fact, T cells - mainly T-helper cells - constitue up to 20% of the cells in the fibrous cap of atherosclerotic plaques (Jonasson et al., 1986).

In Kawasaki arteritis, T cells are apparently even more frequent than in atherosclerosis, and it appears likely that the smooth muscle population may contain class II antigen-expressing cells. If this is the case, it could be important for autoimmune responses to vascular antigens.

Recent studies indicate that gamma interferon can exert other effects on target cells than induction of class II antigens. Amento et al. (1985) have found that recombinant gamma inter-feron, when added to cultured fibroblasts, inhibit the synthesis of collagens. If this is the case also for smooth muscle cells, it could hamper the resistance of the vessel to mechanical strain, and this could explain the occurrence of aneurysms in Kawasaki disease.

The pathogenetic mechanisms described in this article are summarized in Figure 1, which is a cartoon with a very significant speculative component. The initiating event may be a viral or bacterial infection, or perhaps an allergic reaction. These etiolo-gical factors are discussed in other chapters of this volume. The activation of the T-helper cells results in the secretion of lymphokines, among them gamma interferon (γIFN), which in turn induces the expression of specific endothelial antigens. An anti-body response to such antigens results in a complement-mediated cytolysis of endothelial cells (EC). This is followed by the binding of platelets and monocytes to the injured endothelium, possibly due to Fc-dependent mechanisms.

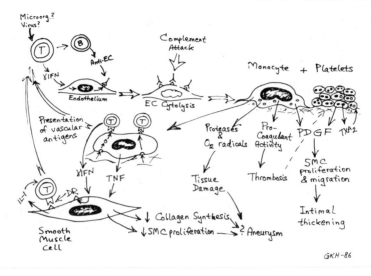

Figure 1. Pathogenetic mechanisms.

Both platelets and monocyte/macrophages release PDGF, which stimulate the migration and proliferation of smooth muscle cells (SMC) in the forming intimal thickening. In addition, the release of thromboxane A_2 (TxA_2) by platelets and of procoagulant activity by monocytes could increase the tendency to thrombus formation, and monocytes may induce tissue damage via free radicals and proteases. Finally, monocytes can serve as antigen-presenting cells, which could amplify an autoimmune reaction.

T lymphocytes may be recruited to the arteritis by mechanisms such as chemotactic attraction by interleukin-1 (IL-1) released from monocytes (Cavender et al., 1986) and possibly also smooth muscle cells (Libby et al., 1986), and binding to gamma-interferon-induced endothelial cells (Masuyama et al., 1986).

Vascular autoantigens, or exogenous, microbial antigens, may be presented to T cells both by monocytes and by smooth muscle and endothelial cells, which seem to acquire antigen-presenting capacity after exposure to gamma interferon. In addition, gamma interferon could reduce collagen synthesis by smooth muscle cells, which could promote the development of aneurysms. Other monokines and lymphokines, such as tumour necrosis factor (TNF) and the interleukins, might perhaps also modulate functions of the vascular cells.

It would be interesting to test these hypotheses by intervening with T cell activation, lymphokine-target cell interactions, and growth factor-induced smooth muscle proliferation. This obviously requires good experimental animal models, and it is important to develop and refine such models for the study of Kawasaki disease. The ultimate goal of this work would be to improve the therapeutic potential offered to Kawasaki disease patients.

ACKNOWLEDGEMENT

My work has been supported by the Swedish Medical Research Council (proj. 6816) and the Swedish National Association against Heart and Chest Disease.

REFERENCES

Amento EP, Bhan AK, McCullagh KS, Krane SM (1985). Influences of gamma interferon on synovial fibroblast-like cells. Ia induction and inhibition of collagen synthesis. J Clin Invest 76:837-848.

Bondjers G, Brattsand R, Bylock A, Hansson GK, Björkerud S (1977). Endothelial integrity and atherogenesis in rabbits with moderate hypercholesterolemia. Artery 3:395-408.

Cavender DE, Haskard DO, Joseph B, Ziff M (1986). Interleukin 1 increase the binding of human B and T lymphocytes to endothelial cell monolayers. J Immunol 136:203-207.

Davies PF, Remuzzi A, Gordon EJ, Dewey CF, Gimbrone MA (1986). Turbulent fluid shear stress induces vascular endothelial cell turnover in vitro. Proc Natl Acad Sci 83:2114-2117.

DiCorleto PE, Bowen-Pope DF (1983). Cultured endothelial cells produce a platelet-derived growth factor-like protein. Proc Natl Acad Sci 80:1919-1923.

Fry DL (1968). Acute vascular endothelial changes associated with increased blood velocity gradients. Circul Res 22:165-197.

Fujiwara H, Fujiwara T, Kao T-C, Ohshio G, Hamashima Y (1980). Pathology of Kawasaki disease in the healed state. Relationships between typical and atypical cases of Kawasaki disease. Acta Pathol Japon 36:857-867.

Hansson GK, Bondjers G (1980). Endothelial proliferation and atherogenesis in rabbits with moderate hypercholesterolemia. Artery 7:316-329.

Hansson GK, Schwartz SM (1983a). Endothelial cell dysfunction without cell loss. In: Cryer A (ed): "Biochemical Interactions at the Endothelium", Amsterdam, Elsevier, pp 343-361.

Hansson GK, Schwartz SM (1983b). Evidence for cell death in the vascular endothelium in vivo and in vitro. Am J Pathol 112:278-286.

Hansson GK, Starkebaum GA, Benditt EP, Schwartz SM (1984). Fc-mediated binding of IgG to cytoskeletal intermediate filaments in vascular endothelial cells. Proc Natl Acad Sci 81:3103-3107.

Hansson GK, Chao S, Schwartz SM, Reidy MA (1985). Aortic endothelial cell death and replication in normal and lipopolysaccharide-treated rats. Am J Pathol 121:123-127.

Hansson GK, Bondjers G (1986). Unpublished observations.

Hansson GK, Jonasson L, Holm J (1986). Unpublished observations.

Harlan JM, Harker LA, Reidy MA, Gajdusek CM, Schwartz SM, Striker GE (1983). Lipopolysaccharide-mediated bovine endothelial cell injury in vitro. Lab Invest 48:269-274.

Heldin C-H, Westermark B (1984). Growth factors: mechanism of action and relation to oncoogenes. Cell 37:9-20.

Hopkins PN, Williams RR (1981). A survey of 246 suggested coronary risk factors. Atheroscler 40:1-52.

Japan MCLS Research Committe (1980). Kawasaki disease, diagnosis, pathology, treatment and epidemiology. Tokyo: Institute of Public Health.

Jonasson L, Holm J, Skalli O, Gabbiani G, Hansson GK (1985). Expression of class II transplantation antigen on vascular smooth muscle cells in human atherosclerosis. J Clin Invest 76:125-131.

Jonasson L, Holm J, Skalli O, Bondjers G, Hansson GK (1986). Regional accumulations of T cells, macrophages, and smooth muscle cells in the human atherosclerotic plaque. Arteriosclerosis 6:131-138.

Jonasson L, Stemme S, Hansson GK (1986). Unpublished observations.

Leung DYM, Collins T, Lapierre LA, Geha RS, Pober JS (1986). IgM antibodies present in the acute phase of Kawasaki syndrome lyse cultured vascular endothelial cells stimulated by gamma interferon. J Clin Invest 77:1428-1435.

Libby P, Ordovas JM, Birinyi LK, Auger KR, Dinarello CA (1986). Inducible interleukin-1 gene expression in human vascular smooth muscle cells. J Clin Invest 78:1432-1438.

Masuyama J-i, Minato N, Kano S (1986) Mechanisms of lymphocyte adhesion to human vascular endothelial cells in culture. T-lymphocyte adhesion to endothelial cells through endothelial

HLA-DR antigens induced by gamma interferon. J Clin Invest 88:1596-1605.

Moyer CF, Reinish CL (1984). Ia expression and antigen presentation by vascular smooth muscle cells in arteritis of MRL mice. Am J Pathol 117:380-390.

Nathan CF, Murray HW, Cohn ZA (1980). The macrophage as an effector cell. New Engl J Med 303:622-626.

Nerem RM, Cornhill JF (1980). Hemodynamics and atherosclerosis. Atherosclerosis 36:55-65.

Newburger JW, Takahashi M, Burns JC, Beiser AS, Chung KJ, et al. (1986). The treatment of Kawasaki syndrome with intravenous gamma globulin. New Engl J Med 315:341-347.

Niwa Y, Sohmiya K (1984). Enhanced neutrophilic functions in mucocutaneous lymph node syndrome, with special reference to the possible role of increased oxygen intermediate generation in the pathogenesis of coronary thromboarteritis. J Pediatrics 104:56-60.

Pober JS, Collins T, Gimbrone MA, Cotran RS, Gitlin JD, Fiers W, Clayberger C, Krensky AM, Burakoff SJ, Reiss CS (1983). Lymphocytes recognize human vascular endothelial and dermal fibroblast Ia antigen induced by recombinant immune interferon. Nature 305:726-729.

Reidy MA, Schwartz SM (1981). Endothelial regeneration. III. Time course of intimal changes after small defined injury to rat aortic endothelium. Lab Invest 44:301-308.

Reidy MA, Schwartz SM (1983). Endothelial injury and regeneration. IV. Endotoxin: A nondenuding injury to aortic endothelium. Lab Invest 48:25-34.

Reidy MA (1985). A reassessment of endothelial injury and arterial lesion formation. Lab Invest 53:513-520.

Ross R, Glomset J, Harker LA (1977). Response to injury and atherogenesis. Am J Pathol 86:675-684.

Ross R (1986). The pathogenesis of atherosclerosis - an update. New Engl J Med 314:488-500.

Ross R, Raines EW, Bowen-Pope DF (1986). The biology of platelet-derived growth factor. Cell 46:155-169.

Schwartz SM, Benditt EP (1973). Cell replication in the aortic endothelium: a new method for study of the problem. Lab Invest 28:699-707.

Schwartz BS, Edgington TS (1981). Immune complex-induced human monocyte procoagulant activity. I. A rapid unidirectional lymphocyte-instructed pathway. J Exp Med 154:882-906.

Shimokado K, Raines EW, Madtes DK, Barrett TB, Benditt EP, Ross R (1985). A significant part of macrophage-derived growth factor consists of at least two forms of PDGF. Cell 43:277-286.

Kawasaki Disease, pages 395-399
© 1987 Alan R. Liss, Inc.

DISCUSSION:

CARDIOLOGIC ASPECTS OF KAWASAKI DISEASE

Dr. D. Leung (Boston) inquired about the basis for Dr. Kato's estimate of 2% incidence for aneurysms of vessels other than coronary arteries. Dr. Kato (Kurume) indicated that this figure is derived from peripheral angiographic data. Dr. M. Takahashi (Los Angeles) noted that Dr. Kato's data are the most comprehensive long-term data available and that his own data confirm that a high percentage of coronary aneurysms regress with time. The frequency of such regression is related to the configuration of the aneurysm, the severity of the initial illness, and the age at onset, with younger infants more likely to resolve their aneurysms. Dr. Takahashi emphasized the great importance of giant aneurysms and asked if any special therapy was useful for this subclass. Dr. Kato suggested that aspirin alone was probably inadequate to prevent thrombi for this group. Dr. S. Shulman's (Chicago) inquiry about the relationship of Kawasaki Disease to Moya-moya suggested on one of Dr. Kato's slides led to the disclaimer that this was only a postulated relationship.

Dr. Burns (Boston) emphasized that aneurysms represent only the end of the spectrum of coronary involvement and expressed concern that there may be potential long-term consequences of milder degrees of arteritis as a result of withholding IVGG therapy. Dr. Newberger (Boston) pointed out that data show that many resolved aneurysms do not respond normally to nitroglycerin. Dr. Nakano (Shizuoka) recommended IVGG in the early stages of severe cases because it is so important to prevent giant aneurysm formation. He expressed concern about long-term consequences of Kawasaki Disease since it is nearly always complicated by coronary arteritis histologically.

Dr. Jacobs (New York) pointed out that the U.S. gamma globulin trial showed that coronary "dilatations" rather aneurysms specifically were prevented. Drs. Takahashi and Newberger agreed that the U.S. trial used the term coronary abnormalities rather than aneurysms because of the variable interpretation of ectasia or aneurysms.

Dr. Nakano (Shizuoka) emphasized the importance of classifying the severity of coronary aneurysms and uses a scale of grade I-III based on the size of the vessel, with I <4mm, II 4-8mm, and III >8mm. He believes there is a correlation between aneurysm grade, patient prognosis, and cardiac function, with a very good prognosis in the patient with a small aneurysm that regresses, in contrast to the patient with a giant aneurysm (III) that doesn't regress or that develops obstruction.

Dr. Nakano (Gifu) discussed the difficulty of detection of those at highest risk of developing coronary lesions. He has studied levels of α_1 anti-trypsinogen, retinol-binding protein, pre-albumin, albumin, and cholinesterase levels as predictors. Dr. Benson (Toronto) pointed out that review of the sensitivity and specificity of suggested predictors of risk for development of coronary abnormalities leads him to conclude that the most conservative course is to treat all Kawasaki patients with gamma globulin and that interfering with arteritis may be very important for all patients. He emphasized that coronary anatomy and physiology changes with age, pointing out that 6mm is a normal left main coronary diameter for a 17-year-old and that it is important to define normality before one can define abnormality.

Dr. Koren (Toronto) suggested that risk factors for coronary disease may differ between Caucasian and Japanese patients since in Canada young age did not appear to be a risk factor. He noted that widespread use of IVGG will tend to obscure variables by changing the natural history of the disease.

Dr. Nakano (Shizuoka) noted that he has reported six cases of aortic regurgitation in the Journal of Pediatrics and believes it is not rare. He asked about the mechanism

and pathogenesis of late onset valvular disease. Dr.
Gidding (Chicago) responded that there was no laboratory
evidence of chronic inflammation even in the patient with
histologic evidence of chronic valvulitis, normal
coronaries, and lack of ischemic changes of papillary
muscles.

Dr. Naoe (Tokyo) indicated that the basic pathologic
process is an endocarditis that can involve the valve but
doesn't produce a verrucous endocarditis. He speculated
that the more frequent involvement of the mitral valve may
relate to its proximity to the left coronary artery. In
response to Dr. Kato's question about the duration that
acute valvulitis may persist, Dr. Naoe indicated that 30-40
days or less would be the maximum.

Dr. Suzuki (Osaka) studied 17 acute, febrile patients
with daily Doppler echos and then twice weekly Dopplers
until the 28th day of illness and documented 8/17 (43%) to
have mitral regurgitation (MR), 9/17 (53%) to have tricuspid regurgitation and none to have aortic or pulmonic
regurgitation. All were mild and without murmur. She also
found 86% of those with MR but none without to have an
abnormal gallium scintigram. In addition, MR in the acute
phase was associated with a low ejection fraction by M-mode
echocardiography. MR was detectable, on average, from days
7.5 to 11.9 of illness, suggesting that it is a result of
acute carditis.

Commenting on the CASS data in adults, Dr. Bierman
noted that in Kawasaki Disease stenosis is usually distal
to a coronary aneurysm, but that the adult data may reflect
post-stenotic dilatation rather than aneurysms per se.

Dr. Melish (Honolulu) asked if any of Dr. Naoe's
patients who had died of other causes had had angiographic
evidence of aneurysms or dilatation 3 or 8 weeks after
their acute illness. Dr. Naoe indicated that the 5
patients had been collected over a 15-year period so that
clinical data were not necessarily accurate. In case 2,
the Asai score was 1. Echo and angiographic data were not
available at this time. Dr. Brown (New York) noted that
4/5 deaths from other causes seemed to have an immunologic
basis (2 infections, 2 cancers). Dr. Chung (San Diego)
asked if the coronary endothelium appeared normal at
autopsy (yes) and if similar changes were seen in the

pulmonary or cerebral arteries. Dr. Naoe reported mild
intimal thickening at the junction of the 4th and 5th
branches of the pulmonary artery, while of 85 autopsied
cases only one showed cerebral angiitis (none in these 5
cases). Dr. Kamiya (Osaka) noted that few patients who
have had angiography have subsequently died and had
autopsies. Dr. Lehman (Los Angeles) asked if serial
angiography had been performed in IVGG recipients. Dr.
Kamiya indicated not.

Dr. Rauch (Atlanta) pointed out the problems of case
definition raised by the occurrence of atypical cases of
Kawasaki Disease, particularly with the availability of
IVGG therapy. Dr. Rowley (Chicago) responded that one must
individualize case management and that she has treated some
atypical cases with IVGG and others with aspirin and
follow-up echocardiograms. Dr. Sonobe (Tokyo) indicated
that the decision to give IVGG to a patient with incomplete
Kawasaki Disease depends on the signs and symptoms and is
based on the echographic and clinical findings. Dr.
Kawasaki (Tokyo) emphasized how very difficult it is to
diagnose atypical cases early in their course. Dr. Cremer
(Heilbrunn) noted that atypical cases have been seen in
Germany and that he believes a normal white blood count and
sedimentation rate (ESR) rules out Kawasaki Disease. Dr.
Melish agreed that an elevated ESR was a must for the
diagnosis and suggested that a decreased number of T8
suppressor cells may be a useful marker. She emphasized
that it is not necessary to have a full 5 days of fever and
that she believed that some children can be diagnosed on
the second or third day of illness, with effective therapy
therefore instituted early. Dr. Shulman suggested that it
will not be possible to construct a clinical case
definition for atypical Kawasaki Disease for use by the
general medical community.

Dr. Kamiya asked how many Kawasaki patients had had
myocardial metabolic studies by MRI. Dr. Chung indicated
that a few patients had had normal MRI studies but that
spectroscopic studies reflecting myocardial energy changes
had not yet been done. Dr. Takahashi suggested that there
may be evidence of prolonged derangement of endothelial
metabolism. He also suggested that intimal proliferation
is involved in aneurysm regression but could also lead to
adverse effects such as accelerated atherosclerotic
disease. Dr. Naoe indicated that a simpler interpretation

of the data is that intimal thickening occurs as a repair mechanism in an area of disrupted and damaged media.

Dr. Hansson (Goteberg) noted that it is unclear why intimal thickening persists and progresses in some cases but regresses without scars in others. He suggested that it is important to look at the effects of growth factors released by blood-borne cells.

Kawasaki Disease, pages 401-413
© 1987 Alan R. Liss, Inc.

EFFICACIES AND RISKS OF ASPIRIN IN THE TREATMENT OF THE
KAWASAKI DISEASE

Sanji Kusakawa and Katsunori Tatara

Department of Pediatrics, Tokyo Women's Medical
College, Daini Hospital, 2-1-10, Nishiogu, Ara-
kawa-ku, Tokyo 116, Japan

This paper will discuss the efficacies and risks of
using Aspirin in the treatment of the Kawasaki Disease.
But, prior to going into that, the author will review when
and how Aspirin came to be used in treating the Kawasaki Disease in Japan.

In 1967, when Dr. Kawasaki made his first report on the
50 cases of this disease, he did not say anything about Aspirin in the clinical discussion of his disease. He had
referred to only prednisolone as being anything in the
report -- that is, as having been antipyrectic in some
cases -- but had never held steroid hormone as effective for
anything in the studies.

We, too, at our Tokyo Women's Medical College Daini Hospital, had treated many cases of our own--many clinical cases
involving that disease. At no time, however, in those early
days had we ever, as a matter of fact, used anything, not
even close to prednisolone, in any case. The reason for
that was simply that we didn't know the cause of the ailment,
that no bacterium or virus had been found   responsible for
it or that none of the antibiotics we had tried had shown
any effect. While on the other hand, the Erythrocyte sedimentation rate was "very fast", the CRP was "strongly positive" and all other symptoms, including body temperature
and rash, and all other laboratory findings resembled
Juvenile Rheumatoid Arthritis or the like of a connective
tissue disease. Steroid hormone seemed to be the most logical drug to use at that time.

Then, over the years, while the number of patients gradually increased across the country, the Health and Welfare Ministry, in 1970, took to setting up a committee named the Japan Kawasaki Disease Research Committee, to mark the launch of an official effort to probe into its causes and to initiate fullscale research into its therapies, linking that effort to the nation's therapeutic endeavors to overcome cardiovascular diseases.

Orthodoxies in efficacy   evaluation for drugs have largely consisted of the efforts to shorten the duration of an attack of fever, the duration of any specific symptom or the duration of abnormal laboratory findings. The Kawasaki disease is essentially self-limited inflammation that gives rise, in some patients, to the development of coronary aneurysms. Further, it was discovered that occlusion tended to invite myocardial infarction, resulting in patients' deaths. Ever since, the therapeutic aims directed to this disease have mainly focused on the ability to minimize the frequency of occurrence of aneurysms in the patients. Hence a drug's efficacy has also come to be measured on the basis of its abilities to curtail that frequency. It is not an exaggeration to say that the entire research on the treatment of the Kawasaki disease has heretofore hinged on the sole purpose of that point.

In 1975, five years after the organization of the research committee, we made surveys with patients in a total of 7 hospitals (A through G) in order to examine the frequencies at which aneurysms were affecting the coronary arteries in those patients. By then, we were considerably advanced in research techniques surrounding cardiac ailments to make this type of survey a worth-while project. The results are shown in Table 1.

TABLE 1. Comparison of incidence of cases with coronary aneurysm in different hospitals

Hospital	A	B	C	D	E	F	G
No. of cases	9 0	1 5	2 6	5 0	3 1	4 1	6 3
Cases with aneurysm (%)	1 9 (21.1)	3 (20.0)	6 (23.1)	5 (10.0)	6 (19.4)	1 3 (31.7)	1 3 (20.6)

Japan Kawasaki Disease Research Committee (1975)

Most hospitals in those days were treating such patients with therapeutic measures centered to the use of steroid hormone, as stated earlier in this paper. But, as it turned out, and came to our knowledge later, one hospital, identified as "D", among those covered by our surveys had used Aspirin instead and to the exclusion of other drugs. Since our surveys were principally directed at knowing the total rate of incidence of aneurysms by coronary angiography taken of all patients -- and not at discerning why the rate of incidence varied from one hospital to another, we did not take note of the fact, at the time, that the occurrence at Hospital "D" had been much lower than at others where the incidences averaged at a high 20 to 30 %.

Another important point was that those we had made were all 'retrospective' surveys, and we did not use 2-D-ECHO; therefore, the rate of incidence referred not to the actual incidence being measured but those data show the retained incidence after some months or years from the onset. It is to be noted that the coronary aneurysm left by Kawasaki disease is, in over 50% of the case, known to spontaneously regress in a matter of about a year. Hence, we must make distinction between the rate of incidence in the normal sense of the word and that which was meant to refer only to a rate of 'retained' incidence.

A retrospection of the thinking that underlay the therapeutic activities for this disease may be useful before going further in this discussion. Treatment of the disease had started in this disease when what caused it was unknown. For that reason, the physicians invented treatments depend-

ing on their observations of the symptoms. They used agents
and treatments, derived from their studies of symptoms and
laboratory findings, which they thought would give the best
cure of all in their unending series of trials and errors.
As earlier stated, their first agents consisted of antibiotics and steroid hormone.

But, in 1972, not long after the research had started
on this disease, Prof. Nagayama of Kyushu University is
said to have reported his insistence regarding the nature
of the disease: That this was a disease resulting from infection , that the use of the steroid could result in over-
modifying the patient conditions and, finally, that, inas-
much as many deaths from this disease had been caused by
aneurysmal thrombotic obstructions, the steroids, in view
of their tendency to promote blood coagulation, should be
contra-indicated for use in this disease. The Professor
is reported to have insisted, further, that Aspirin be used
instead to treat the patients to control the inflammation.

A hospital that had abided by the Professor's instruc-
tions happened to be the "D" Hospital referred to earlier.
The results achieved by this hospital were significantly
different from those which had relied on the steroid. This
distinction between the two major therapies came to be clearly recognized in about 1978.

In about 1974, or 4 years earlier than that, we, in
the Tokyo Women's Medical College Daini Hospital, had done
our versions of studies, namely, a mixed drug therapy, on
one hand, in which we tested steroids in different combinations with Warfarin and, on the other, a dosage response
test in which we compared therapeutic effects between the
steroid dosage of 2 mg/kg/day and 4 mg/kg/day. Results of
those tests are shown in Table 2.

TABLE 2. Therapeutic evaluation on coronary lesions (1)

Therapy	No.	Cases with aneurysm
prednisolone (4mg/kg/day)	3 1	7 (22.6%)
" (2mg/kg/day)	3 4	8 (23.5%)
aspirirn	1 4	1 (7.1%)

Asai, Kusakawa et al. Tokyo Women's Medical College Daini Hospital (1977)

These tests revealed to us that the therapeutic effect was not necessarily better if the steroid was used in the higher dosage. The results were rather better with tests in which Aspirin had been used, as the control, than those in which the steroid had been used.

The same had held with the results of Prof. Nagayama discussed earlier and the same was holding with the results that Prof. Kato and his associates, who had succeeded to the research work of Prof. Nagayama.

Such being the general developments, the research committee under the Health and Welfare Ministry made in 1977 a comparative study and review again of all the data then available from around the country. Though it was a 'retrospective' survey, this study covered the data from a total of 691 cases. Table 3 shows the results of the first such studies made by Prof. Kato and Table 4, the results announced by the Health and Welfare Ministry committee.

TABLE 3. Therapeutic evaluation on coronary lesions (2)

Therapy	No.	Cases with aneurysm
steroid	1 6	1 0 (62.5%)
steroid + warfarin	7	2 (28.6%)
steroid + aspirin	7	0
warfarin	1	0
aspirin	2 5	1 (4.0%)
antibiotics	2 1	5 (23.8%)

Kato et al. Kurume Univ (1977)

TABLE 4. Therapeutic evaluation on coronary lesions (3)

Therapy	No.	Cases with aneurysm
steroid	9 4	4 2 (44.7%)
steroid + aspirin	7 5	2 4 (32.0%)
aspirin	2 1 9	4 8 (21.9%)
others including unknown	3 0 3	4 9 (16.2%)

Japan Kawasaki Disease Research Committee (1979)

As all of these data indicate, the results were the best with Aspirin group. And results were the worst with steroid. With this much revealed by test results, the Ministry's research committee had no choice but to make Aspirin its recommendation for the treatment and control of the disease since about 1978, and formalized its policies in that direction to publish them in a set of standards in 1980.

These standards concede that nothing has yet been es-

tablished as the true cause of the present disease and recommended that drugs that combine anticoagulating and at the
same time antiinflammatory effect be used as the first step
to cope with the disease and that a steroid of any type is
not be used as a rule to combat the disease. As drugs to
provide such effective controls, the Ministerial Committee
has selectively named, firstly, Aspirin and, secondarily,
such agents as Flurbiprofen.

Regarding the best dosages at which Aspirin may be
used, the Health and Welfare Ministry team was divided in
opinions with some recommending a dosage of 100 mg/kg/day
or even higher, in order to most importantly suppress the
inflammation as in the case of dosages for arthritis,
while others did not advise such dosages for fear of high dose
Aspirin's ability to restrain prostacyclin effects as well
as to accelerate blood coagulation. The team's final recommended dosages were documented as ranging from 30 to 100
mg/kg/day for patients with fever and 30 mg/kg/day for 2
months for those in post-fever   stage. This therapeutic
procedure rapidly spread to all parts of the country to
become in no time the therapy of 'first choice' among all
therapists.

The therapies advocated before the advent of above Ministerial recommendations had included one which went by the
name of 'steroid pulse therapy'. The appearance of the
present Ministerial therapy marked the beginning of a long
period in which no other such propositions appeared to introduce a new approach or procedure for the disease. This
blank period continued until 1983, in which year Dr. Furusho and his associates introduced their gamma-globulin therapy.

During this period, in 1981, prospective randomized
studies on the therapeutic effects of Aspirin for the Kawasaki disease were carried out by the Kawasaki Disease Research Committee. This group of studies took place on a
joint, concurrent basis, under the direction of a control-
ler, in a total of 8 hospitals, following 3 therapeutic procedures. The first procedure, which used Aspirin alone,
started at a dosage of 50 mg/kg/day to run for 30 days and,
after that period, was allowed to go down to 10 mg/kg/day.
The second, which was a flurbiprofen group, went at 4 mg/
kg/day for 30 days but was allowed to switch to Aspirin
after that period. The third procedure prescribed 2 mg/kg/

day of prednisolone, and 5 mg/kg/day of Dipyridamole, each for 7 days, followed by the same dosage of Dipyridamole alone for 30 days, and a switch thereafter to Aspirin. All of these procedures stipulated the patients to be no older than 4 years, to be capable of joining the test, at the latest, on their 7th day of illness and, further, to have had no intake of either an Aspirin or steroid prior to that day.

These series of research were initiated in July, 1981, and were concluded in October, 1982. The total cases studied ran up in number to 345. But 39 of them had for various reasons dropped out from the program before it concluded, 15 months later, with a net count of cases at 306. Results of those studies are summed up in Table 5.

TABLE 5. Cases with coronary lesion in groups treated with three different protocols.

Protocol	No.	initial exam	I Mo	2 Mo	I Yr	2 Yr	3 Yr
aspirin	I O I	I 6 (15.8)	2 2 (21.8)	I I (10.9)	I (1.0)	I (1.0)	I (1.0)
flurbiprofen	I O 4	I 3 (12.5)	4 O (38.5)	2 7 (26.0)	I 2 (11.5)	I O (9.6)	7 (6.7)
prednisolone dipyridamole	I O I	I 4 (13.9)	2 7 (26.7)	2 O (19.8)	9 (8.9)	6 (5.9)	5 (5.0)

(%)

Japan Kawasaki Disease Research Committee (1981~1982)

The ECHO tests immediately after hospitalization had found coronary abnormalities with 15.8%, 12.5%, and 13.9% of patients in the three respective groups, which were practically no different in age and sex. One month after the initiation of studies, the Aspirin-dosed group showed somewhat lower than the other groups but there was practically no statistical difference between the three groups. The same generally held with the groups after 2 months of observation, but whatever variances existed were now more visible than before. The same tendencies were observed more clearly each year thereafter, during the next 3-year period in which the same observation was continued. With the Aspirin group the dilatation or aneurysms were observable with 1% of the patients in 3 years, but the percentages were 6.7% and 5%, respectively, with the Flurbiprofen and prednisolone groups.

An analysis of such results seems to permit a summation that the 3 groups compared without much difference between them until the end of their 1st month of observation, but that the Aspirin group began to stand out, better and clearly, over the others the second month and onward. While coronary inflammation regressed sharply in the Aspirin group during those periods, such signs of normalization were not remarkable in either of the other groups. That is to say, in other words, that Aspirin helped little to prevent the occurrence of aneurysms but that it helped to rapidly normalize the affected coronary arteries once the disease had left its acute phase.

Early in this year, 1986, therapeutic data were collected on up to one year of gamma-globulin usage by Furusho and his associates. These data are believed to evidence Aspirin's visible effects on patients who are in the process of recovering from the disease. (Table 6)

TABLE 6. Incidence of coronary lesion in cases treated with aspirin

	No.	initial exam	1 Mo	2 Mo	1 Yr	2 Yr	3 Yr
Jul. '81 ~Oct. '82	101	15.8	21.8	10.9	1.0	1.0	1.0
Oct. '83 ~Feb. '84	75	9.3	20.3	14.9	4.1	——	——

Japan Kawasaki Disease Research Committee   aspirin 50 mg/kg/day

	No.	initial exam	1 Mo	2 Mo	1 Yr	2 Yr	3 Yr
Apr. '83 ~Apr. '84	45	0	31.1	26.7	6.7	——	——

Furusho et al.   aspirin 30～50 mg/kg/day

※ Exclusion of cases that were confirmed coronary lesion by the initial examination at admission

As will be seen, this collection of information included data, also, from the first 3 years of research made
by the Ministry's Research Committee No. 1 and, further,
part of data from the Ministry's Research Committee No. 2,
conducted by Ohkuni and others, each referring to the results from their respective Aspirin groups. Those shown
at the bottom are the results from Furusho's Aspirin group.
It will be seen that, despite the results that somewhat differed from one another between these groups, and, further,
despite their incidence on coronary dilatation or aneurysms
are different in each group from the others for about two
months, the data came to agree, from group to group, in
showing a conspicuous reduction within the period of a year
thereafter.

There is another problem in using Aspirin for K.D.
This is the problem of time when Aspirin is started to be
used during the acute stage. There is one study. This
shows when Aspirin is used within 7 days of illness, the
incidence is 17% while the others 24% (Table 7).

TABLE 7. Incidence of coronary lesion in cases treated with
aspirin

within 7th day of illness	after 8th day of illness
2 1 / 1 2 3 (17%)	2 1 / 8 8 (24%)

P < 0.1

Japan Kawasaki Disease Research Committee (1979)

I would like to consider why Aspirin has such efficacy. Two factors can be considered in trying to answer
that question: First, Aspirin's potential effect to control arterial inflammation and, second, its effect as a control of blood coagulation. The former is hard to validate,
considering the rates of incidence of the aneurysms for the
Aspirin group shown in the results. Gamma-globulin can be
credited far better on that potential as these results

duly bear out. The factor to consider, then, is the latter, which is blood coagulation. The question to ask here is about the degree to which intravascular coagulation could occur in the aneurysms, and adhere to the endothelium.

With so much input as background, we shall attempt to take a fresh look at the potential efficacy of Aspirin as a control of the Kawasaki disease. First, I shall assess Aspirin's potential to control inflammation. Its anti-inflammatory effect, orally, can never be said too high or remarkable, because it is not easily absorbed in the intestines. Recently, Aspirin has come to be dosed by intraveneous injection but its effect still remains unclarified. If this intraveneous attempt is to meet with success, it is still premature to project when it will ever become a reality.

Any hope that seems to remain will then be with the agent's anti-coagulation potential. As the available test results indicate, such potential if any can be derived, it seems, only from dosing at the lower levels. What must be argued in this connection is, firstly, the conventional thinking that Aspirin has not been much of a control for inflammation in the area of the coronary artery.

It is true that the gamma-globulin will admittedly serve to curtail the incidence of the aneurysms sharply in the first month it is used. It must be noted, however, retained incidence of aneurysms, not occurring incidence, will not be significantly better than Aspirin in the years after that. Some contend, and to a degree we can agree to the contention, that this disease can best be checked at stage of incidence than later, because its aftereffects can damage vascular wall and eventually invite arteriosclerosis.

That argument need, however, be discounted against the fact that the gamma-globulin is an agent very expensive to use clinically. Further, it should be noted that the agent associates with a danger of overuse, which can invite loss in immune functions, and with the danger of producing occasional shock. The question we want to ask here is whether it is already safe enough to use the gamma-globulin with every patient that comes our way with the disease. I do not know yet. So I believe gamma-globulin should not be used for every patient, but should be used only for severe cases if it could be predicted.

Side-effects of the Aspirin were limited in the scope of appearance in our experience, the hepatic disturbances being the most important of them all, except Reye syndrome. About Reye syndrome I don't want to speak today. There is no relation among K.D. and Aspirin and Reye. As will be seen from Table 8, 9 cases of a total 80 had shown a GOT level of 500 or higher. Those symptoms resolved rapidly as soon as the dosing was stopped. None was considered to be serious in nature.

TABLE 8. Maximum GOT level in groups treated with three different protocols

GOT (K.U.)	aspirin		flurbiprofen		prednisolone dipyridamole	
0~ 49	44	55	59	75	66	80
50~ 99	13	16	7	9	11	13
100~199	7	9	7	9	4	5
200~299	4	5	0		1	1
300~399	3	4	1	1	1	1
400~499	0		1	1	0	
500~999	9	11	3	4	0	
1000~	0		1	1	0	
Total	80	100%	79	100%	83	100%

Japan Kawasaki Disease Research Committee (1981 - 1982)

Considering both merits and demerits, we have compared Aspirin with gamma-globulin in our case studies to draw a semblance of conclusions to the effect that they come to perform about the same in controlling the Kawasaki disease, given the timeframe of about a year. We reason that, while the gamma-globulin goes far in curtailing the incidence of the aneurysm, Aspirin proves strong in repairing the disturbances. When we consider the effort of combatting the Kawasaki disease with an international perspective, we cannot help the view that the number of countries that can financially afford the use of gamma-globulin is still limited but that such is not the case with the use of Aspirin. It already permits universal usage. Its efficacy should be termed high and great -- measured on that yardstick.

REFERENCES

Kato H, Koike S, Yokoyama T (1979). Kawasaki Disease:
Effect of Treatment on Coronary Artery Involvement. Pediatrics 63:175-179.
Kawasaki T (1967). M.C.L.S.-clinical observation of 50
cases (in Japanese). Jap J Allergy 16:178-222.
Kusakawa S (1983). Long-term Administrative Care of Kawasaki Disease. Acta Pediatrica Japonica Overseas Edition
25:205-209.
Kusakawa S (1983). Therapeutic study of Kawasaki disease
in acute stage (in Japanese). Acta Ped Jap 87:2486-2491.

Kawasaki Disease, pages 415–424
© 1987 Alan R. Liss, Inc.

SALICYLATES IN KAWASAKI DISEASE – A REVIEW OF CLINICAL
PHARMACOKINETICS AND EFFICACY

Gideon Koren* M.D., ABMT

Division of Clinical Pharmacology, Research
Institute and Department of Pediatrics, The
Hospital for Sick Children, Toronto

Salicylates are the corner stone of drug therapy in
Kawasaki Disease (KD) because of their potential antiplatelet effects (Pedersen et al, 1984) and anti-
inflammatory properties (Goodman and Gillman, 1985).
Whereas very low doses of salicylates are needed to
achieve acetylation of platelet cyclooxygenase (Pedersen
et al, 1984), much higher doses are needed to maintain
effective anti-inflammatory serum concentrations.

During the last few years evidence has accumulated
that the disposition of salicylates in KD is very different from healthy or febrile children. In this communication, I wish to present the unique characteristics of
salicylate pharmacokinetics in KD and to critically
review studies which evaluated its clinical efficacy.

Difficulty in Achieving Therapeutic Serum Concentrations:

In 1979, Jacobs documented that during the acute,
febrile phase of KD, it is very difficult to achieve serum
concentrations of salicylates within the therapeutic range
extrapolated from rheumatoid arthritis (15–30 mg/dl).
Doses as high as 180 mg/kg are often not capable of
achieving theraputic serum concentrations (Fig. 1). For
comparison, in healthy children accidently exposed to
salicylates, or in febrile children, therapeutic concentrations are generally achieved with 30–40 mg/kg/day
(Wilson et al, 1982), whereas doses in the range of

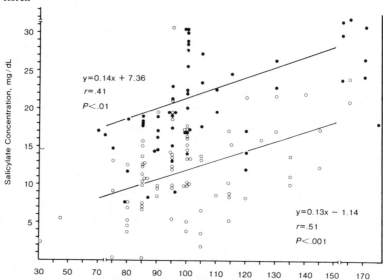

Figure 1. Salicylate serum concentrations during febrile phase (open circles) are on average twofold lower than those achieved with same dose during subsequent normothermic phase (closed circles) (Reprinted with the permission of the American Medical Association from Koren et al, JAMA 254:767-769, 1985).

100-180 mg/kg are usually associated with various degrees of toxicity (Goldfrank, 1982).

Under steady state conditions, serum concentrations of a drug are governed by its systemic bioavailability (F) and clearance (Cl) according to Equation I (Gibaldi and Perrier, 1982):

$$\text{Conc.} = \frac{\text{Dose x F}}{\text{Cl x Dose interval}} \qquad (I)$$

Hence, the lower salicylate concentrations in KD may potentially result from impaired bioavailability, enhanced clearance or both.

Impaired Bioavailability

Bioavailability of a drug is defined as the fraction of the parent drug which enters   the systemic circulation (Gibaldi and Perrier, 1982). If all the drug given

orally arrives at the systemic circulation, then concentrations over time (AUC) with the oral dose should equal
those achieved with a similar IV dose. In such a case
bioavailability is considered to be complete (100%).

A drug may not fully arrive at the systemic circulation either because it is not absorbed, or because it is
metabolized during its first pass through the liver. In
the latter case, the metabolites can be recovered in the
blood.

In the case of salicylates, the systemic bioavailability is considered to be almost complete (Goodman and
Gillman, 1985); if one collects 24 hr urine, one should be
able to recover almost all the given dose either as salicylic acid or as one of its metabolites. Studies by
Jacobs and from our laboratory have shown that during the
febrile phase of KD less than half of the administered
dose of aspirin is absorbed (Jacobs, 1982; Koren and
MacLeod, 1984) and recovered in the urine. In a small
number of subject, Jacobs could recover the non-absorbed
salicylates in the feces.

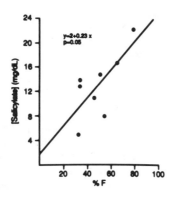

Figure 2. Correlation between salicylate bioavailability
(F) and mean steady state serum concentrations in the
febrile phase of KD.

In a controlled study completed by us recently, we could show the changes in salicylate absorption using children as their own control. During the acute phase the mean dose recovered in the urine was 47.7 $\pm$ 6.6%, whereas during the subsequent subacute phase it increased to 75.1 $\pm$ 9.3% (p < 0.01). These changes are consistent with the signficantly lower steady state serum concentrations achieved with a given dose (8; Fig. 1) during the acute phase compared to the subacute phase.

In the 8 children studied, there was a good correlation between systemic bioavailability in the acute phase and steady state mean serum concentrations (Fig. 2).

The mechanisms leading to malabsorption of salicylates in KD are not clear. This illness is not usually characterized by gastrointestinal symptoms and signs, and therefore no studies on absorption of nutrients or other pharmacological agents have been reported. Of interest, we could show in a small group of children, that despite salicylate malabsorption, adequate serum concentrations of other drugs were achieved (theophylline, digoxin and barbiturates). High gastric pH is known to modulate salicylate absorption in two different ways: Dissociation of the tablets is more rapid on the one hand, but absorption of the ionized molecules is slower on the other hand. It is believed that these two factors cancel each other in a way that the extent of absorption of aspirin is only marginally affected (Levy et al, 1979).

Changes in Salicylate Clearance

We recently showed the changes in elimination of salicylates during the febrile phase by comparing salicylate renal clearance during the acute phase (15.8 $\pm$ 2.8 ml/kg/ hr) to the subacute phase (7+1.6 ml/kg/min) (p < 0.05). Salicylates are unique in that two of the main metabolic patterns (glucuronidation to salicyluric and salicyl phenolic) are of limited capacity and therefore saturable (Levy et al, 1972). Characteristically, at higher concentrations, the elimination of salicylates from the serum follows zero order kinetics, whereas at lower concentrations it follows first order kinetic behaviour. Consequently, at higher serum concentrations clearance values of salicylates are lower (Fürst et al, 1979).

This fact is of great importance in interpreting our comparison of clearance values. Under normal circumstances, clearance values should be lower in the same child during higher serum concentrations. The fact that during the acute phase clearance rates are faster is, therefore, a unique characteristic of KD.

Several mechanisms control the clearance rate of salicylates:

The hepatic metabolic rate: Most of the body load of salicylates is metabolized in the liver to salicyluric acid (SUA) or phenolic glucuronide (Gluc). A small percentage is metabolized by other pathways and yet another portion is excreted by the kidney as unchanged salicylic acid (SA) (Levy, 1977).

We recently compared the secretion of salicylate metabolites in the urine of children with KD and found it to be similar to that in children with juvenile rheumatoid arthritis. This suggests that the enhancement of salicylate clearance during the acute phase of KD is not due to change in the metabolic rate of salicylates.

Urinary pH: Alkalinization of the urine results in ionization of the weak salicylic acid. Consequently, less SA is available for reabsorption and salicylate clearance will increase (Furst et al, 1979). In alkaline urine, significantly more salicylate will be secreted as SA. During the febrile phase of KD we could show a correlation between renal clearance and urinary pH. Moreover, high clearance values corresponded to larger percentage of SA in the urine. However, urinary pH did not differ in the acute and subacute phase and therefore it is unlikely to be the mechanism of increased clearance.

Protein binding: Salicylates have a high protein binding in the serum (Goodman and Gilman, 1985). Lowering their protein binding in uremic patients has been shown to enhance clearance (Furst et al, 1979; Borga et al, 1976). Other highly protein-bound drugs such as corticosteroids and phenytoin have been shown to have a higher clearance in patients with nephrotic syndrome due to lower albumin concentrations (Gugler and Azarnoff, 1983). By lowering protein binding, more drug is in its free form and is available for metabolic and renal elimination. In our patients with KD studied during the acute febrile phase and the subsequent subacute phase, we found significant changes in serum albumin concentrations: The febrile phase was characterized by hypoalbuminemia (2.7 ± 0.23 gr/dl), with an improvement after the fever has subsided (3.78 ± 0.21 gr/dl) (p < 0.05). The mean 30% drop in serum albumin during the acute phase may be very significant in terms of salicylate binding capacity and may lead to the enhanced clearance seen in our patients during the febrile phase.

In summary, an increase in salicylate clearance during the acute febrile phase of KD is a determinant, not recognized previously, which may lead to the difficulty in achieving therapeutic serum concentrations.

More studies are needed to explain the hypoalbuminemia seen during the acute phase of the disease.

Clinical Efficacy of Salicylates in Kawasaki Disease:

The main goal of salicylate therapy in KD is to prevent hypercoagulability and coronary vasculitis leading to coronary aneurysms and infarcts. In a broader context, an effective anti-inflamatory therapy may prevent or shorten involvement of other systems. Initial studies have shown that aspirin doses in the range of 100 mg/kg/day are needed to shorten the febrile phase of the disease (Mellish et al, 1982). Calabaro presented a typical picture in a febrile patient with KD, showing that 100 mg/kg/day caused a rapid drop of temperature to normal (Calabaro et al, 1983). In an analysis of a large number of patients with KD we could not confirm this observation (Koren et al, 1985). Typically, the drop in fever is not immediate, and it appears that only after the temperature settles, there is a gradual increase in salicylate serum concentration (Fig. 3). This suggests that the pathological process governs the absorption and clearance of salicylates and not vice versa.

Does aspirin change the natural course of Kawasaki Disease? This is undoubtedly the main question to try to answer when dealing with a disease with a high rate of coronary involvement. Only few studies tried to address

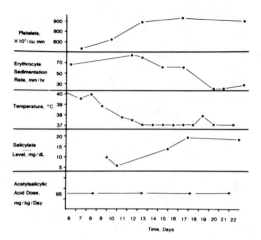

Figure 3. A typical case, showing that with fixed dose
(95 mg/kg), initial levels were subtherapeutic and subsequently increase during normothermia. Decrease in
erythrocyte sedimentation rate follows normothermia;
platelet count settles last (Reprinted with permission of
the American Medical Association from Koren et al, JAMA
254:767-769, 1985).

this question in a controlled manner and all of them have
methodological problems.

Kato and colleagues compared low dose salicylate therapy (30 mg/kg/day) to other modalities (steroids, steroids
plus salicylates and antibiotics) in small subgroups and
could not detect any advantage to salicylates over antibiotics (Kato et al, 1979). With current knowledge it is
clear that the 30 mg/kg/day given by Kato may suffice for
the antiplatelet effect but cannot be expected to reverse
coronary vasculitis.

Two studies have recently assessed the effect of high
dose salicylates versus no salicylates in patients with
KD.

We studied prospectively the disposition of salicylates in 36 children with KD. At the same time period, an
additional cohort of 18 children with comparable age and
sex distributions were hospitalized, who had not been
treated with salicylates during the acute phase because

diagnosis had not been established in time. The two
groups were comparable in the clinical and laboratory picture (Koren et al, 1985). In the treated group, the rate
of coronary disease was 17%, similar to the results of a
recent large collaborative study (Newberger et al, 1986).
In the untreated group, 50% of the children (9/18) had
coronary aneurysms. The main problem with such a study
is the non-randomized allocation of patients into the two
groups. However, it was thought unethical in our institution to prevent salicylates from some children. Even a
dose of 30 mg/kg/day was ruled unjustified knowing the
difficulties in achieving meaningful serum concentrations.

A new study from Cincinnati has arrived at similar
conclusions using a different methodological approach.
Daniels and colleagues (1986) compared the characteristics of 9 patients with coronary aneurysms to 68 without
aneurysms. They found that in the children with aneurysms,
aspirin was started significantly later (14.7 $\pm$ 3.9 days
after the onset of fever vs 9.4 $\pm$ 3.8 days, p < 0.001).
The two groups were comparable in their age and sex distributions as well as in the prescribed doses of
salicylates.

Conversely, Melish et al (1986) feel that the fact
that different groups, treated with salicylate doses
between 5-100 mg/kg·day, have aneurysm rates around 20%,
proves that high dose of salicylates may not be effective
in preventing coronary involvement. It is clear that this
controversy can be settled only through large prospective,
randomized studies.

Pathological studies from Japan have clearly indicated
that in lethal cases, coronary arteritis is present after
less than one week of fever (Fijuiwara et al, 1978).
Therefore, it is conceivable to treat patients vigorously
with high dose ASA once the diagnosis of KD has be confirmed. In many cases, treatment is postponed for several
days because the diagnosis is still controversial. Based
on current knowledge it is conceivable that the risk of
not treating the disease during the febrile phase may
overweigh the risks of high dose (but poorly absorbed)
salicylates.

As shown above, the "therapeutic range" of salicylates is not achieved in most cases even with 100 mg/kg/day. However, this range is extrapolated from rheumatoid arthritis and was never objectively proven in this disease either (Levy, 1977). Moreover, with lower albumin concentrations and presumably lower protein binding of salicylates in KD, it is possible that a higher free fraction of salicylic acid would produce an adequate anti-inflammatory effect even in the presence of lower total concentrations (Marcus et al, 1986).

CONCLUSIONS

In this review I have tried to identify several trends characteristic of salicylate disposition and effect in KD. More research is needed to identify the mechanisms leading to these peculiarities.

Because of the erratic absorption and enhanced clearance of salicylates in KD and the large interpatient variability, careful monitoring of salicylate serum concentration must accompany the course of therapy.

REFERENCES

Borga O, Odar-Cedarlof J, Ringberger VA, Norlin A (1976). Protein binding of salicylate in uremic and normal plasma. Clin Pharmacol Ther 20:464-475.

Calabro JJ, Kostylo F, Williamson PK (1983). Kawasaki disease. In Clinical Medicine. JA Spittle Jr(ed). Philadelphia, Harpers Row, 4:1-6.

Daniels SR, Specker B, Capannari TE, Schwartz DC, Burke MJ, Kaplan S (1986). Correlates of coronary artery aneurysm formation and prevention in patients with Kawasaki disease. Pediatr Res 20:169A.

Fijuiwara H, Hamashima Y (1978). Pathology of the heart in Kawasaki disease. Pediatrics 61:100-107.

Furst DE, Tozer TN, Melmon KL (1979). Salicylate clearance, the resultant of protein binding and metabolism. Clin Pharmacol Ther 26:380-389.

Gibaldi M, Perrier D (1982). "Pharmacokinetics." New York: Marcel Dekker.

Goldfrank LR (1982). "Toxicologic emergencies." New
    York: Appleton-Century-Crafts New York, pp 50-59.
Goodman LS, Gilman AG (1985). The pharmacological basis
    of therapeutics. New York: MacMillian, pp 674-689.
Gugler R, A Zarnoff LD (1983). Drug protein binding and
    the nephrotic syndrome. In: "Handbook of Clinical
    Pharmacokinetics" (Eds: Gibaldi M, Prescott L.), ADIS
    Press New York Section III, pp 96-108.
Hicks RV, Melish ME (1986). Kawasaki syndrome. In:
    Pediatric Rheumatology (Ed. Miller ML), Ped Clin N
    Amer 33:1151-1176.
Jacobs JC (1982). Pediatric rheumatology. New York:
    Springer-Verlog, pp 418-422.
Kato H, Koike S, Yokoyama T (1979). Kawasaki disease:
    Effect of treatment on coronary artery involvement.
    Pediatrics 63:175-179.
Koren G, MacLeod SM (1984). Difficulty in achieving
    therapeutic serum concentrations of salicylates in
    Kawasaki Disease. J Pediatr   :991-995.
Koren G, Rose V, Louis, Rowe R (1985). Probable efficacy
    of high-dose salicylates in reducing coronary
    involvement in Kawasaki disease. JAMA 254:767-769.
Levy G, Lampman T, Kamath BL, Garretson LK (1975).
    Decreased serum salicylate concentrations in children
    with rheumatic fever treated with antacid. N Engl J
    Med 293:323-325.
Levy G, Tsuchiya T, Amsel LP (1972). Limited capacity
    for salicyl phenolic glucuronide formation and its
    effects on the kinetics of salicylate elimination in
    man. Clin Pharmacol Ther 13:258-268.
Levy G (1977). Clinical Pharmacokinetics of aspirin.
    Pediatrics 62:(Suppl) 867-872.
Marcus SM, Bekersky J, Popick AC (1986). Pharmacokinetics
    of aspirin in Kawasaki disease. Ped Res 20:207A.
Melish MF, Hicks RV, Reddy V (1982). Kawasaki syndrome:
    an update. Hosp. Practice 17:99-111.
Newberger JW, Takahashi M, et al (1985). The treatment
    of Kawasaki disease with intravenous gamma gloublin.
    N Engl J Med 315:341-347.
Pedersen AK, Fitz Gerald GA (1984). Dose related
    kinetics of aspirin. N Engl J Med 311:1206-1211.
Wilson JT, Brow RD, Bocchini JA, Keans GL (1982).
    Efficacy, disposition and pharmacodynamics of
    aspirin, acetaminophen and choline salicylate in
    young febrile children. Ther Drug Monit 4:147-192.

Kawasaki Disease, pages 425–432
© 1987 Alan R. Liss, Inc.

JAPANESE GAMMA GLOBULIN TRIALS FOR KAWASAKI DISEASE

Kenshi Furusho, Tetsuro Kamiya, Hiroyuki Nakano,
Nobuyuki Kiyosawa, Keisuke Shinomiya, Tadashi
Hayashidera, Tokio Tamura, Osamu Hirose, Yutaka
Manabe, Tatsuo Yokoyama, Masaharu Kawarano,
Kunizo Baba, Kiyoshi Baba, Chuzo Mori, Kunitaka
Joho, and Shiro Seto

Department of Paediatrics, Kokura Memorial,
Kyoto National, Mimihara General, Wakayama Red
Cross, and Kohga Public Hospitals, National
Cardiovascular Centre, Kyoto Prefectural Univer-
sity of Medicine, Faculty of Medicine, Kyoto
University, Heart Institute, Kurashiki Central
Hospital and Shimane Medical University; Division
of Paediatric Cardiology, Shizuoka Children's,
Tenri, Kobe General, Kyushu Koseinenkin Hospi-
tals, and Osaka Medical Centre for Maternal and
Child Health; and Department of Paediatric Car-
diology, Kinki University School of Medicine,
Japan

INTRODUCTION

Kawasaki disease (KD) is self limiting but a serious
consequence is the possibility of coronary artery lesion
(CAL), and clinical research has concentrated on attempts
at preventing such lesions. Aspirin (ASA) therapy is usually advised, this being the recommendation of the Kawasaki
Disease Research Committee of Japan, but it has not been
proved to reduce the occurrence of CAL.

In 1984, we reported in a multicentre controlled trial
that high-dose intravenous gammaglobulin therapy (IVGG),
given in the acute stage of KD, is followed by a decreased
frequency of CAL. Thereafter, we completed additional two
controlled studies of IVGG in KD comparing different doses
of gammaglobulin infused, to see if lower doses than those
in first study are also effective.

We report here the results of a series of our multi-centre controlled trials of IVGG on the frequency of CAL in the children with KD.

PATIENTS AND METHODS

Sixteen institutes took part. All patients were cared by specialists in paediatric cardiology and two-dimensional echocardiograph and selective coronary arteriography were available. Patients admitted with KD in study 1 from April 1983 to April 1984, in study 2 from May 1984 to September 1985 and in study 3 from October 1985 to June 1986 were studied. Patients with incomplete or with recurrent KD were excluded, as were those whose treatment could not begin within 7 days of the onset of KD and those with CAL on admission.

Design

Study 1: Eligible patients were allocated at random to treatment with aspirin (ASA) or IVGG plus ASA. While a fever was present, ASA was administered orally at a daily dosage of 30 - 50 mg/Kg in three divided doses. From the time that the fever went until the acute reaction had also disappeared ASA was given at a dose of 10 - 30 mg/Kg once a day. The other group was given ASA (as previously) plus IVGG (S-sulphonated intact gammaglobulin; 'Venilon', Teijin Ltd, Japan) as a 5 % solution, the infusion rate being 50 drops/min at a dose of 400 mg/Kg daily, for 5 days from day 1 of treatment.

Study 2: Eligible patients were allocated at random to three treatment groups. The first group was given on IVGG at a dose of 100 mg/Kg daily, for 5 days, the second group IVGG at a dose of 200 mg/Kg daily, for 5 days, the third group IVGG at a dose of 400 mg/Kg daily, for 5 days, from day 1 treatment respectively. Each group was given ASA as previously.

Study 3: Eligible patients were allocated at random to three treatment groups. The first group was given IVGG at a dose of 200 mg/Kg daily, for 5 days, plus ASA (as previously), the second group IVGG at a dose of 200 mg/Kg daily, for 5 days, without ASA., the third group was given ASA alone as previously, from day 1 treatment respectively.

Evaluation

Two-dimensional echocardiography was done three times a week for 60 days after the onset of KD. A positive echocardiographic case was followed continuously twice a month until 12 months of the illness. The development of even a transient dilatation of coronary artery was regarded as indicating CAL. The echocardiographic criteria used were those of the Kawasaki Disease Research Committee. A positive echocardiographic report was followed by selective coronary arteriography to confirm the presence of a lesion.

Statistical Analysis

A chi square test (with Yates' correction) was used for intergroup comparison of the frequency of CAL.

RESULTS

Exclusion

100 patients in study 1, 165 patients in study 2 and 163 patients in study 3 were randomized but data from 15 cases in study 1, 20 cases in study 2 and 12 cases in study 3 not managed according to the trial protocols were excluded from the analysis, respectively.

Matching

These left 45 in ASA group and 40 in IVGG (400 mg/Kg x 5) group in study 1, 41 in IVGG (100 mg/Kg x 5) group, 51 in IVGG (200 mg/Kg x 5) group and 53 in IVGG (400 mg/Kg x 5) group in study 2, 49 in IVGG (200 mg/Kg x 5) plus ASA group, 53 in IVGG (200 mg/Kg x 5) alone group and 49 in ASA alone group in study 3. The groups in each study did not differ significantly in respect of sex ratio, age distribution, or the duration of illness before entry into the trials (Table 1, 2, 3).

TABLE 1. Distribution by sex and age and time of entry into trial in study 1

	ASA group (n = 45)	IVGG group (n = 40)
Sex		
Male	25	24
Female	20	16
Age (mo)*		
< 12	14	11
12 - 24	13	9
24 - 36	7	11
36 - 48	6	5
> 48	3	4
Time of entry to trial (days)	5.2±1.6(2-7)	5.2±1.1(3-7)

* Mean ages (± SD) were 22 ± 16 months for the ASA group and 27 ± 20 months for the IVGG group

TABLE 2. Distribution by sex and age and time of entry into trial in study 2

	IVGG (100mg/Kg x 5) (n=41)	IVGG (200mg/Kg x 5) (n=51)	IVGG (400mg/Kg x 5) (n=53)
Sex			
Male	21	30	36
Female	20	21	17
Age (mo)*			
< 12	13	15	12
12 - 24	15	13	16
24 - 36	6	8	4
36 - 48	2	9	11
> 48	5	6	10
Time of entry to trial (days)	5.3±1.1(3-7)	5.6±1.2(3-7)	5.4±1.1(3-7)

* Mean ages(±SD) were 23.7 ± 23.3 months for IVGG(100mg/Kg x 5) group, 25.7 ± 21.6 months for IVGG (200mg/Kg x 5) group, and 29.7 ± 23.6 months for IVGG (400mg/Kg x 5) group

TABLE 3 Distribution by sex and age and time of entry into trial in study 3

	ASA + IVGG (200mg/Kg x 5) (n=49)	IVGG (200mg/Kg x 5) (n=53)	ASA (n=49)
Sex			
Male	28	27	26
Female	21	26	23
Age (mo)*			
< 12	15	16	15
12 - 24	17	19	15
24 - 36	5	6	8
36 - 48	4	3	7
> 48	8	9	4
Time of entry to trial (days)	4.9±1.3(1-7)	4.9±1.3(3-7)	4.9±1.2(3-7)

* Mean ages(± SD) were 24.3±21.2 months for the ASA+IVGG group, 24.1 ± 20.0 months for the IVGG alone group, and 21.9 ± 15.1 months for the ASA alone group

Echocardiographic Findings

Echocardiographic evidence of the patients in each group of 3 studies evaluated before day 30 of the illness and on day 30 were illustrated in Fig. 1.

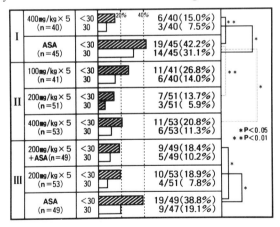

Figure 1. Echocardiographic evidence of CAL in the each treatment group of the three studies before day 30, and on day 30 of the onset of KD.

In study 1 echocardiographic evidence of CAL was significantly lower in IVGG (400 mg/Kg x 5) group than that in ASA before day 30 of the illness and on the day 30 respectively.

In study 2 three groups did not differ significantly in respect of echocardiographic evidence with each other before day 30 of the illness and on the day 30 respectively. However, as compared with the evidence of CAL of ASA group in study 1 (42.2%), the evidence in IVGG (200 mg/Kg x 5) group or in IVGG (400 mg/Kg x 5) group was significantly low, but did not differ in IVGG (100 mg/Kg x 5) group.

In study 3, as compared with ASA group both IVGG (200 mg/Kg x 5) plus ASA group and IVGG (200 mg/Kg x 5) group differed significantly in respect of echocardiographic evidence before day 30 of the illness but did not on day 30.

In long term follow up observation of CAL in study 1 the echocardiographic evidence of CAL in both ASA group and IVGG group regressed gradually. But at twelve months of the illness the lesion was still recognized in 3 of 45 cases (6.7%) in ASA group and 2 of 40 cases (5.0%) in IVGG group (Table 4).

TABLE 4. Long-term follow up observation of CAL

	Number of cases with CAL	
	ASA group (n=45)	IVGG group (n=40)
Months since onset		
1	14 (31.1)	3 (7.5)
2	12 (26.7)	2 (5.0)
3	11 (24.4)	2 (5.0)
6	8 (17.8)	2 (5.0)
9	6 (13.3)	2 (5.0)
12	3 (6.7)	2 (5.0)

( ) = %

The difference of the evidence of CAL between the two groups was significantly low in IVGG group until three months of the illness; however, thereafter it was not.

Side-effects

None of the patients had serious side-effects from receiving IVGG. One child had shaking chills with fever on day 3 of treatment with IVGG, which disappeared rapidly on discontinuation of IVGG. One child treated with IVGG had neutropenia (absolute granulocyte count < 500) with mild anemia for several months after IVGG.

DISCUSSION

We carried out a series of multicentre controlled trials of IVGG for KD from April 1983 to June 1986 to confirm the efficacy of the treatment and to decide on adequate dose of gammaglobulin infused. In KD symptoms can change rapidly, so in controlled studies matching is important. We achieved this for sex, age, duration of disease until the start of treatment, and disease severity in all three studies (Table 1, 2 and 3).

According to the results of a series of our studies some evidence in the relation between the occurrence of CAL and the treatments used would be conducted as follows: (1) The echocardiographic evidence of CAL was found in 39 % - 42 % of patients when treated by ASA alone, before day 30 of the illness (study 1 and study 3). (2) The echocardiographic evidence of CAL was decreased to 26.8% of patients when treated by IVGG (100 mg/Kg x 5), before day 30 of the illness, but this did not differ significantly as compared with ASA treatment in study 1 (study 1 and study 2). (3) The echocardiographic evidence of CAL was further reduced to 13.7 % - 20.8 % of patients when treated by IVGG (200 mg/Kg x 5) or IVGG (400 mg/Kg x 5) with or without ASA, before day 30 of the illness. This was significantly low as compared with that in ASA treatment (study 1, study 2 and study 3). (4) The echocardiographic evidence of CAL during first 3 months of the illness was significantly low in patients treated by IVGG (400 mg/Kg x 5) as compared with ASA treatment; however, thereafter the difference between the two groups did not differ significantly.

These facts suggest that when using IVGG for KD, we should select a dose of intact gammaglobulin, 1000 mg/Kg in total or more, to prevent the occurrence of CAL. Both our trials and US-trial have demonstrated not only a significant reduction in the occurrence of CAL in patients treated with IVGG but a reduced frequency of persistent dilatation beyond 30 days compared with those on ASA alone.

It is unlikely that the coronary artery damaged once by KD would normalize pathologically, even if the appearance of the coronary artery seems to be normal by echocardiography as seen in a follow up observation of CAL in study 1. Accordingly we would like to emphasize that it is most important for us to prevent the occurrence of CAL in the acute stage of KD.

It would be ideal if, before undertaking therapy of IVGG, clinicians could identify prospectively the patients in whom CAL would ultimately develop, because IVGG is very expensive and CAL do not develop in approximately 60 % of patients. However, at the present time, we can not identify any definite risk factors for the development of CAL in the initial stage of KD. Therefore, we recommend that all patients with KD should be treated, in the present time, by IVGG as soon as possible after diagnosis.

REFERENCES

Feigin RD, Barron KS (1986). Treatment of Kawasaki Disease. New Eng J Med 315: 388-390.
Furusho K, Kamiya T, Nakano H, Kiyosawa N, Shinomiya K, Hayashidera T, Tamura T, Hirose O, Manabe Y, Yokoyama T, Kawarano M, Baba K, Baba K, Mori C (1984). High-dose intravenous gammaglobulin for Kawasaki Disease. Lancet 2: 1055-1058.
Newburger JW, Takahashi M, Burns JC, Beiser AS, Chung KJ, Duffy E, Glode MP, Mason WH, Reddy V, Sanders SP, Shulman ST, Wiggins JW, Hicks RV, Fulton DR, Lewis AB, Leung DYM, Colton T, Rosen FS, Melish ME (1986). The treatment of Kawasaki Syndrome with intravenous gamma globulin. New Eng J Med 315: 341-347.

Kawasaki Disease, pages 433–439
© 1987 Alan R. Liss, Inc.

INTRAVENOUS GAMMA GLOBULIN THERAPY IN KAWASAKI DISEASE--
TRIAL OF LOW DOSE GAMMA GLOBULIN

Masahiko Okuni, Kensuke Harada, Hideo Yamaguchi,
Hiroshi Yanagawa, Tomoyoshi Sonobe,
Tomisaku Kawasaki
Research Committee of Kawasaki Disease, Tokyo,
JAPAN
Japanese Red Cross Medical Center
4-1-22 Hiroo Shibuya-ku Tokyo 150, JAPAN

INTRODUCTION

Kawasaki Disease is an acute febrile illness of unknown
cause. The optimal therapy has not yet been established.
Furusho et al (Furusho et al., 1984) and Newberger et al
(Newberger et al., 1986) reported that high dose intravenous gamma globulin (IVGG) reduces the prevalence of
coronary artery lesions of Kawasaki Disease.

A trial was organized in Japan to study whether low
dose IVGG therapy is effective for the prevention of
coronary artery lesions in Kawasaki Disease. We report
here the results of a multi-center randomized trial of low
dose IVGG plus aspirin as compared with aspirin alone upon
the development of coronary artery abnormalities.

MATERIALS AND METHODS

Patients were assigned to receive aspirin alone
(aspirin group) or gamma globulin plus aspirin (gamma
globulin group).

In the first phase, a single dose of 100mg/kg IVGG was
administered from October 7, 1983 to February 14, 1985.

In the second phase, 100mg/kg/day of IVGG for 5
consecutive days was given from February 15, 1985 to March
31, 1986.

Two kinds of gamma globulin (pepsin-treated and intact gamma globulin) were used in these studies.

Aspirin 50mg/kg/day was given to both the aspirin group and the gamma globulin group until the temperature became below 37.5°C, and aspirin 30mg/kg/day was continued after that.

To be eligible for this study, patients had to be enrolled within 7 days of illness onset.

Echocardiograms were obtained at enrollment and at least once every week in the acute phase and at 30 days, 60 days and one year of illness.

Coronary artery findings were classified into three groups, i.e. normal, dilatation and aneurysm, by the classification standard by Research Committee of Kawasaki Disease (Research Committee of Kawasaki Disease, 1984).

RESULTS

(I) IVGG 100mg/kg single dose study

Of 236 eligible cases, 217 cases were enrolled in this study. The data for eligible cases at enrollment is shown in Table 1.

TABLE 1. Data at enrollment (gamma globulin 100mg/kg single dose)

Variable		Treatment group		
		Aspirn	Pepsin treated γ-gl	Intact γ-gl
Number		75	73	66
Sex (M : F)		47 : 28	40 : 33	36 : 30
Age (months)	0~11	25	21	22
	12~23	19	25	23
	24~35	16	14	11
	36~47	7	7	7
	48~	8	6	3
	Mean± S.D.	22.1± 15.0	21.6± 14.7	19.2± 15.4
Start of treatment (Days after onset)		4.9± 1.3	5.5± 1.2	5.5± 1.2

Echocardiograms were obtained for all patients. The echocardiographic results of the coronary arteries are shown in Table 2. No significant difference was found among these three groups. This includes the cases with coronary artery lesions upon enrollment in the study. Excluding the patients with coronary artery lesions at enrollment, again no statistical difference was noted among these three groups.

TABLE 2. Number of children with coronary artery lesions on echocardiography, including children with coronary artery lesions at enrollment (gamma globulin 100mg/kg single dose)

		Aspirin (75)	Pepsin treated γ-gl (77)	Intact γ-gl (66)
At Enrollment	Normal	68	65	61
	Dilation	7(9.3)	8(11.0)	5(7.6)
Before Day 30 of Disease	Normal	46	39	42
	Dilation	22(29.3)}(38.7)	26(35.6)}(45.2)	18(27.3)}(33.3)
	Aneurysm	7(9.3)	7(9.6)	4(6.1)
	Drop-out	0	1	2
30 Days after onset	Normal	59	56	52
	Dilation	9(12.2)}(20.3)	11(15.1)}(23.3)	10(15.2)}(21.2)
	Aneurysm	6(8.1)	6(8.2)	4(6.1)
	Drop-out	1	0	0
60 Days after onset	Normal	63	59	56
	Dilation	9(12.2)}(14.9)	9(12.3)}(19.2)	7(10.6)}(15.1)
	Aneurysm	2(2.7)	5(6.8)	3(4.5)
	Drop-out	1	0	0
6 Months after onset	Normal	66	64	60
	Dilatation	7(9.5)}(10.8)	7(9.6)}(12.3)	5(7.6)}(9.1)
	Aneurysm	1(1.4)	2(2.7)	1(1.5)
	Drop-out	1	0	0
1 Year after onset	Normal	70	67	62
	Dilation	2(2.7)}(4.1)	4(5.5)}(8.2)	2(3.0)}(4.5)
	Aneurysm	1(1.4)	2(2.7)	1(1.5)
	ND†	1	0	1
	Drop-out	1	0	0

†ND:Not Done

(II) IVGG 100mg/kg/day for 5 days study

Of 309 eligible cases, 295 cases were enrolled in this study. Echocardiograms were obtained on all patients. The data for eligible cases at enrollment are shown in Table 3. The result of coronary artery lesions by echocardiogram is shown in Table 4.

TABLE 3. Data at enrollment (gamma globulin 100mg/kg/day x 5 days).

Variable		Treatment group		
		Aspirn	Pepsin treated γ-gl	Intact γ-gl
Number		99	96	100
Sex (M : F)		58 : 41	63 : 33	59 : 41
Age (months)	0~11	37	29	42
	12~23	31	32	31
	24~35	21	23	8
	36~47	8	5	7
	48~	2	7	2
Mean± S.D.		18.5±12.1	21.0±13.4	17.7±11.3
Start of treatment (Days after onset)		4.4±1.4	5.3±0.9	5.4±1.1

TABLE 4. Number of children with coronary artery lesions on echocardiography, including children with coronary artery lesions at enrollment (gamma globulin 100mg/kg/day x 5 days.

		Treatment group		
		Aspirin (99)	Pepsin treated γ-gl (96)	Intact γ-gl (100)
At Enrollment	Normal	88	90	89
	Dilatation	11(11.1)	6(6.3)	11(11.0)
Before Day 30 of Disease	Normal	47	52	62
	Dilatation	32(33.0)	32(34.0)	31(31.6)
	Aneurysm	18(18.6) (51.5)	10(10.6) (44.7)	5(5.1) (36.7)
	Drop-out	2	2	2 ※※
30 Days after onset	Normal	65	75	77
	Dilatation	16(16.8)	8(8.6)	14(14.7)
	Aneurysm	14(14.7) (31.6)	10(10.8) (19.4) ※	4(4.2) (18.9)
	Drop-out	4	3	5 ※
60 Days after onset	Normal	70	82	83
	Dilatation	12(13.2)	2(2.2)	7(7.5)
	Aneurysm	8(8.8) (22.0)	9(9.7) (11.8)	3(3.2) (10.8)
	ND†	1	0	0
	Drop-out	8	3	7

†ND:Not Done
※ $P < 0.05$
※※ $P < 0.01$

Comparing the prevalence of coronary artery abnormalities in these groups before 30 days of illness, we detected 36.7% with coronary abnormality (dilatation 31.6% and aneurysm 5.1%) in the intact gamma globulin group, as compared with 51.5% (dilatation 33.3% and aneurysm 18.6%) in the aspirin group (p<0.01).

There was no statistical difference between the aspirin alone group and pepsin treated IVGG group.

At 30 days after the onset of illness, there were 18.9% (dilatation 14.7% and aneurysm 4.2%) in the intact gamma globulin group, and 19.4% (dilatation 8.6% and aneurysm 10.8%) in the pepsin treated gamma globulin group, as compared with 31.6% (dilatation 16.8% and aneurysm 14.7%) in the aspirin group (p<0.05).

At 60 days after the onset of illness, no statistical difference was recognized among these three groups.

Table 5 is the summary of the results of coronary artery lesions by echocardiogram excluding the patients who had coronary artery lesions at enrollment.

TABLE 5.   Number of children with coronary artery lesions on echocardiography excluding children with coronary artery lesions at enrollment (gamma globulin 100mg/kg/day x 5 days)

| | | Treatment group | | |
		Aspirin (88)	Pepsin treated γ-gl (90)	Intact γ-gl (89)
At Enrollment	Normal	88	90	89
	Dilatation	0	0	0
Before Day 30 of Disease	Normal	47	52	62
	Dilatation	25(29.1) (45.3)	27(30.7) (40.9)	22(25.3) (28.7)※
	Aneurysm	14(16.3)	9(10.2)	3(3.4) ※※
	Drop-out	2	2	2
30 Days after onset	Normal	64	70	74
	Dilatation	11(12.9) (24.7)	8(9.2) (19.5)	8(9.5) (11.9)※
	Aneurysm	10(11.8)	9(10.3)	2(2.4) ※
	Drop-out	3	3	5
60 Days after onset	Normal	68	77	77
	Dilatation	7(8.6) (16.0)	2(2.3) (11.5)	3(3.7) (6.1)
	Aneurysm	6(7.4)	8(9.2)	2(2.4)
	ND[†]	0	0	0
	Drop-out	7	3	7

[†]ND:Not Done
※ P<0.05
※ ※ P<0.01

Before 30 days of illness, the incidence of coronary artery abnormality was 28.7% (dilatation 25.3% and aneurysm 3.4%) in the intact gamma globulin group, as compared with 45.3% (dilatation 29.1% and aneurysm 16.3%) in the aspirin only group (p<0.01). At 30 days of illness, the incidence of coronary abnormality was 11.9% (dilatation 9.5% and aneurysm 2.4%) in the intact gamma globulin group, as compared with 24.7% (dilatation 12.9% and aneurysm 11.8%) in the aspirin only group (p<0.05). There was no statistical difference between the aspirin group and the pepsin-treated gamma globulin group before 30 days of illness or at 30 days of illness. In addition, there was no statistical difference detected among the three groups at 60 days of illness.

DISCUSSION

Furusho et al initially studied the effect of gamma globulin therapy in Kawasaki disease and reported that high dose IVGG therapy reduces the prevalence of coronary artery lesions.

Newberger et al also made an attempt to treat with high doses of IVGG and reported similar results to those of Furusho et al.

Concerning the effect of gamma globulin therapy for Kawasaki disease, several problems have to be considered:

1. Is gamma globulin therapy superior to aspirin therapy?
2. Is gamma globulin effective regarding the acute phase symptoms or coronary artery lesions, or both?
3. Does gamma globulin have only a therapeutic effect or only a preventive effect, or both, for coronary lesions?
4. How much is the minimum dose? Is the effect dose-dependent?
5. How should gamma globulin be given and how much should the total dose of gamma globulin be?
6. What type of gamma globulin is effective?
7. What is the cost-benefit balance?
8. What are the adverse effects of gamma globulin (including long-term effects)?

These are the problems we have to consider. In order to clarify these problems, we have carried out this study.

The data demonstrate that administration of 100mg/kg/day for 5 days IVGG is more effective in reducing the prevalence of coronary lesions than aspirin therapy alone. However, the effect of 100mg/kg IVGG as a single dose is almost identical to therapy with aspirin alone. Pepsin-treated gamma globulin is not as effective as intact gamma globulin. Nevertheless, we are not sure whether the 100mg/kg/dose is optimal. The prevalence of coronary abnormalities in the high dose (400mg/kg) gamma globulin group and 100mg/kg/day for 5 days group has not been studied. If the prevalence of coronary abnormalities between these two doses is identical, it would be possible to say that 100mg/kg/day for 5 days is so far the ideal minimal dose of gamma globulin for Kawasaki disease. A comparison of coronary artery abnormalities between high dose gamma globulin and 100mg/kg/day gamma globulin for 5 days will be necessary.

Although the prevalence of coronary artery abnormalities is less in the 100mg/kg/day for 5 days group than the aspirin group before 30 days of illness and at 30 days of illness, there is no statistical difference at 60 days of illness. This evidence may suggest that there is no significant difference in long-term prognosis between the gamma globulin group and aspirin group. Further long-term follow-up is necessary to clarify the long-term prognosis of coronary artery abnormalities.

REFERENCES

Furusho K, Kamiya T, Nakano H, et al (1984). High-dose intravenous gamma globulin for Kawasaki Disease. Lancet 2:1055-1058.

Newberger JW, Takahashi M, et al (1986). The treatment of Kawasaki disease with intravenous gamma globulin. New Engl J Med 315:341-347.

Research Committee on Kawasaki Disease. Report of subcommittee on standardization of diagnostic criteria and reporting coronary artery lesions in Kawasaki disease. Tokyo, Japan, Ministry of Health and Welfare (1984).

Kawasaki Disease, pages 441–443
© 1987 Alan R. Liss, Inc.

U.S. GAMMA GLOBULIN TRIAL

Jane W. Newburger, M. D.

For the U.S. Multicenter Kawasaki Study Group.
From the Departments of Pediatrics and
Cardiology, Children's Hospital and Harvard
Medical School, Boston; the Department of
Pediatrics, Children's Memorial Hospital and
Northwestern University School of Medicine,
Chicago; Children's Hospital, The University of
Colorado Health Sciences Center, and the
University of Colorado School of Medicine,
Denver; Children's Hospital of Los Angeles and
the University of Southern California School of
Medicine; Children's Hospital, the University
of California, San Diego, Medical Center, and
the University of California, San Diego, School
of Medicine; Tufts-New England Medical Center
and Tufts University School of Medicine,
Boston; Kapiolani-Children's Medical Center and
John A. Burns School of Medicine, Honolulu;
and the Epidemiology and Biostatistics Section,
Boston University School of Public Health.

In Phase I of the NIH-sponsored United States
multicenter randomized gamma globulin trial, we compared
the efficacy of intravenous gamma globulin (IVGG) plus
aspirin (ASA) to that of ASA alone in reducing the
frequency of coronary artery abnormalities in children
with acute Kawasaki Syndrome (Newburger et al., 1986).
Children randomized to the IVGG arm received IVGG, 400
mg/kg/day, for four consecutive days; both treatment
groups received ASA, 100 mg/kg/day through the 14th day
of illness, then 3-5 mg/kg/day. The presence of
coronary artery abnormalities were ascertained by
two-dimensional echocardiograms, interpreted blindly and

independently by two or more readers. Two weeks after enrollment, abnormalities were present in 18 of 78 children (23%) in the ASA group and in 6 of 75 (8%) in the IVGG group (p=.01, Fisher's exact test). Seven weeks after enrollment, coronary artery lesions were present in 14 of 79 (18%) in the ASA group and in 3 of 79 (4%) in the IVGG group (p=.005). At two and seven weeks, the estimated relative prevalence rates (IVGG:ASA) of coronary artery abnormalities, adjusted for age/sex strata, were 0.36 (95% confidence limits 0.16, 0.79) and 0.22 (95% confidence limits 0.07, 0.64), respectively. Children in the IVGG group also had significantly greater declines in fever (p<.001), white blood cell count (p<.0001), absolute granulocyte count (p<.0001), and serum alpha-1-antitrypsin level (p=.05). No child suffered serious adverse effects from IVGG. We concluded that high-dose IVGG is a safe and effective therapy for reducing the prevalence of coronary artery abnormalities and duration of systemic inflammation when administered early in the course of Kawasaki syndrome.

Further investigation is needed to determine the ideal dose, frequency, and duration of IVGG therapy. The original choice of a four-day regimen for IVGG administration was based on the success of investigators in Japan with three to five day regimens of similar daily dose (Furusho et al., 1984; Nakano, 1984). The four-day protocol used in Phase I is also similar to those originally used for the treatment of immune thrombocytopenic purpura (ITP) (Imbach et al., 1981; Bussell et al., 1984). However, recent data indicate that a single higher dose of IVGG is a similarly effective and safe therapy for ITP (Bussell et al., 1984), and this regimen has now entered clinical practice. We hypothesize that a single higher dose of IVGG may also be effective for the treatment of Kawasaki syndrome. The single-dose regimen would have the advantage of reducing the total number of days of hospitalization, resulting in substantially reduced financial cost, decreased morbidity from long-term intravenous therapy and nosocomial infection, and psychological benefits for both families and patients. As in the case of ITP, single infusion, if proven effective, might eventually be given as an out-patient infusion for some children, thus eliminating the need for hospitalization altogether.

Phase 2 of our trial is currently comparing a single large dose of intravenous gamma globulin (2.0 g/kg over 10 hours) to that of smaller doses (400 mg/kg/day over 2 hours) given on four consecutive days with regard to: 1) the prevalence of coronary artery abnormalities; 2) resolution of acute inflammation as reflected in laboratory indexes; 3) serum IgG level; and 4) frequency of adverse side effects.

REFERENCES

Bussell JB, Goldman A, Imbach P, Schulman I, Hiltgartner MW. Treatment of acute idiopathic thrombocytopenia of childhood with intravenous infusions of gamma globulin. J Pediatr 1984; 106:886.

Bussell JB, Hiltgartner MW. Usage and mechanism of action of intravenous gamma globulin treatment of autoimmune hematologic disease. Br J Hematol 1984; 56:1.

Bussell JB, Hiltgartner MW, Barandum S. Intravenous use of gamma globulin in the treatment of chronic immune thrombocytopenic purpura as a means to defer splenectomy. J Pediatr 1983; 103:651.

Furusho K, Nakano H, Shinomiya K, et al. High-dose intravenous gamma globulin for Kawasaki disease. Lancet 1984; 2:1055.

Imbach P, Barandum S, Wagner HP, et al. High-dose intravenous gamma globulin for idiopathic thrombocytopenic purpura in childhood. Lancet 1981; 1:1228.

Nakano M. The correlation between the activated oxygen production in neutrophiles and high-dose therapy of intact gamma-globulin in Kawasaki Syndrome. Exerpta Medica Fujii Conference, Tokyo, Japan, November, 1983 (abstract).

Newburger JW, Takahashi M, Burns JC, Beiser AS, Chung KJ, Duffy CE, Glode MP, Mason WH, Reddy V, Sanders SP, Shulman ST, Wiggins JW, Hicks RV, Fulton DR, Lewis AB, Leung DYM, Colton T, Rosen FR, Melish ME. The treatment of Kawasaki Syndrome with intravenous gamma globulin. N Engl J Med 1986;315:341.

Kawasaki Disease, pages 445–454
© 1987 Alan R. Liss, Inc.

INTRACORONARY THROMBOLYTIC THERAPY IN KAWASAKI DISEASE :
TREATMENT AND PREVENTION OF ACUTE MYOCARDIAL INFARCTION

Hirohisa Kato, Eisei Ichinose, Osamu Inoue,
Teizi Akagi

Department of Pediatrics, Division of Pediatric
Cardiology, Kurume University School of Medicine,
Kurume, Japan

INTRODUCTION

The main cause of death in Kawasaki disease is acute
myocardial infarction due to thrombotic occlusion of a
coronary aneurysm (Kato et al., 1985). At the present
time, antithrombotic agents such as aspirin are primarily
used in the treatment for Kawasaki disease (Kato et al.,
1979). However myocardial infarction has occurred in some
patients, particulary in those with giant coronary aneurysms though the patients had been given such drugs (Kato
et al., 1986). Recently, intracoronary thrombolytic
treatment or percutaneous transluminal coronary revascu-
lization (PTCR) has been used for the treatment of adult
myocardial infarction, and its efficacy has been reported
(Rentrop et al., 1979). The initial experience of PTCR in
Kawasaki disease was attempted by us in 1982 for a 2 year-
old girl who had suffered acute myocardial infarction
(Ichinose et al., 1983). This study reports our experiences of PTCR in nine patients with Kawasaki disease who
had thrombotic occlusions in coronary aneurysms.

PATIENTS AND METHODS

We conducted PTCR with use of urokinase in nine
patients, whose ages were in the range from 1 to 8 years.
There were 7 boys and 2 girls. In a 2-year-old girl with
acute myocardial infarction, PTCR was performed 3 hours
after the attack. Another patient had had several episodes of angina attack. The seven other patients had not
developed myocardial infarction but showed significant

evidence of massive thrombus formation in coronary aneurysms on serial two-dimensional echocardiography or coronary angiography. All cases had giant coronary aneurysms in acute stage which were over 8 mm in diameter. PTCR was performed within 48 hours when massive thrombus formation was detected by 2-D echocardiography, which detection was undertaken from 21 days to 5 years from the onset of illness. Diagnosis of massive thrombus formation was made by the observed presence of newly-appearing cloud echo in giant coronary aneurysms in serial echocardiographic studies which were taken once each month at the clinic. Repeat PTCR was performed in 3 cases who had suffered a subsequent massive thrombus formation at 3 months, 6 months, and at 9 months after the 1st PTCR, respectively.

Table 1.

PATIENTS PROFILES (PTCR)

Case (Sex)	Age (yr)	Size of Aneurysm[1]	Time of Procedure[2]	Symptom	Dose of UK(IU)	Thrombus by 2-D echo Before PTCR	After PTCR	Effect of PTCR
K.S. (F)	2.0	R:18mm	21 day of	AMI	R:2,000	massive	diminish	+
		L:11mm	illness		L:2,000	small	no change	−
M.K. (M)	8.4	R:24mm	5 year of	angina	R:96,000	massive	no change	−
		L:17mm	illness					
N.O. (M)	1.7	R:11mm	1st: 9mo	none	R:48,000	massive	diminish	+
		L:4mm						
			2nd: 1.5yr	none	R:96,000	massive	diminish	+
T.W. (M)	1.7	R:14mm	1st: 9mo	none	R:72,000	small	invisible	+ +
		L:21mm						
			2nd: 1.6yr	none	R:120,000	massive	no change	−
K.H. (M)	2.1	R:12mm	1.6yr	none	R:48,000	small	invisible	+ +
		L:10mm						
T.T. (M)	6.8	R:14mm	1st: 1.11yr	none	R:120,000	massive	invisible	+ +
		L:7mm						
			2nd: 2.2yr	none	R:240,000	massive	no change	−
T.I. (M)	4.7	R:5mm	1.11yr	none	L:150,000	massive	diminish	+
		L:12mm						
R.U. (F)	1.1	R:8mm	2mo	none	L:60,000	massive	no cange (evaluated by CAG)	−
		L:8mm						
M.M. (M)	3.0	R:8mm	7mo	chest pain	L:120,000	small	diminish	+
		L:5mm						

R: RCA,　L: LCA,　AMI: acute myocardial infarction.　1: Size of aneurysm at acute phase.
2: PTCR was performed within 48 hours when massive thrombus was noted by 2-D echo.

Prior to urokinase infusion, 100 units/kg of heparin was administered intravenously. Selective coronary angiography was performed by usual method using specially designed catheters by us. 60,000 units of urokinase was diluted with 10 to 20 ml of 5% glucose solution, and then urokinase was infused directly into the coronary aneurysms that had massive thrombus as a bolus of 8,000 to 10,000 units per kilogram via catheter over 10 to 20 minutes. After completion of the infusion, repeat coronary angiography was performed. Continuous IV heparin infusion was begun after the procedure at 500 Units/kg/day to maintain the PTT at 2 to 3 times the level in controls and this infusion was continued for 12 to 24 hours. The efficacy of thrombolysis was evaluated by repeat coronary angiography and follow-up echocardiography to detect recanalization of the coronary artery or decrease in the massive thrombus echo. Coagulation studies were obtained in 5 patients before and after the procedure. These studies included platelet counts, fibrinogen, prothrombin time (PT), PTT, thrombotest, fibrinogen degradation products (FDP) and alpha 2 plasmin inhibitor.

RESULTS

We performed a total of 13 procedures of PTCR on the 9 patients which were summarized in Table 1. Details of clinical data on some representative cases are presented here.

CASE K.S.: A 2-year-old girl visited our hospital at 20 days of illness after fever and acute manifestations had subsided. Aspirin had not been administered to this patient during the acute stage. Early on the 21st morning, she had experienced sudden onset of acute myocardial infarction and developed cardiac arrest. Fortunately, she was well resuscitated, and was then immediately taken into the heart catheterization laboratory. Coronary angiography was performed 3 hours after the onset of the myocardial infarction, and this demonstrated giant aneurysms in both right and left main coronary arteries. The right coronary artery aneurysm was completely occluded by a massive thrombus. In the left coronary aneurysm a small thrombus was recognized. Electrocardiogram showed inferior wall infarction. We decided to perform PTCR on this patient. However, this was a precedent for a patient with Kawasaki disease to undergo PTCR and a suitable dosage of urokinase was unknown at that time. So we used a cautious amount of about 2,000 units of urokinase for each of both the right and left coronary aneurysms. After 20 minutes, then partial recanalization of the right coronary artery was determined. The thrombus was less prominant but significant filling defect persisted. During the procedure the vital signs remained stable and no arrhythmias occurred. The patient was returned to the ICU and was continued to receive intravenous urokinase infusion for the next 6 hours. This patient has been followed for more than 4 years to date and has not revealed reinfarction or angina and is doing well now.

The abnormal deep Q waves have eventually disappeared and are no longer present.

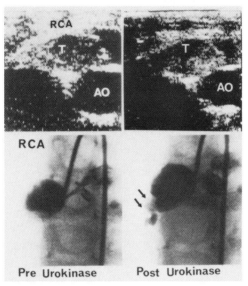

Fig. 1. Two-dimensional echocardiograms and coronary angiograms in a case of Kawasaki disease with myocardial infarction (Case K.S.: 2-year-old girl).
Massive thrombus formation (T) is detected in a right coronary aneurysm (RCA: upper left panel). Coronary angiography shows complete obstruction of the right coronary aneurysm (lower left panel). After Urokinase injection (right panels), partial coronary recanalization is observed (black arrow).

CASE N.O. : This patient had been diagnosed as having Kawasaki disease at 10 months of age and had giant, diffuse right coronary aneurysm. A massive thrombus echo was detected at 9 months of illness and this was confirmed by angiography. No ischemic symptoms or signs were presented. After PTCR for the right coronary aneurysm the massive thrombus echo did not completely disappear and decreased only partially.

CASE T.W. : In this patient, a small thrombus was recognized in the large right coronary aneurysm at 9 months of illness. This thrombus was difficult to detect by angiography. After PTCR the thrombus echo disappeared completely.

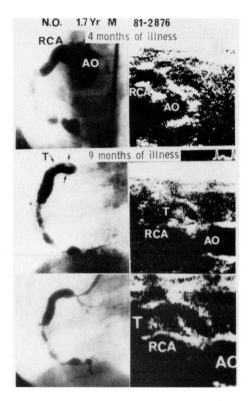

Fig. 2. Serial two-dimensional echocardiograms and coronary angiograms in a case with intracoronary thrombus (Case N. O. : 1. 7-year-old boy).
A coronary aneurysm can be seen first at four months illness (upper panel). Massive thrombus formation(T) is visualized in the right co-ronary aneurysm at nine months illness. In this patient, there is no clinical sign of myocardial infarction. After PTCR in the right coro-nary aneurysm the massive thrombus echo did not completely disa-ppear and decreased only partially.

CASE M.K. : This patient had been diagnosed as having Kawasaki disease at 3 years of age, and had giant aneu-rysm in both the right and left coronary arteries. Two years later there were several episodes of transient chest pain, but electrocardiograms and enzyme studies did not demonstrated any evidence of myocardial infarction. Echo-cardiography revealed the presence of a massive thrombus formation which completely occluded the right coronary artery. We performed PTCR on this patient. The thrombus echo, however, did not change. We speculate that this may not have been a fresh thrombus since the procedure was done late at 2 months after the first attack of angina. Subsequent coronary bypass surgery was undertaken in this case.

Table 1. shows the summary of our experiences. We performed a total of 13 procedures of PTCR on the 9 patients. In 3 patients the thrombus echo completely disappeared, in 5 it diminished, but in 5 patients it was unaffected. We performed repeat PTCR in three patients which resulted in disappearance in only one case, and was unchanged in the other two.

We noted no adverse effect or side effect such as bleeding tendency, arrhythmias, or any allergic effect during or after PTCR. Coagulation studies were performed in five cases. Hemoglobin, platelet count, PT, and PTT, showed no significant change. Fibrinogen, FDP and alpha 2 plasmin inhibitor changed significantly just after PTCR and then returned to normal levels by 24 hours later.

Fig. 3. COAGULATION VARIABLES BEFORE AND AFTER PTCR

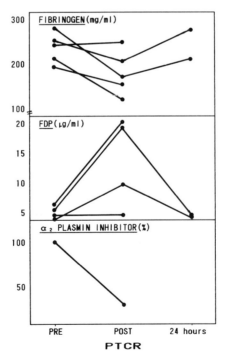

DISCUSSION:
The main cause of death in Kawasaki disease is acute myocardial infarction due to the thrombotic occlusion of coronary aneurysms. Currently, antithrombotic agents such as aspirin are primarily used for treatment in Kawasaki disease. However, myocardial infarction has occurred in some patients, particulary in those with giant coronary aneurysms despite administration of such drugs. Systemic intravenous infusion of urokinase or streptokinase in Kawasaki disease has been reported previously, but the efficacy was uncertain (Igarashi and Ishibashi, 1981, Terai et al., 1985, Burtt et al., 1986). Recently, PTCR has been used for the treatment of adult myocardial infarction, and its efficacy has been determined (TIMI Study Group, 1985). In adult patients it is generally performed immediately following acute myocardial infarction, and its efficacy is established by the observed recanalization of the occluded coronary artery by angiography or otherwise by survival of the patient (Rutsh et al., 1981). In our study, we performed PTCR in one patient at 3 hours after the onset of acute myocardial infarction, and recanalization of the coronary artery was obtained. In a further 8 patients who had not revealed acute myocardial infarction but had massive thrombus formation in giant coronary aneurysms, then PTCR was performed within 48 hours after our detecting massive thrombus by serial echocardiographic studies which had been routinely performed in every one month at the clinic (Tanino and Yanagisawa, 1982). PTCR was effective in 6 out of 8 patients. Successful PTCR was determined by the disappearance or decrease of the thrombus echo in 2-D echocardiography. This suggests that PTCR in Kawasaki disease may be effective not only in the treatment but also in the prevention of acute myocardial infarction, and also in the withholding progression to ischemic heart disease. The indication for, and the evaluation of, PTCR in Kawasaki disease may be different from such in coronary artery disease in adults.

The goal of thrombolytic therapy in acute myocardial infarction is reduction of infarct size, which is dependent upon the appearance of coronary reperfusion and the interval between the onset of infarction and reperfusion. The critical time period is thought to be within 6 hours in myocardial infarction of an adult; however it remains unknown in infants and children. In case M.K. where chest pain occurred repeatedly, we had performed PTCR 2 months after the onset of angina pectoris. PTCR resulted uneffective, which may be due to the lateness of PTCR. If we could have determined the existence of the thrombus earlier, then PTCR might have been effective in this case.

A recommended dosage of urokinase in Kawasaki disease is uncertain; however from our experiences 10,000 IU/kg may be adequate for thrombolysis. We studied alpha 2 plasmin inhibitor levels before and after PTCR which resulted a significant reduction after the administration of urokinase. This indicates that our dosage of urokinase for neutralization of circulating plasmin may be sufficient; however, no bleeding tendency was recognized.

Systemic intravenous infusion of urokinase or streptokinase in Kawasaki disease has been reported previously though with unknown efficacy. We undertook systemic infusion of urokinase in one patient (case T. T.), which resulted in slight decrease in the thrombus echo. The subsequent PTCR demonstrated complete disappearance of the thrombus echo. This suggests that intracoronary infusion is more effective than systemic intravenous infusion. However the selective coronary angiography and PTCR for infants or small children can only be performed in the specialized medical centers. Further investigations on procedures such as intravenous administration and drugs or dosage used for thrombolysis such as tissue plasminogen activator are necessary(De Werf et al., 1984).

As post-urokinase treatment we used systemic infusion of heparin of 500 U/kg per day for 6 to 12 hours, and then continued with usual oral aspirin administration. However massive thrombus occurred subsequently in three patients several months later, and on whom a 2nd PTCR was therefore then performed. In such patients the use of heparin or warfarin in combination with aspirin may be necessary after PTCR over the long-term. If massive thrombus reappears in the serial 2-D echocardiography, then we recommend repeat PTCR. If the repeat PTCR is not effective and patient remains at high risk to possible myocardial infarction, then coronary bypass surgery is recommended.

In conclusion, PTCR is effective in some patients with Kawasaki disease. By this method patients may survive acute myocardial infarction. If patients have massive thrombus formation in the coronary aneurysms we can prevent the occlusion of the artery and withhold the progression to ischemic heart disease. In Table 2. we summarize the indication and prospective methods for PTCR in Kawasaki disease from our experiences. We must further investigate which drug is best, how much constitutes the proper dosage and determine the long-term outcome following PTCR in Kawasaki disease.

Table 2.

INTRACORONARY THROMBOLYTIC TREATMENT

INDICATION:

   1. Acute myocardial infarction (within 6 hours from onset)

   2. Massive thrombus formation detected by serial two-dimensional echocardiography or coronary angiography

METHOD:

   1. Heparin 100 units/kg IV, before PTCR

   2. Urokinase 60,000 IU diluted with 10~20ml 5% glucose solution, intracoronary infusion for 10~15 minutes. Repeat infusion of urokinase, if necessary. Maximal dosage 10,000 IU/kg.

   3. Systemic heparin infusion 500 units/kg/day after PTCR.

EVALUATION:

   1. Repeat Coronary Angiography

   2. Follow-up 2-D Echocardiography

REFERENCES

Burtt DM, Pollack P, Bianco JA(1986). Intravenous streptokinase in an infant with Kawasaki disease complicated by acute myocardial infarction. Pediatr Cardiol 6 : 307-311

De Werf FV, Fox KA, De Geest H, Verstraete M, Collen D, Sobel BE (1984). Coronary thrombolysis with tissue-type plasminogen activator in patients with evolving myocardial infarction. N Engl J Med 310 : 609-613

Ichinose E, Kato H, Kawakami N, Yoshioka F, Matsunaga S (1983). Intracoronary thrombolytic treatment in Kawasaki disease. (in Jpn). Shonika 24 : 385-389

Ichinose E, Kato H, Inoue O, Hirata K, Ito Y, Yoshioka F (1985). Intracoronary thrombolytic therapy in Kawasaki disease and the usefulness of two-dimensional echocardiography in detecting intracoronary thrombi. J Cardiography 15 : 79-86

Igarashi K, Ishibashi M (1981). High dose urokinase administration in a Kawasaki disease patient with myocardial infarction. Med Postgraduates 19 : 225-229

Kato H, Koike S, Yokoyama Y (1979). Kawasaki disease : Effect of treatment on coronary artery involvement. Pediatrics 63 : 175-179

Kato H, Ichinose E, Yanagawa Y, Kawasaki T (1985). Clinical analysis of 104 fatal cases in Kawasaki disease. (in Jpn) Shonika 26 : 1017-1021

Kato H, Ichinose E, Kawasaki T (1986). Myocardial infarction in Kawasaki disease : Clinical analyses of 195 cases. J Pediatr 108 : 923-927

Rentrop KP, Blanke H, Karsch KP, Wiegand V, Kostering H, Oster H, Leitz K (1979). Acute myocardial infarction : Intracoronary application of nitroglycerin and streptokinase. Clin Cardiol 2 : 354-360

Rutsch W, Schartl M, Mathey D, Kuck K, Merx W, Dorr R, Rentrop P, Blanke H (1981). Percutaneous transluminal coronary recanalization : Procedure, results, and acute complications. Am Heart J 102 : 1178-1183

Tanino S, Yanagisawa S, Ito G (1982). Follow-up study of coronary aneurysms in Kawasaki disease by two-dimensional echocardiography. Med Ultrasound 9 : 223-227

Terai M, Ogata M, Sugimoto K, Nagai Y, Toba T, Tami K, Aotsuka H, Niwa K, Nakajima H (1985). Coronary arterial thrombi in Kawasaki disease. J Pediatr 106 : 76-78

TIMI Study Group (1985). The thrombolysis in myocardial infarction (TIMI) trial. N Engl J Med 313 : 932-936

Kawasaki Disease, pages 455–458
© 1987 Alan R. Liss, Inc.

SURGICAL TREATMENT FOR CORONARY ARTERIAL LESIONS IN
KAWASAKI DISEASE

Soichiro Kitamura

Division of Thoracic and Cardiovascular Surgery
Nara Medical College

The national survey of surgical treatment for Kawasaki
Disease (KD) was conducted by the research group supported
by the Japanese Ministry of Public Welfare in 1984. Surgical treatment of KD has had a history of more than a decade
since our first successful report of coronary artery bypass
in pediatric patients in 1974, but the number of patients
at each institution is not sufficient to allow any meaningful analysis. Therefore, it was considered that a collection of the nation-wide surgical experience might enable
significant analysis. We are grateful to the doctors who
kindly responded to the survey.

The results of the survey showed that coronary artery
bypass surgery for KD had been performed in 43 patients
whose mean age was 10 years, including 35 males and 8
females. The mean number of arterial grafts was 1.6 per
patient and the mean pre-operative left ventricular ejection fraction was 0.53. Coronary bypass is certainly the
most common form of surgery, with other cardiac procedures
for mitral valve regurgitation secondary to papillary
muscle dysfunction and/or valvulitis. Seven patients with
a mean age of 7.7 years (6 males and 1 female) underwent
either mitral valve replacement or mitral valve repair.
The mean left ventricular ejection fraction of this group
of patients was 0.43, 0.1 lower than the coronary bypass
group.

Analysis of the distribution of coronary arterial
lesions in 43 surgical patients shows that both dilata-
tional and occlusive lesions exist primarily in the

proximal coronary arteries, particularly in the left
coronary artery. Obstructive lesions, which are certainly
more important in ischemic heart disease of children, were
observed in the proximal right and left anterior descending
and left circumflex arteries. The distribution pattern of
this lesion suggests that surgery can be undertaken for all
occlusive lesions except when the diameter of the artery is
too small, probably <1 mm.

In 43 patients, 70 grafts were inserted. The LAD and
the RCA were the two most common arteries grafted. In 8 of
the 43 patients, left ventricular ejection fraction was
<0.4.

First, I would like to compare the graft patency of the
autologous saphenous vein graft in patients below and above
8 years of age. The saphenous vein grafts in younger
patients showed a statistically significantly higher
closure rate, 35% in younger patients and 13% in the older
age group. The incidence of early graft occlusion within
one month of surgery was 13%. In contrast, occlusion
occurring later than one month or even later than one year
is frequently seen in saphenous vein grafts in pediatric
patients, with an overall closure rate of 87%. This may
mean that pediatric saphenous vein grafts close slowly due
to degenerative changes. This fact is very important when
considering surgical treatment for KD.

Four of the 43 grafted patients (9%) died four months
to three years and three months after operation. Details
regarding the graft status were not available for all
patients, but at least in one patient, late graft closure
appeared to be the cause of death. Their mean left ventricular ejection fraction was 0.43, less than that of the
total group by 0.1.

Next, I would like to talk about my personal surgical
experience with 15 KD patients from 2.5 to 26 years old.
These included 13 males and 2 females. Myocardial
infarction had occurred in 9/15 (60%) of the patients.
Their left ventricular ejection fraction ranged from 0.35
to 0.66, with a mean of 0.51.

Coronary artery bypass grafts were performed in 14
patients. The number of grafts placed per patient ranged
from one to four, with a mean of 2.2 per patient. Mitral

valve replacement was performed on two patients, one of whom had concomitant bypass surgery. Nineteen autologous saphenous vein grafts and 12 internal mammary artery grafts were utilized in 14 patients. There has been no operative, hospital or late mortality observed during the follow-up period from six months to 12 years. Six children had surgery at the Osaka University Hospital, and nine patients had their operation at the Nara Medical College, my current location.

I would like to focus particularly on the use of the internal mammary artery (IMA) grafts in pediatric patients. We first successfully used the IMA in 1984 in the treatment of KD. Nine patients (8 males and 1 female) in this series underwent myocardial revascularization utilizing the IMA generally to the left anterior descending, with saphenous vein grafts to other arteries. All patients had multiple vessel involvement and six had so-called giant aneurysms. Left main coronary trunk involvement was seen in five. Two to four grafts (mean of 2.4) per patient were placed, with no mortality.

In surgery, the IMA was used for 12 coronary arteries, particularly for the LAD. Bilateral IMA grafts were placed in three patients. Simultaneously, ten autologous saphenous vein grafts were used for ten coronary arteries, particularly the right and left circumflex. The rate of early graft patency for saphenous vein grafts is 84% and the late potency is 68%. In contrast, both early and late patency rates of the IMA grafts are 100%, although the number of grafts studied at the late period is small.

I must stress, however, that some saphenous grafts are nicely open for a long time. However, generally speaking, saphenous grafts tend to close rather often in pediatric patients, more often than in adults. With surgery, exercise EKG improved, and thallium 20 myocardial scintigraphy during exercise improved if there were abnormalities prior to the operation.

Although comparisons of LVEDP and EF at rest before and after operation showed no change, the response of stroke volume to the increase of EDP during exercise is more favorable after surgery compared to before.

The growth possibility of the IMA grafts should be mentioned. In contrast to adults who undergo CABG, pediatric
CABG surgery has another big problem, i.e., graft length in
response to the child's body growth. In other words, do
grafts become too short inside the chest when the body and
heart approach adult size? We have performed angiograms at
two different times after surgery in three patients, at one
month after and more than one year after surgery. We
measured the diameter of the IMA graft and the IMA left
intact as well as tracing the entire length of the IMA
grafts. We found a definite increase in both the diameter
and the length of the IMA grafts. In contrast, the saphenous vein grafts showed a tendency to shorten somewhat with
time. Although the number of cases studied in this way is
still limited, these findings are new and very important,
particularly with respect to pediatric CABG for KD. I
believe that the IMA graft is a live conduit with the
possibility of growth along with the patient's body growth,
quite different from the saphenous vein graft.

Kawasaki Disease, pages 459–470
© 1987 Alan R. Liss, Inc.

STATISTICAL ISSUES IN THE DESIGN AND EVALUATION OF
CLINICAL TRIALS IN KAWASAKI DISEASE

A. Lawrence Gould, Ph.D.

Merck, Sharp, and Dohme Research Laboratories
West Point, PA 19486   U. S. A.

INTRODUCTION

The statistical issues arising in the design and
evaluation of clinical trials in general also arise in the
design and evaluation of clinical trials in Kawasaki Disease. Since there is much yet to learn about the etiology, mechanisms, and therefore, definitive treatment of
Kawasaki Disease, it seems appropriate to lay out the
basic statistical issues, to form a framework for evaluating the trials that have been done and to provide guid-
ance for the design and analysis of future trials.

The issues discussed here (see in Table 1) are
important because of their relationship to the three
objectives of an ideal intervention trial, i.e., a trial
aimed at evaluating the effect on the course of an illness
of a therapeutic or other intervention. These objectives
are (Sackett, 1980): (1) validity, i.e., the results are
true; (2) generalizability, i.e., the results are widely
applicable; and (3) efficiency, i.e., the trial is
affordable and that resources remain for patient care and
other health research. Several books address these issues
in depth (e.g., Mainland, 1963; Bradford Hill, 1962, 1971;
Feinstein, 1977; Bulpitt, 1983; Friedman, Furberg and
DeMets, 1983). Here, we present them as a checklist. At
the design stage, the aim of the checklist is to assure
that these objectives are met; at the evaluation stage,
its aim is to evaluate the degree to which the objectives
have been met.

TABLE 1. Checklist of Key Points for Designing/
Evaluating Clinical Trials

1. What questions is the trial designed to answer?

2. Which results/conclusions reflect the questions the trial was designed to answer, and which reflect associations suggested by the data?

3. What is the target patient population?

4. What population does the trial sample represent?

5. How is/was the randomization carried out?

6. How is/was blinding employed?

7. Were clinically relevant treatment regimens used?

8. Are the observations/measurements appropriate?

9. What is the justification for the sample size, including effect on sensitivity for detecting treatment differences?

10. Were appropriate statistical methods used?

11. Were all patients randomized to treatment accounted for, either in the analyses or separately?

12. What kinds of bias might affect the results, and what steps are/were taken to control them?

QUESTIONS THE TRIAL IS DESIGNED TO ANSWER

This is the foundation on which the validity and generalizability of a clinical trial rest. The first step in the design of a trial is a clear and precise definition of the questions it is to answer (Mainland, 1963, pp. 19–28; Bradford Hill, 1971, pp. 253–254; Feinstein, 1977, pp. 28–37; Bulpitt, 1983, pp. 28–34; Friedman, Furberg, and De-Mets, 1983, pp. 8–17). For intervention trials, the questions will address the differences between the intervention strategies (e.g., treatments) that will emerge during the course of the trial. Not all trials are intervention trials: a trial may consist of the accumulation of data on a particular group of patients (or normal people), to obtain expected ranges of various clinical parameters.

Precision and detail are important. For example, the major question addressed by a trial in Kawasaki Disease might be: "Do children treated with gamma globulin plus high dose aspirin have a lower incidence of coronary artery lesions than children treated with high dose aspirin alone?". This apparently clear statement still requires specifying the dosage regimen of gamma globulin, the dosage regimen of "high-dose" aspirin, the duration of treatment, the definition of "coronary artery lesion", the duration of follow-up to see if coronary artery lesions develop, the difference in coronary artery lesion incidence between the two treatment groups that will be considered clinically meaningful, the diagnostic criteria the children must satisfy for entry into the trial, etc.

Clearly specifying the primary questions the trial is intended to answer also can help to identify the kinds of data needed. For example, a question pertaining to the length of time until fever abates focusses attention on the need to schedule temperature measurements sufficiently frequently to be able to discern precisely enough when the fever has abated. Thus, if the difference of a day in the time to abatement of fever is important, then temperature measurements should be taken at least daily; if the relevant margin of time is a week, then measurements once or twice a week should suffice. The timing issue is not peculiar to clinical trials; how soon and how often cell culture supernatant fluids are sampled markedly affects the findings from in vitro experiments.

Specifying the secondary questions clearly at the outset also is important, to be sure that the kinds of data needed to answer them can be collected. Thus, a secondary question such as "is gamma globulin plus aspirin more effective than aspirin alone in children presenting with acute inflammatory signs?" signals a need to stratify (allocate children to treatment separately) on the presence or absence of acute inflammatory signs at entry.

Clearly and precisely specifying the questions also greatly simplifies the tasks of analyzing the data from a trial and evaluating the findings of a completed trial.

Focusing on analyses that directly address the relevant
questions is much more effective and efficient than per-
forming a series of analyses in the hope that the results
will answer useful questions. A knowledge of the target
questions makes determining whether or not they have been
answered a straightforward process, in evaluating the findings from completed trials. Knowing the answers, but not
the questions, makes evaluating the validity of the conclusions of the trial very difficult, if not impossible.

A PRIORI QUESTIONS VS DATA-GENERATED ASSOCIATIONS

"Seek and ye shall find" is a very old expression
that well describes the usual consequence of intensively
analyzing the data to find between-group differences or
other associations. Even if there really are no treatment
differences or other associations, there is a 64% likelihood that 20 independent, 5% level ad hoc analyses performed on the data will yield one or more "significant"
results by chance alone, and a 26% likelihood that by
chance alone two or more will be found. In other words,
significant results are almost certain if enough analyses
are carried out, and there is no predicting beforehand
where they will occur. This is why it is important to
distinguish between the findings pertaining to questions
asked at the design stage, and those reflecting the result
of intensive analysis. The only conclusions that can be
reached from the analysis of a trial's data are those pertaining to hypotheses specified when the trial was designed. Any other findings, no matter how provocative or
fascinating they might be, must be regarded as provisional
until they can be confirmed by a subsequent trial addres-
sing the questions they seem to answer. Sackett (1979)
refers to coincidental findings as "data dredging bias",
and asserts that "the results are suitable for hypothesis-
forming activities only."

TARGET POPULATION

The target population of a clinical trial consists of
the people with the target illness or condition for whom
the proposed intervention will provide clinical benefit
now or ever. Specificity in the definition of this target
population is important. For example, identifying the

target population for a trial in Kawasaki Disease requires careful definition of what the term "Kawasaki Disease" means. Children may present with the symptoms of Kawasaki Disease very shortly after onset or several days after onset; they may or may not have fever; they may or may not have acute inflammatory signs; they may or may not have evidence of coronary artery lesions; they may be infants or not infants; and so on. If the success of a treatment depends on these and other prognostic factors, then the outcome of a trial will depend on how the population for the trial is defined.

The definition of the target population determines the generalizability of the conclusions from the trial. Thus, if the population in which a treatment effectively diminishes the risk of a coronary artery lesion consists of children without acute inflammatory signs who start therapy within two days of onset of symptoms, then the results of the trial may not be very generalizable if in practice few children satisfy these criteria.

TRIAL POPULATION

The trial population, comprising the patients included in a clinical trial, represents only the patients nominally satisfying the target population criteria who happen to have been selected by an investigator participating in the trial. Since the investigators undertaking clinical trials are not randomly selected from the universe of physicians who would treat patients with the target condition, their patients may not be a random, or even representative, selection from the universe of patients now or in the future. This fact alone does not necessarily render the trials invalid; if it did, there would be no valid intervention trials. In practice, the relevant target population is assumed not to differ greatly from the population actually represented by the patients selected for the trial. The degree to which this assumption is justified depends on how precisely the target population and patient selection criteria were defined, and how well these criteria were met by the patients entered into the trial.

RANDOMIZATION

The basic objective of an intervention trial is to
provide valid inferences about how the patients in the
target population would respond to the intervention strategies studied in the trial. Since the entire target population cannot be included in the trial, these inferences
must be based on random samples of the observations that
would result from applying the intervention strategies to
the target population (Mainland, 1963, pp. 72-78; Feinstein, 1977, pp. 105-120; Bulpitt, 1983, pp. 45-46, 48;
Friedman, Furberg, and DeMets, 1983, pp. 29-36). Randomization is the process for assigning the patients to the
treatment groups to assure that the patients in the trial
who receive a treatment can be regarded as a truly random
sample from the target population. The absence of randomization almost always renders suspect the validity of a
trial's conclusions; overcoming this suspicion requires
very dramatic findings (Bradford Hill, 1962, pp. 603-4).

Randomization can be accomplished in various ways.
Simple randomization would assign the patients entering
into the trial to the various groups without regard to
factors that might be present at entry. However, the
prognosis for the effectiveness of a treatment regimen
often depends on factors present at the onset of treatment. For example, in Kawasaki Disease the likelihood of
developing coronary artery lesions may depend on how long
the symptoms have been present before starting treatment,
the intensity of the inflammatory process, the age of the
patient, etc. Although randomization guards in principle
against systematic differences among the patients in the
various treatment groups with respect to these factors, it
does not guarantee similarity of the patients actually
entered into the treatment groups. Chance dissimilarity
of important prognostic factors among the treatment groups
can make it difficult or impossible to distinguish between
the effects of the treatments and the effects of the prognostic factors. Stratification, or random assignment of
the patients to the treatment groups separately within
strata defined by combinations of important prognostic
factors, is a simple way to protect against severe imbalance of important prognostic factors among treatment
groups (see, e.g., Friedman, Furberg, and DeMets, 1983,
Chapter 5). As a simple example, if a child's age (e.g.,
< 1 year of age, $\geq$ 1 year of age) were an important

prognostic factor for outcome in Kawasaki Disease, then separate randomization schedules should be used for the younger and the older children.

BLINDING

Blinding, the concealing of the identity of an assigned treatment in a trial, is as important as randomization. Randomization assures that the process of assigning patients to the various treatment groups does not cause systematic differences among the patients in the treatment groups. Blinding assures that there are no conscious or unconscious systematic differences in how the observations are made on the patients in the different treatment groups. Although the potential for observational bias with unblinded subjective evaluations is obvious, the objectivity of an observation is itself no guarantee against bias (Kahn, et al, 1969; Bulpitt, 1983, pp. 61-63).

Blinded trials do not require fixed treatment regimens. Using double observers (one person treats the patient and adjusts dosages, and another assesses the patient's response) or double dummies (each patient is supplied apparently with each treatment, but one of the treatment forms is a placebo, so that both treatments can be adjusted without revealing the identity of the active treatment) allows dosing flexibility without compromising the blindedness of the trial (Bulpitt, 1983, pp. 70-71). In a trial involving IV gamma globulin, for example, maintaining the blind would require that the children not receiving gamma globulin be treated with the same IV solution, but without the gamma globulin.

TREATMENT REGIMENS

The treatment regimens (route of administration, duration, timing, and frequency of treatment, etc.) that a trial employs directly affect the conclusions and their relevance. The efficacy and/or tolerability demonstrated by patients on a fixed regimen different from the usual usage of a treatment may be very different from what would occur were dosage adjustments allowed (Feinstein, 1977, pp. 108, 113). The interpretation of the results even of a trial that distinguished between two treatments could be equivocal if the regimens differed materially from the normal clinical use of the treatments. Regimen variations between otherwise similar trials often may help to explain differences in outcomes and conclusions.

Especially in Kawasaki Disease, it may be important to define the treatment regimen in terms of blood levels rather than in terms of dosage administered. Salicylate absorption in particular seems to be markedly depressed during the initial phase of the disease, when fever is present, so that ordinarily therapeutic dosages of aspirin may not yield blood levels of salicylate high enough for clinical effect.

OBSERVATIONS AND MEASUREMENTS

The questions the trial is designed to answer govern the timing of the observations on each patient, the kinds of measurements that are made (including procedures and techniques), who makes them (e.g., the investigator, a consulting specialist, the patient), etc. Careful consideration has to be given to the source of the data (designed case report forms, hospital records, etc.); the accuracy and reproducibility of the recording techniques (especially true when interpretations are involved, as with echocardiograms); the sensitivity and specificity of the key response variables; whether the response variable measures a relevant quantity; precisely how the measurement is obtained (e.g., if a measurement is an interpretation, is it obtained by the same person each time?); baseline evaluations; frequency of observation (too seldom may miss important within-patient variations); etc. Also important are the quality control procedures built into the trial, to assure that the data are recorded on schedule, that all required observations are made, that the data are being obtained properly, etc. Mainland (1963, Chapter 9) illustrates why these considerations are important.

SAMPLE SIZE

The number of patients entered into a trial represents a balance between sensitivity for detecting clinically meaningful treatment differences and not exposing patients needlessly to an inferior treatment. An inadequate sample size may lead to an appreciable probability of failing to detect even clinically worthwhile differences: Freiman et al (1978) found that most of 71 published trials had a greater than 10% chance of missing a 50% therapeutic improvement because of inadequate sample size.

The sample size needed for a trial depends on the clinically meaningful difference to be detected in the "key" response variable, the acceptable risk of concluding that a real difference exists when it does not (the Type 1 error rate), the acceptable risk of concluding that a real difference does not exist when it does (the Type 2 error rate), and the likelihood that a patient will not complete the trial. Unfortunately, published reports of clinical studies seldom discuss the Type 2 error rate, even though it is closely related to the sample size.

The Type 2 error rate and sample size are related through the magnitude of the clinically meaningful difference in the "key" response variable the investigator wishes to have a reasonable chance of detecting. Since the required sample size increases directly with the variability of the "key" response variable, it should be measured as precisely as possible. Although the value of the "clinically meaningful difference" the investigator wishes to detect often is chosen because of the outcome of a similar previous trial, the magnitude of the difference observed in the previous trial cannot be assumed to be the value that a new trial would achieve (Gould, 1983).

STATISTICAL METHODS

The statistical methods used to analyze the data from a trial should reflect the design of the trial and the nature of the variables analyzed. For example, if many clinics participate in the trial, the analysis should be one appropriate for a multiclinic trial (see also Fleiss, 1986). Likewise, if the data tend not to be symmetrically distributed, or if "extreme" values are not uncommon, then methods that do not assume a normal or Gaussian underlying distribution, such as nonparametric procedures, should be used instead of methods that do require this assumption, such as the analysis of variance. Subject to these general principles, the methods used to analyze the data are not nearly as critical to the credibility of the results as are the more fundamental issues of the questions the trial is intended to answer, the distinction between questions identified in advance and associations suggested by the data, proper definition of the trial population, and conscientious execution of the trial.

ACCOUNTING FOR ALL PATIENTS

Patients may withdraw from a clinical trial before completing the course of observation prescribed in the protocol for a number of reasons, some of which may be related to their treatment. Often, patients withdraw because of treatment intolerance or because they are not experiencing sufficient therapeutic effect. Ignoring these withdrawals can seriously bias the conclusions of the trial, especially if withdrawals occur heavily or at different rates in the treatment groups, since the remaining patients no longer may represent random representatives from the same population. Regardless of how withdrawals are addressed analytically (Gould, 1980), all patients randomly assigned to treatment must be accounted for either in the analysis or in the discussion. Finally, some provision should be made in the design of the trial for following up withdrawn patients, at least to be sure that no untoward events have occurred since they withdrew.

ACCOUNTING FOR BIAS

Many sources of bias can afflict a clinical trial. Sackett (1979) provided a catalog of 35 sources of bias; most, but not all, of these pertain to case-control and retrospective trials rather than prospective intervention trials. Randomization and blinding (with stratification if necessary), when executed properly, avoid the serious biases. However, it is worth noting that some biases can occur even in well-designed and executed studies: Compliance bias occurs when strict adherence to therapy is required, but not achieved, leading to confounding of efficacy and compliance; Expectation bias occurs when observers err systematically in measuring and recording observations to concur with prior expectations.

BRIEF DISCUSSION OF TRIALS PRESENTED AT THE SYMPOSIUM

The preceding discussion has covered many aspects of the application of statistical principles to clinical trials in Kawasaki Disease, so these need not be repeated here. The considerations listed in Table 1 clearly have figured into the planning and execution of the two large-scale clinical trials described at this Symposium. However, the similarity, but not identy, of the designs and findings of the two trials reinforces the necessity of specificity in defining the target population and treatment strategy. The three studies of the ongoing Japanese Gamma Globulin Trial (Dr. Furusho) reflect an evolving view of the most appropriate dosage regimen; 200 mg/kg/day of gamma globulin for 5 days either alone or in combination with adequate doses of aspirin appears to be as effective as 400 mg/kg/day of gamma globulin with aspirin and, in the short term, more effective than aspirin alone. The U.S. trial (Dr. Newberger) also reflects an evolving view about the most appropriate dosage regimen (2 gm/kg/day of gamma globulin for 1 day vs 400 mg/kg/day for 5 days); the only difference appears to be the greater reduction in maximum temperature during the first day with the single-dose regimen.

The conclusion from both trials is that an early course of an adequate dosage of IV gamma globulin along with large initial doses of aspirin (which might not be necessary) provides at least a short-term benefit in reducing the risk of vascular lesions. However, certain important issues remain to be resolved, as pointed out by Dr. Okuni: minimum effective dosage of gamma globulin; identification of alternative, equally effective dosing strategies, along with their costs and benefits; whether gamma globulin is prophylactic or therapeutic for coronary artery lesions; long-term consequences of alternative therapeutic strategies; safety, including adverse effects that may have a long latency; etc.

Some evidence suggests that drug therapy may not greatly benefit patients in whom lesions have already emerged, and that lesions may be inevitable regardless of the short-term effectiveness of various regimens. It may be appropriate to consider a trial to confirm Dr. Kitamura's findings on the results of alternative surgical interventions. Such a trial should study the short- and long-term consequences of various surgical interventions on patients who have developed lesions, both those in whom the prognosis without surgery would be poor, and those for whom surgery might be beneficial, but not currently needed.

REFERENCES

Bradford Hill, A. (1962). Statistical Methods in Clinical and Preventive Medicine (E. & S. Livingston, Ltd., Edinburgh).

Bradford Hill, A. (1971). Principles of Medical Statistics, 9th edition. (Oxford University Press, New York).

Bulpitt, C.J. (1983). Randomized Controlled Clinical Trials (Martinus Nijhoff, The Hague).

Feinstein, A.R. (1977). Clinical Biostatistics (C.V. Mosby, St. Louis).

Fleiss, J.L. (1986). Analysis of data from clinical trials. Controlled Clinical Trials 7, 267-275.

Freiman, J.A., Chalmers, T.C., Smith, H., and Kuebler, R.R. (1978). The importance of beta, the type II error, and sample size in the design and interpre- tation of the randomized control trial: survey of 71 "negative" trials. New England Journal of Medicine 299, 690-694.

Friedman, L.M., Furberg, C.D., and DeMets, D.L. (1983). Fundamentals of Clinical Trials (John Wright PSG, Inc., Boston).

Gould, A.L. (1980). A new approach to the analysis of clinical drug trials with withdrawals. Biometrics 36, 721-727.

Gould, A.L. (1983). Sample sizes required for binomial trials when the true response rates are estimated. Journal of Statistical Planning and Inference 8, 51-58.

Kahn, H.A. et al (1969). Serum cholesterol: Its distribution and association with dietary and other variables in a survey of 10,000 men. Israel Journal of Medical Science 5, 1117-1127.

Mainland, D. (1963) Elementary Medical Statistics, 2nd edition. (W. B. Saunders, Philadelphia).

Sackett, D.L. (1979). Bias in analytic research. Journal of Chronic Diseases 32, 51-63.

Sackett, D.L. (1980). The competing objectives of random- ized trials. New England Journal of Medicine 303, 1059-1060.

Kawasaki Disease, pages 471–474
© 1987 Alan R. Liss, Inc.

DISCUSSION:

THERAPY OF KAWASAKI DISEASE

Dr. Pachman (Chicago) asked if the proportions of free and bound salicylate differ in those with and those without hypoalbuminemia; it was thought not. Dr. Jacobs (New York) indicated that his salicylate regimen includes 150mg/kg/day on the first day, then 120mg/kg/day within 36 hours and 100mg/kg/day within another 36 hours. He noted that he had no data re the efficacy of aspirin in prevention of coronary lesions, and said that 5% of his patients have residual coronary lesions. Dr. Levin (London) pointed out that the Japanese studies show steroids to be worse than salicylates but that they do not demonstrate aspirin to be superior to no therapy.

Dr. Kato (Kurume) reported that there was no initial difference between his no aspirin group and the 30mg/kg/day group, but that aspirin appeared both to promote regression of coronary lesions and to prevent thrombus formation, with better results at 1-2 years in the aspirin group. He found in a comparison of 100mg/kg/day v. 30 mg/kg/day of aspirin that there was little difference in maximal sedimentation rate, fever, platelet count, or coronary problems but that platelet aggregation did not decrease in the 100mg/kg group but did with 30mg/kg, and there was about 80% with liver dysfunction in the high-dose group.

Dr. Tada (Tokyo) cautioned that high-dose IVGG might have unexpected results on the immune system, and he calculated that at 400mg/kg/day for five days the amount of immunoglobulin given is equivalent to 2000ml whole blood. He suggested that, if IVGG contains a neutralizing antibody

or antitoxin, convalescent serum could be used. Dr. Rosen
(Boston) suggested that in fact IVGG may provide anti-
idiotype antibody or may block Fc receptors on mononuclear
cells. Dr. Leung (Boston) pointed out that the failure of
pepsin-treated gamma globulin is important, since a cheaper
recombinant preparation could be used if only an intact Fc
portion were necessary.

Dr. Rauch (Atlanta) asked about the degree of center-
center variability in the U.S. IVGG trial; Dr. Newberger
(Boston) indicated that there was none with respect to the
aneurysm rate.

Dr. Yanase (Tokyo) reported that 8 patients had been
given pepsin-digested convalescent Kawasaki sera at doses
from 1-10mg/kg with unclear results. Three cases appeared
to show diminished fever and 5 had unchanged clinical
signs.

Dr. Benson (Toronto) emphasized that the experience in
Japan with endomyocardial biopsies showed abnormalities in
virtually all of 800-900 cases and that echo data show a
high frequency of functional abnormalities. He asked if
there were long-term implications even in those without
coronary aneurysms. Dr. Newberger responded that by echo
all the U.S. trial patients resolved systolic function
abnormalities and that diastolic function abnormalities
were more persistent; no differences were observed between
the IVGG and aspirin alone groups. In this regard, Dr.
Suzuki (Osaka) stated that, while IVGG prevents coronary
lesions, it doesn't prevent carditis more than aspirin, as
indicated by endomyocardial biopsy or gallium studies.

Dr. Takahashi (Los Angeles) asked if there had been any
attempt to standardize the echo equipment or readings in
the Japanese studies. Dr. Okuni (Tokyo) indicated that
they used standard criteria as did Dr. Furusho's group.
Dr. Onouchi (Aichi) reported a 20% rate of discrepancy in
echo readings done blindly. Dr. Nakano (Shizuoka) stated
that there is no uniform opinion regarding the classification of coronary lesions by echo and asked Dr. Newberger if
any information regarding the size of coronary lesions in
the U.S. trial was available, rather than merely presence
or absence. Dr. Newberger responded that no such information was available.

Dr. Lewis (Los Angeles) asked if there had been analysis of patients by the day of disease on which therapy had been begun in any of the GG trials. Dr. Newberger, speaking for the U.S. study, indicated that all children who had abnormalities on enrollment had been enrolled on Day 7 or later of illness. When those were excluded from analysis, there was no effect of day of enrollment on subsequent development of new aneurysms. Dr. Bierman (New York) emphasized that echocardiography is an inexact science and asked if there had been an attempt to separately analyze ectatic and aneurysmal lesions (defined, for example, as 1.5 times the adjacent vessel) with respect to mode of treatment. Dr. Newberger indicated that that had not been done. Dr. Nakano (Shizuoka) indicated that in the Japanese classification the mild form of coronary lesion is ectasia and the more severe form aneurysm, a subjective distinction. He feels it is more objective to classify vessels as <4mm or >4mm.

Dr. Levin (London) raised the issue of safety of IVGG re risk of AIDS or hepatitis. Dr. Rosen indicated that hepatitis has been reported only with British preparations of IVGG, and that normal liver tests have been documented in recipients of 34 lots of the preparation used in the U.S. trial. This preparation is also safe re HIV in that recipients have not seroconverted and spiking experiments show this agent to be readily destroyed in the manufacturing process. Dr. Nakano (Gifu) questioned whether IVGG should be used in all Kawasaki Disease patients because the side effects and mechanism are not known. He has administered IVGG to 50 of the last 100 patients he has seen with Kawasaki Disease and has seen two IVGG recipients develop coronary dilatation >4mm; the remainder remained normal. He believes the indications for IVGG therapy are: 1) serum albumin <3gm/dl; 2) cholinesterase <0.50ΔpH; or 3) an echo-enhanced coronary lesion. He also administers vitamin E 100mg/day orally to all patients.

Dr. Kusukawa (Tokyo) asked how long after formation of a thrombus urokinase would be effective in lysis, since chest pain is not necessarily the first sign. Dr. Kato agreed that it is difficult to determine when a thrombus forms, even using echo and angiography. Since patients with giant aneurysms easily form thrombi, he recommends outpatient echo evaluation to inspect the inside of the aneurysm every two weeks. Dr. Wiggins (Denver) asked about the optimal anticoagulants for patients with giant aneurysms and thrombus formation. Dr. Kato reported on three such patients who developed thrombi despite aspirin and persantine. Dr. Takahashi cautioned against too great reliance on the echo for early thrombus detection and indicated that one must change the gain for detection. Dr. Kato felt that old thrombus is more difficult to detect than early thrombus.

Dr. Nakano (Gifu) reported a 5-year-old who was followed by echo every two weeks and who suffered a myocardial infarct despite warfarin and aspirin. Within 5 hours PCTR was performed and 30,000u/kg urokinase was given. Almost immediately the EKG showed improvement, although echo showed persistent large thrombus. Despite discontinuation of urokinase, the thrombus completely resolved by echo within two weeks. He postulated that the new thrombus responded to PCTR and a new channel formed within the thrombus while in vivo thrombolysis led to complete resolution. This patient had a massive nasal hemorrhage as a consequence of urokinase and had had a minor nasal hemorrhage prior to this therapy. Dr. Kato emphasized that the bleeding tendency is much less with use of urokinase than with streptokinase.

Dr. Wedgewood (Seattle) asked about the cost of coronary bypass surgery and how many patients could be treated with IVGG for that cost. Dr. Kitamura (Nara) indicated that the Japanese government currently supports care of Kawasaki patients including surgery but will not cover IVGG cost.

Dr. Chung (San Diego) asked about the bypass experience in children under 4 years old. Dr. Kitamura indicated that he has operated on a 2 1/2-year-old and a 4-year-old with two saphenous vein grafts that were patent at one month but not at one year. He uses dipyrimadole and coumadin post-bypass. In response to Dr. Takahashi's question about whether he had noted any internal mammary artery abnormalities, Dr. Kitamura indicated not and emphasized they use only the distal portion. Dr. Suzuki reported on 12 patients with six saphenous and 10 internal mammary grafts. These include a 2-year-old and two 3-year-olds with patent internal mammary grafts. She believes that saphenous grafts occlude after one year. Dr. Cheatham (Omaha) agreed that internal mammary is the graft of choice and that most saphenous grafts occlude. He asked what the options were for children with occluded venous grafts. Dr. Kitamura emphasized the substantial degree of collateral formation or recannalization that occurs in such children.

Kawasaki Disease, pages 475-484
© 1987 Alan R. Liss, Inc.

IS KAWASAKI HLA ASSOCIATED?

Noel Maclaren, M.D.and Nicos Skordis, M.D.
Department of Pathology, University of Florida College of Medicine, Box J-275, JHMHC, Gainesville, Florida 32610

Kawasaki syndrome (K.S.) or mucocutaneous lymph node syndrome, characteristically afflicts infants and young children with fever, conjunctivitis, stomatitis, cheilitis, glossitis, cervical adenitis, polymorphous rash, erythema and induration of the palms and soles and desquamation of the fingertips. Interest in K.S. stems from the aneurysmal dilatation and thromboses within the coronary arteries, in about a third of patients, with sudden cardiac failure and death of a few percent of them.

Is K.S. Genetically Determined?

Etiological data strongly suggest that an etiological agent is involved in K.S. since clusters of cases are seen especially in Winter and Spring, superimposed upon a sporadic endemic occurrence. One recent study implicated a retrovirus in the pathogenesis (1). Whereas some reports of familial occurrences of K.S. has been forthcoming, the number has been small perhaps due to the relative rarity of K.S. One argument for an inherited predisposition comes from the strong predeliction of orientals and especially Japanese for K.S. Thus one could suppose that this ethnic group had predisposition genes not often present among others. Alternatively, it could be argued that epidemiological factors peculiar to orientals could provide the explanation. The same discussion might equally apply to acquired immuno deficiency disease or AIDS which has been identified in only a handful of Japanese living in Japan. Are factors involved in the contagion of HTL-III virus so different in Japan versus the USA or could genetic predispositions be involved?

More males than females have been reported to develop K.S. Since K.S. typically afflicts prepubertal children, hormonal differences between the sexes may not explain this effect of gender. Whereas newborn males secrete augmented levels of testosterone for several weeks to months after birth, estradiol and testosterone levels are not different between the sexes after this until the onset of puberty. Could a predisposition gene be located on the x chromosome to account for the male excess seen? In insulin dependent diabetes (IDD) there is a clear excess of males over females for those developing the disease in early life, but these gender differences disappear in patients presenting after 5 years of age. It might be interesting to learn whether a similar age related gender affect, occurs in K.S.

Perhaps the most compelling evidence for an inherited predisposition to K.S. comes from the limited HLA studies reported to date. Whereas these findings will be discussed later, it may be important to acknowledge at this point that K.S. may be heterogeneous and that HLA associations may be applicable to only one subtype.

The Human Leukocyte Antigen (HLA) System:

Immune response genes include those of the HLA system on chromosome 6, the immunoglobulin complex on chromosomes 2, 14 and 22, and T lymphocyte receptor genes on chromosomes 7 and 14. Whereas all are possible candidates for explanation for associations with immunologically mediated disorders, the most striking findings to date have been with the HLA complex. To discuss possible HLA associations with K.S., some overview of the HLA system may be helpful.

Class I HLA molecules (A, B, C, antigens) have distinctive heavy chains encoded by separate loci on the short arm of chromosome 6, which combine with an invariant light β_2 microglobulin chain to form a trans membrane molecule present on the surface of all nucleated body cells. Structural homologies to immunoglobulin molecules are evident. In functional terms, HLA molecules aid the distinction of self from non self. Class I molecules are also important in T lymphocyte mediated cytotoxicity responses. Class II molecules (D related) consist of two glycopeptide chains which form transmembrane dimers on the surfaces of only certain immunocompetent cells such as macrophages, B lymphocytes and activated T lymphocytes. Whereas somatic cells with the exception of certain endothelia and dendritic cells do not usually express class II antigens, they may be induced to do so by lymphokines such as gamma interferon. In a number of autoimmune disorders, aberrant expression of class II HLA on target tissues may be an important pathogenic event since an important function of these molecules is to present antigens to initiate immune responses. Thus autoantigen presentation may also be facilitated by such aberrant class II antigen expression, although cause and effect in this regard has yet to be proven. Class II antigens are also important in cell-cell interactions as part of the immune response.

Structurally, each class II HLA chain consists of two extracellular domains, a connecting piece, a transmembrane portion and a small intracellular tail. The first class

II allelic series of genes was designated DR;
however with the aid of molecular genetic and
other techniques, two further subregions
designated DQ and DP have been identified.
The DR subregion consists of one locus
encoding invariant DR chains and two
polymorphic ß chain encoding loci and one DRß
pseudogene. The DR specificities 1 through
W10 (DR5 and DRW6 are further split into two:
DRW11 and 12; 13 and 14) are determined by the
polymorphic $ß_1$ locus, while the DR $ß_2$ encodes
for one ß chain component of DRW52 associated
with DR3, 5 and W6 specificities, and one ß
chain component of DRW 53 associated with DR4,
7 and 9. DR1 and DR2 chromosomes lack $ß_2$
locus expressivity. Immediately centromeric
are the DQ and DQß loci. Three DQ molecules
are produced. DQWI is found on DR1, DR2 and
some DR5 chromosomes, DQW2 is found on DR3 and
most DR7 chromosomes while DQW3 is associated
with DR4, DR6 and DR9, and some DR5 and DR7
chromosomes. More centromeric again are DX ,
DXß, DOß and DZ loci followed by one DP and
DPß locus and one DP and DPß pseudogene.
(figure 1).

Recombinant events are non random through
the HLA complex genome, but occur in 3 hot
spot regions; the DQ subregion, between the DQ
and DP subregions and between class I B and C
loci. Class III alleles encode complement
(C_2, C_4 properdin factor B) allotypes. Class
III loci reside near the class I HLA-B locus.
The line up of HLA alleles on a six chromosome
is an HLA haplotype, and usually such
haplotypes are inherited completely with a few
percent recombinant events. However over the
aeons, such recombinations have not reached
equilibrium between alleles at different loci,
for reasons which remain unclear. Rather,
alleles at difference loci occur in non
randomly distributed statistical haplotypes, a
phenomenon termed linkage disequilibrium.

HLA and Disease Susceptibility:

Particular HLA gene products are associated with susceptibility to certain diseases, notably those with autoimmune features. For some diseases, class I HLA associations are primary. Examples include the relationship between HLA-B27 and diseases such as Reiter's syndrome and ankylosing spondylitis, in which presence of HLA-B27 is a genetic requirement but interaction with an environmental factor such as the organism Shigella flexneri, is necessary to trigger it.

In most instances however, the primary associations are to class II antigens (table I). Whereas for most of these diseases, weak associations with class I HLA were initially reported, primary associations with class II antigens were subsequently realized. In the case of insulin dependent diabetes, initial reports linked the disease to HLA B8, B18, B15, B40 etc. while subsequently it was discovered that the primary associations were with DR3 (linkage disequilibrium to B8 and B18) and DR4 (linkage disequilibria to B15[62], B40[60] and B12[44]).

In a recent study by Ayoub and colleagues from Florida, Caucasian patients with rheumatic fever were found to have increased frequencies of DR4, with a relative risk value of 3.6 for the antigen (2). Relative risk (RR) is the number of times risk of disease is increased or decreased in individuals with a certain HLA in comparison to those without the marker. A RR of 1.0 indicates no association, while significantly negative or positive associations indicate protective or susceptibility effects respectively. In Ayoub's study, the strength of associations to DR4 was even higher in patients with clinical associations such as chorea (RR 4.1) and persistent mitral insufficiency (RR 8.8).

There was also a positive correlation between DR4 and persistent antibody to streptococcal carbohydrate antigen (RR 4.3). For black patients, DR4 was only slightly more increased than controls (RR 1.3); however DR2 was strikingly more common (RR 10.7).

In other studies of rheumatoid arthritis (RA) among U.S. and European Caucasians, it became evident that an association with DR4 was present.(3) DR4 positive chromosomes can be split into subtypes by primed lymphocyte reactions. The DW4 subtype so defined is strongly associated with susceptibility to RA but this is so for not the DW10 subtype. Whereas DR4 associations with RA holds for many other ethnic groups such as Chippewa Indians and Japanese, DR4 is present in only 23% of Black Americans with RA. Among Asian Indians living in the UK and Ashkenazi Jews living in Israeli, the HLA association with RA is to DR1. A monoclonal antibody (109d6) which defines DR4 specificity was found to react with 90% of Caucasian patients with RA, a considerable excess over that for conventional DR4 reactive alloantiserum. The antibody reacted with DR1 positive RA patients also.(4) In very recent studies, a common domain in DRß coding genes was identifiable in DR1 and DR4 chromosomes conveying susceptibility to RA, suggesting that the antibody 109d6 was reacting to a common epitope on both DR molecules.

There are two monoclonal antibodies A 10/13 and II B3 which recognize the DQW3 related specificities TA 10 and 2 B3 respectively and thus can split DR4 chromosomes (5). It was further shown that the TA 10 occurred less frequently in IDD DR4 patients than DR4 normal controls (6).

HLA Associations with Kawasaki Syndrome:

Virtually all studies performed to date have involved class I alleles, and interpretation of the results (table 2) is difficult because of the different ethnic groups represented.(7) By analogy with the disease associations (table 1) described above, primary linkage to DR antigens would be most likely for KS also.

Among Japanese, positive associations with the Japanese variant of B22 have been reported.(8,9) Based upon studies of IDD in Japanese, this variant, now designated as B54, is the one primarily involved. This B54 antigen is in strong linkage disequilibrium with DR4 and DR9. Thus one might guess that KS among Japanese might similarly have positive associations with DR4 and DR9 and/or DQW3, as is the case for insulin dependent diabetes among Japanese (table I).

Table 1

Some Disease Associations With
Certain HLA-DR/DQW

DR2	:	Narcolepsy Goodpasture's Syndrome
		Multiple sclerosis DIOADM syndrome
DR3	:	Graves disease Myasthenia Gravis Sjögrens syndrome Chronic active hepatitis
		Gold/Penicillamine nephritis
DR2 or DR3	:	SLE
DR4	:	Pemiphigus vulgaris
DR4 or (DR1)	:	Rheumatoid Arthritis-(In Jews)

Continued

Table 1 continued

DR4 or (DR2)	:	Rhematic Fever-(In Blacks)
DR4 or DR3	:	Insulin dependent diabetes and
or DR1 or (DR9)	:	Addison's disease-(In Japanese)
DR5	:	Juvenile chronic polyarthritis Hodgkins
DQW2 (DR3/DR7)	:	Celiac disease Dermatitis herpetiformis
DQW3 (DR5/DR4)	:	Chronic lymphocytic leukemia

In another report from Israel (10) BW51 was found to be increased, while in New England, B5 and its BW51 split were more common among patients with KS than local controls.(11) In the Boston area, 80% of patients were HLA-B5 and 70% were HLA BW51 during endemic periods; however there were no HLA-B5 individuals identified during an epidemic period. Rather, the epidemic patients had an increased incidence of BW44.(12) DR linkage disequilibria with B51 include DR2, DR3 and DR5. In other reports an association with B44 has been reported, especially with the A2 B44 CW5 haplotype.(13) Thus one might suspect that a primary association between KS and DR4 might be uncovered by specific studies. Taken together, the studies to date would suggest an important association with DR4 to be probable (perhaps including DR9 among Japanese) while another antigen such as DR2 may be associated in other patients such as Ashkenazi Jews. To prove such speculations, however, specific studies are now required.

References

Ayoub E, Barrett D, Maclaren N and Krischer J (1986). Association of class II human histocompatibility leukocyte antigens with rheumatic fever. J Clin Invest 77:2019-2026.

Bontrop RE, Schreuder GMTh, Mikulski MA, van Miltenburg RT, Giphart MJ (1986). Polymorphisms within the HLA-DR4 haplotypes: various DQ subtypes detected with monoclonal antibodies. Tissue Antigens 27:22-31.

Kaslow R, Railowitz A, Feng Y, et al. (1985). Association of epidemic Kawasaki syndrome with the HLA-A2, B44, CW5 antigen combination. Arthritis and Rhematism 28:938-940.

Kato S, Kimura M, Tsuji K, et al. (1978). HLA antigens in Kawasaki disease. Pediatrics 61:252-255.

Keren G, Danon Y, Orgad S, et al. (1982). HLA B51 is increased in mucocutaneous lymph node syndrome in Isaeli patients. Tissue Antigens 20:144-146.

Krensky A, Berenberg W, Shanley K and Yunis E (1981). HLA antigens in mucocutaneous lymph node syndrome in New England. Pediatrics 67:741-743.

Krensky A, Grady S, Shanley K, et al. (1983). Epidemic and endemic HLA-B and DR associations in mucocutaneous lymph node syndrome. Human Immunol 6:75-77.

Lee S, Gregersen P, Shen H, et al. (1984). Strong association of rheumatoid arthritis with the presence of a polymorphic Ia epitope defined by a monoclonal antibody: comparison with the allodeterminant DR4. Rhematol Int 4, Suppl. 17.

Matsuda, I., Hattori, S., Nagata, N., et al.: HLA antigens in mucocutaneous lymph node syndrome. Clinical memoranda. Am J Dis Child 131:1417-1418.

Shulman S and Rowley AH (1986). Does Kawasaki disease have a retroviral aetiology? Preliminary Communication. Lancet 2:545-546.

Tait BD and Boyle AJ (1986). DR4 and
  susceptibility to type I diabetes mellitus:
  discrimination of high risk and low risk DR4
  haplotypes on the basis of TA10 typing.
  Tissue Antigens 28:65-71.
Winchester R (1986). The HLA system and
  susceptibility to diseases: an
  interpretation.   Clinical Aspects of
  Autoimmunity 1, 1:9-26.
Woodrow J (1986).   Analysis of the HLA
  association with rheumatoid arthritis.
  Disease Markers 4:7-12.

Kawasaki Disease, pages 485–491
© 1987 Alan R. Liss, Inc.

KAWASAKI SYNDROME
FURTHER ETIOLOGIC PURSUITS - NOT TRIVIAL

Karl M. Johnson, M.D.
Vice President, Medical Affairs
Viratek
3300 Hyland Avenue
Costa Mesa, CA 92626

I have been asked to comment on current hypotheses
regarding the etiology of Kawasaki Syndrome and to suggest
some further endeavor. Before I do, I should emphasize
that:
1. I was unable, due to unavoidable acute responsi-
bilities, to have the benefit of presentations and discussion during this important and useful symposium.
2. I am not a pediatrician and have never worked
directly on the problem.
3. I am not a retrovirologist.
4. I have had a reasonably high "stumble quotient" in
the past when it came to discovery of etiologic agents of
"new" viral disease and of discerning the broad outlines of
epidemiology and ecology which define their behavior.

Think, then, that the following sense are offered in
the spirit of an attempt to sense an emergent forest in a
rapidly expanding thicket of trees. I well remember how
pleased we all were at the 1st International Symposium
nearly three years ago to discover general consensus that
Kawasaki Syndrome is most probably an infectious disease
for which host genetics plays a significant role in disease
expressions. Where are we today?

IS KAWASAKI A SYNDROME OR A DISEASE? (KS OR KD?)

You may think that this question is merely semantic.
After all, we have sound clinical criteria laid down by
both the Japan MCLS Research Committee (1978) and the

Centers for Disease Control (Morens, 1981), and these have been used to plot occurrence of the illness throughout the world with the result that age, race, and season have all been implicated as important variables in its natural history. My own concern is that when we use Disease rather than Syndrome to describe a <u>clinical</u> entity, we begin to assume, consciously or otherwise, that the process has a single necessary etiologic entity; in this case, one infectious agent. It has frequently turned out to be so in the past, but not always. We won't know until any putative agent is finally isolated, shown to replicate and to be convincingly associated with both infection and disease.

Part of what prompts this gentle admonition is the apparent emergence of "endemic", as well as "epidemic", Kawasaki Syndrome. As you see, I strongly support "syndrome" over "disease" at present. This pattern is nowhere better illustrated than in a recent paper (Salo, et al., 1986) from Finland wherein an epidemic (fall-winter 1982) is placed on a background of clearly endemic illness occurring from 1981-84. All cases were based on the clinical criteria of the Japanese and American oracles. Do all, or nearly all of these cases have the same etiology? If so, I believe that the total pattern has important significance for the type of etiologic agent which is likely, or unlikely, to be the necessary if not the sufficient cause of a single disease. In the meantime, is there anything objective short of an agent in hand that can be used to strengthen the definition of Syndrome in the direction of Disease? I am personally impressed by the recent paper (Leung, et al., 1986) in which the authors demonstrate that acute phase KS sera lyse gamma interferon-activated human endothelial cells. Although the authors showed that this phenomenon is probably not a question of either type I or II histocompatibility antigens and although they suggest that it may be common to acute vascular injury, I believe the latter question, in particular, needs to be elucidated. To be sure, the host has only so many clinical and pathological ways to respond to a larger variety of insult; nevertheless, KS and periarteritis nodosa are very similar in pathological manifestations and rather distinct from other syndromes marked by vascular injury. Further, the technology and clinical samples required for examining this issue are readily available. Thus, epidemic versus endemic KS, active periarteritis nodosa in adults, and other vascular syndromes would be good candidates for determining whether there is anything here of specificity to KS or even epidemic KS. We urgently require a more definitive marker than is presently available.

HAS A CANDIDATE ETIOLOGIC AGENT FOR KAWASAKI SYNDROME BEEN ISOLATED?

If my thoughts on this question are similar to those of Dr. Wade Parks, please be assured that there was absolutely no prior collusion. If not, please remember that Dr. Parks is both pediatrician and retrovirologist!

Very recently research groups in Boston and Chicago (Shulman and Rowley, 1986) (Burns, et al., 1986) have reported that blood mononuclear cells from KS induce detectable increase in reverse transcriptase (RT) activity when co-cultivated with appropriate "activated" continuous cell lines or PHA-stimulated cells from normal donors. Non-KS patients exhibited no such RT activation. The assay is basically that which has become popular, and successful, for detection of human immunodeficiency virus (HIV). Unlike HIV, however, neither KS research team has been able to satisfy the basic requisite for candidacy, namely that there exists a replicating agent. Of special puzzlement is the fact that Burns, et al., were able to transmit RT activity to HUT-78 cells from irradiated positive primary cultures, but apparently only for a single passage (Burns, et al., 1986). The existence of an agent, barring new data presented at this symposium, is tantalizing, but not demonstrated.

IS THE POSSIBLE CANDIDATE KS AGENT A RETROVIRUS?

Perhaps. THe electron micrograph published by the Boston workers shows particles in KS patient mononuclear cells which are compatible with, if not compelling as, a retrovirus. But as Burns, et al., correctly point out, the RT activity on which so much of the current anticipation rests has not yet been shown to depend on an RNA-directed enzyme. Thus, the candidate virus and its "retro" property remain to be proven.

DOES A RETROVIRUS MAKE SENSE AS CAUSE OF KS?

This final question is easily the most interesting. If positive, it has profound implications, not only for KS but also for human vascular disease in a wider sense, and most likely for our biological understanding of the Retroviridae.

Retroviruses are generally species-specific agents which cause chronic infection in their respective hosts. They have the capacity to form a DNA provirus which is integrated into host cell DNA and may be transmitted either endogenously or exogenously. The best characterized exogenously transmitted members are the animal lentiviruses to which HIV belongs. Although infection by some of these agents induces acute disease (HIV and equine infectious anemia (EIA)), subsequent events are dominated by persistence of fully infectious virus in the blood and other tissues, and transmission is generally a direct or indirect consequence of viremia or virocytemia. A possible exception is Visna virus of sheep for which respiratory secretion-based transmission is suspected (Haase, 1986). Thus, venereal and/or vector-borne (whether needles or arthropods) transmission appears to be a hallmark of presently known exogenous retroviruses.

Kawasaki Syndrome is certainly not a venereal infection; unless such infection occurs in utero or during or shortly after birth. In such a pattern chronic exogenous infection would be common among adults or chronic infection could be a phenomenon governed by reproduction in which pre- or peri-natal infection is the epidemiologically controlling event. This second alternative is characteristic of arenaviruses. In either event, however, we must account for the childhood pattern of acute KS, endemic and especially epidemic. The necessary triggering co-factor (or factors) is difficult to postulate.

Less difficult to contemplate is a transmission scheme in which chronic exogenous infection, venereal or not, leads to intermittant shedding of virus from respiratory or gastrointestinal tract. Again, however, the observed descriptive epidemiology of KS dictates that something more than such infection is required to account for seasonal epidemics.

Finally, it could be suggested that KS arises from chronic infection which is transmitted by arthropods. The wide and ecologically diverse distribution of the syndrome argues against this hypothesis if it is based on the concept that virus replicates in both arthropod and vertebrate host because most such cycles have relatively species-specific arthropod reservoirs, and also would be dubious if based on mechanical arthropod transmission because it is difficult to provide a list of flying or crawling "needles" which fit circumstances in Australia, Japan, Hawaii, or Finland, to list a few of the places where KS occurs. In sum, it appears likely that if KS is caused by a retrovirus having the classical property of proviral-induced chronicity, important new virus-host biology must emerge.

Suppose there are retroviruses incapable of pro-viral integration; agents which must survive by means that my former mentor, Dr. Robert Huebner, described in the succinct term "straight". Such a virus would certainly make life easier for the epidemiologist, but probably not the virologist with a sense of evolutionary perspective. Why would a retrovirus give up a fundamental mechanism that guarantees its virtual parasitic perfection? Could such an agent be thought of as a pre-retrovirus, something that had not yet learned how to insinuate itself into host cell DNA; a virus that has only a cytoplasmic existence? The idea is certainly possible, but just as in the foregoing discussion of transmission, I fear that we are stretching the credulity of nature, not to mention our own. Thus, my personal opinion is that it is unlikely that KS is caused by a retrovirus which could be placed into any of the presently recognized genera of that family.

Does the recent demonstration that high-dose gamma globulin therapy reduces the incidence of coronary artery disease in KS mean that antibodies against the unknown etiologic agent are widespread in adult populations in Japan and the United States? Perhaps, but it has been well said that there are several other reasons which might account for the observed effect (Newburger, et al., 1986) (Melish, 1986). There are surely miles to go before we wrest the answer to the mystery.

SOME SUGGESTIONS

What then should be done with the present clues? The evident issues have no doubt been thoroughly discussed. With regard to the "virus" they include:
1. Demonstration that the RT activation is RNA-dependent.
2. Further work to establish replication.
3. Search for antigens in presumably infected mono-nuclear cells. This weapon could be used to define the crucially important issue of infection: morbidity ratio.
4. Determine whether the RT activity observed acutely is also chronic and whether it occurs in family clusters.

With respect to other, perhaps trivial, etiologic pursuits I offer only these small suggestions:
1. Find out whether or not the gamma-interferon-endothelial cell interaction is syndrome specific.
2. Attempt to obtain as many frozen tissues as possible from the occasional child who has the misfortune to die very acutely from KS and use convalescent KS sera to search for agent-specific antigens. Remember that the primary sites of replication of the etiologic agent may not be the disease-targeted vessels. This general approach finally produced Hantaan virus (Lee, et al., 1978), cause of hemorrhagic fever with renal syndrome, after decades of fruitless "straight" searching for that agent.

Finally, let me offer both my thanks and my apologies to you all for the invitation to contemplate the problem and my inability to defend or modify some of my outlandish thought. My purpose was and is to stimulate. What I believe is now evident to us all is the fact that KS has much greater eventual biological significance than the morbidity and mortality it occasions. This problem deserves very significant continuing effort, both intellectual and financial. We must do what we can to ensure that this happens.

REFERENCES

Burns JC, Geha RS, Schneeberger EE, Newburger JW, Rosen FS, Glezen LS, Huang AS, Natale J, Leung DYM (1986). Polymerase activity in lymphocyte culture supernatants from patients with Kawasaki disease. Nature 323:814-816.

Hasse AT (1986). Pathogenesis of lentivirus infections. Nature 322:130-136.

Lee HW, Lee PW, Johnson KM (1978). Isolation of the etiologic agent of Korean hemorrhagic fever. J Inf Dis 137:298-308.

Leung DYM, Collins T, Lapierre LA, Geha RS, Prober JS. (1986). Immunoglobulin M antibodies present in the acute phase of Kawaski syndrome lyse cultured vascular endothelial cells stimulated by gamma Interferon. J Clin Invest 77:1428-35.

Melish ME (1986). Intravenous immunoglobulin in Kawasaki syndrome: a progress report. Pediatr Inf Dis 5:5211-15.

Morens DM (1981). Kawasaki disease. In Feigen RD, Cherry JD (eds): "Textbook of pediatric infectious diseases." Philadelphia: WB Saunders, pp 1637-48.

Newburger JW, Takahaski M, Burns JC, Beisen AS, Chung KJ, Duff CE, Glode MP, Mason WH, Reddy V, Sanders SP, Shulman ST, Wiggins JW, Hicks RV, Fullton DR, Lewis AB, Leung DYM, Colton T, Rosen FS, Melish ME (1986). The treatment of Kawasaki syndrome with intravenous gamma globulin. N E J Med 315:341-77.

Salo E, Palkonen P, Pettay O (1986). Outbreak of Kawasaki syndrome in Finland. Act Paediatr Scand 75:75-80.

Shulman ST, Rowley AH (1986). Does Kawasaki disease have a retroviral aetiology? Lancet 2:545-546.

The Japan MCLS Committee (1978). Diagnostic guidelines of infantile acute febrile mucocutaneous lymph node syndrome. 3rd ed. Tokyo: Japan Red Cross Medical Centre.

Kawasaki Disease, pages 493–508
© 1987 Alan R. Liss, Inc.

CAN CONSENSUS BE REACHED IN CARDIAC MANAGEMENT OF KAWASAKI
SYNDROME?: REVIEW OF A SURVEY AMONG JAPANESE AND U.S. PEDIA-
TRIC CARDIOLOGISTS

Masato Takahashi and Hirohisa Kato

Childrens Hospital of Los Angeles, Los Angeles,
California (M.T.), Kurume University School of
Medicine, Kurume, Japan (H.K.)

INTRODUCTION

Kawasaki syndrome (KS) has become an international disease. In the United States and Japan, it appears to be the
leading cause of acquired heart disease in childhood. Although there is uniformity in the clinical criteria for initial diagnosis of Kawasaki syndrome, controversy abounds in
the areas of diagnosis of cardiovascular lesions and their
management. We conducted a binational bilingual survey on
how the patients are currently managed for their cardiovascular problems. We will review the results of the survey, comparing responses to each question from the two countries followed by some discussion. It is our hope that understanding
areas of consensus as well as areas of controversy will enable us to focus our efforts toward more uniform management
strategies in this syndrome.

METHODS

Between September 1 and September 30, 1986 questionnaires were sent to 220 U.S. cardiologists affiliated with teach-
ing or large community hospitals in the membership roster of
Cardiology Section of American Academy of Pediatrics and 174
Japanese cardiologists belonging to large and medium sized
hospitals on the list of hospitals collaborating with the
Kawasaki Disease Research Committee of the Japanese Ministry
of Health and Welfare. With the hopes of maximizing responses, questionnaires were written in English for the American
cardiologists and in Japanese for the Japanese cardiologists.
With the exception of one additional question in Japanese,

both questionnaires were identical in content. However, pos-
sibilities exist that, due to translation from English to Japanese, some variations in nuance may have arisen between the
Japanese and English versions. Those responses received by
November 25, 1986 were tallied and analysed.

RESULTS AND DISCUSSION

The questions and responses are presented in table format in the order of appearance in the original questionnaire.
The percentages refer to the total number of respondents.
Most questions were phrased to elicit single answers. Other
questions were phrased to permit multiple answers. There
were respondents from both countries who gave more than one
answer to a single-answer question and those who left some
questions unanswered. Thus, the percentages of responses do
not always add up to 100 percent.

TABLE 1.

U.S. - JAPAN SURVEY ON CARDIAC MANAGEMENT
OF KAWASAKI SYNDROME

PERCENT RESPONSE

JAPAN	U.S.A.
155/174 (89%)	86/220 (39%)

P   0.0001

Response rate

Significantly greater percentage of Japanese cardiologists responded to the survey than their American counter-
parts. Those physicians contacted in Japan are accustomed
to such surveys (ankehto in Japanese). In Japan ankehtos are
often utilized as a means of reaching a consensus in mutually
important issues. Americans, on the other hand, have somewhat negative attitudes toward surveys.

TABLE 1.1.

When did you first encounter a patient with Kawasaki syndrome
(KS)?

	Japan	(%)	USA	(%)
Before 1970	76	(49)	4	(4.7)
1970-74	53	(34.2)	19	(22.1)
1975-79	14	(9.0)	48	(55.8)
1980 or later	8	(5.2)	15	(17.4)

TABLE 1.2.

How many new KS patients have you seen in the past 12 months?

	JAPAN	(%)	USA	(%)
Less than 10	23	(14.8)	45	(52.3)
11-20	42	(27.1)	29	(10.5)
21-40	40	(25.8)	7	(8.1)
41-60	25	(16.1)	4	(4.7)
61-80	10	(6.5)	0	
81-100	5	(3.2)	0	
More than 100	7	(4.5)	0	

Questions on overall experience with Kawasaki syndrome

Over 80 percent of the polled Japanese cardiologists have had experience with Kawasaki syndrome dating back before 1975, while only one quarter of American cardiologists have had similarly long experiences. Majority of the responding Japanese cardiologists have seen more than 20 KS patients in the past year while only a handful of American cardiologists can claim this experience. Thus, these Japanese physicians have far greater length and breadth of experience with the disease than the Americans.

TABLE 2.1.

Do you order an echocardiogram in all KS patients or in certain selected patients?

	JAPAN	(%)	USA	(%)
All patients	154	(99.4)	86	(100)
Selected patients	1	(0.6)	0	

TABLE 2.2.

How many echocardiograms do you order on each patient during the first two months of KS?

	JAPAN	(%)	USA	(%)
Once	0		8	(9.3)
2 times	9	(5.8)	30	(34.9)
3 times	23	(14.8)	30	(34.9)
4 times	26	(16.8)	13	(15.1)
5 times or more	96	(61.9)	4	(4.7)

TABLE 2.3.

If a patient has coronary artery abnormalities, how often do you repeat echocardiography?

	JAPAN	(%)	USA	(%)
Every 6 months	75	(48.4)	50	(58.1)
Every 12 months	2	(1.3)	8	(9.3)
Other	74	(47.7)	25	(29.1)

TABLE 2.4.

What echo modalities do you use for evaluation of KS patients?

	JAPAN	(%)	USA	(%)
2D only	20	(12.9)	14	(16.3)
2D and M-mode	83	(53.5)	33	(38.4)
2D, M-mode and Doppler	52	(33.5)	39	(45.3)

TABLE 2.5.

What criteria do you use to determine abnormal coronary arteries? (multiple answers allowed)

	JAPAN	(%)	USA	(%)
Increased perivascular echo brightness	74	(47.7)	23	(26.7)
Increased diameter of coronary artery segment	151	(97.4)	79	(91.9)
Distal diameter greater than proximal diameter	105	(67.7)	57	(66.3)
Irregular or "beady" appearance	105	(67.7)	67	(77.9)

Echocardiography

There is unanimity of opinion on both shores regarding utility of echocardiography in this disease. However, the number of times echocardiography is done during the first two months of illness varies greatly between the two countries. About 80 percent of Japanese cardiologists order echocardiography four or more times during this period. In contrast, 79 percent of U.S. cardiologists ordered echocardiography three times or less during the same time period. Both short-term and long-term follow-up studies have shown that coronary artery disease in this syndrome is dynamic. Coronary arteritis begins early in the disease process and the mean time of appearance of dilatory lesion is the 10th illness day. (1) These dilatory lesions may progress into more lasting aneurysms or may regress rapidly. (2,3) One needs to capture this dynamic disease process by means of serial echo examinations while paying heed to cost-effectiveness. In the opinion of one of us (MT) who participated in the multicenter U.S. study, the optimal number would be four times: at the time of initial diagnosis, 4-6 days later, 2-3 weeks later and 6-8 weeks later. In cases where very large aneurysms threaten rupture or myocardial infarction, however, more frequent echocardiographic examinations may be warranted.

In regard to the frequency with which echocardiography is repeated in case of chronic coronary artery abnormalities (Table 2.3), there appears to be a reasonable consensus on the six-monthly interval.

Combination of M-mode and 2-D echocardiograms is the most often used in Japan, while combination of 2-D, M-mode and Doppler is the one prefered by most cardiologists in the U.S. With recognition that valvular regurgitations frequently accompany the carditis due to KS, Doppler echocardiogram will be used more often in the future.

Criteria used to recognize abnormal coronary arteries in KS were asked in the next question. Multiple choice format of this question may have precluded other criteria physicians may have had. Nevertheless, "increased diameter of coronary artery segment" was most frequently used criterion in both countries. Other criteria such as "distal diameter greater than proximal diameter" and "irregular or beady appearance" were used less often. "Increased perivascular echo brightness" was selected as one of the criteria more often by the Japanese cardiologists than the Americans. This criterion is the most subjective one. Still, in the early stage of disease, intense inflammation affects all layers of the artery before any changes occur in the luminal diameter. (4) Thus, there must be   important information in the periluminal echo itself. The major obstacle is our inability to detect it objectively and measure its intensity.

TABLE 2.6.

What are your echo measurement criteria for normal and dilated coronary arteries?

NORMAL CORONARY ARTERIES	JAPAN	(%)	USA	(%)
No response	0		24	(27.9)
Don't know	0		25	(29.1)
⟨2mm	37	(23.9)	5	(5.8)
⟨3mm	54	(34.8)	21	(24.4)
⟨4mm	5	(3.2)	7	(8.1)
Other criteria*	15	(9.7)	10	(11.6)

*includes cor/ao ratio, BSA-based criteria, age-specific criteria

DILATED CORONARY ARTERIES	JAPAN	(%)	USA	(%)
No response	0		25	(29.1)
Don't know	0		21	(24.4)
⟩2~ 2.5mm	10	(6.5)	2	(2.3)
⟩3 ~ 3.5mm	66	(42.6)	19	(22.1)
⟩4mm	31	(20.0)	6	(7.0)
⟩5mm	1		3	(3.5)
⟩6mm	1		0	
Other criteria	12	(7.7)	4	(4.7)

Luminal diameters of normal and abnormal coronary arteries in infants and children.

There is great divergence of opinions among the Japanese and the U.S. cardiologists in both categories. In Japan about 35 percent and 24 percent of the respondents chose less than 3 mm and less than 2 mm as normal coronary artery diameters, respectively. In the U.S. 57 percent of the respondents did not give any normal values or gave "don't know" answers. Twenty-four percent chose less than 3 mm, 8 percent chose less than 4 mm and six percent chose less than 2 mm as normal values, respectively. Prior to this survey, the only published echo criteria for normal or abnormal coronary arteries were in the 1984 report of a subcommittee of the Research Committee on Kawasaki Disease of Japanese Ministry of Health and Welfare. (5) After stating that there are no sufficient data on echocardiographic measurement of the normal coronary artery size and that the figures mentioned are arbitrary, the authors recommended that an increase of coronary internal diameter to more than 1.5 times the adjacent vessel diameter be considered a dilated lesion (including dilatation and aneurysm). They further stated that, for children under five years of age, coronary arteries with diameter of 3 mm or greater (measured inside to inside of opposing wall echoes) should be regarded as a dilated lesion. Subsequently, Arjunan and coworkers published echocardiographic and angiographic measurements of coronary arteries in 110 children aged 3 months to 16 years. Their measurement was done from the middle of one wall echo to the middle of the other wall echo. (7) There was a wide range of normal diameters for each of the major coronary arteries with the upper limit extending to 4 mm in children under 3 years and 5 mm in children beyond 3 years. Nakano and coworkers published normal coronary artery diameters in children based on angiographic measurements. (8) According to their data, normal coronary artery diameters were 2.5 mm or less in children with body surface area (BSA) under 0.5 m^2, 3 mm or less with BSA from 0.5 up to 1.0, and 3 to 3.5 mm with BSA greater than 1.0 m^2, respectively. Echocardiographic measurement of the coronary artery lumen tends to be slightly greater than the angiographic measurement. Resolution of the echo imaging system is limited by the carrier frequency of ultrasound used, pixel size of the digital image and scan line density of the video image. Using the currently available technique, we cannot achieve accuracy of coronary artery measurement of more than ±0.5 mm, equivalent to 20 to 25 percent of a normal coronary artery diameter. Clearly, there is a need for an improved video system. Echo assessment of the coronary arteries, after all, is the single most important issue confronting the clinician managing KS patients.

TABLE 2.7.

In examining the right coronary artery, how far do you routinely try to visualize the lumen?

	JAPAN (%)	USA (%)
From the origin to the tricuspid valve	90 (58.1)	49 (57.0)
From the origin to the posterior A-V groove	67 (43.2)	32 (37.2)

TABLE 2.8.

In examining the left anterior descending artery, how far do
you routinely try to visualize the lumen?

	JAPAN	(%)	USA	(%)
Just beyond the bifurcation	67	(43.2)	45	(52.3)
Beyond the plane of pulmonic valve	80	(51.6)	36	(41.9)

TABLE 2.9.

In what percentage of patients can you see at least 1cm of
the left circumflex branch?

	JAPAN	(%)	USA	(%)
25–50%	99	(63.9)	41	(47.7)
50–75%	35	(22.6)	18	(20.9)
> 75%	12	(7.7)	11	(12.8)

The techniques of visualizing coronary arteries.

As echocardiography is accepted as the primary and
often the only diagnostic modality for coronary artery lesions in this disease, we feel the need to visualize each
major branch as far distally as possible so as not to miss
any abnormalities. In order to do this, growing numbers of
cardiologists and technicians are shifting away from stereo-
typic view-oriented examinations to structure-oriented approaches, in which each structure such as a coronary artery
is pursued meticulously using multiple and sometimes impro-
vised views. A study should be declared a negative study
only if a normal arterial lumen has been observed from the
origin of that artery, through the entire proximal segment
and at least a portion of the distal segment.

Cardiac catheterization

TABLE 3.1.

How many patients with KS have you done or requested cardiac
catheterization on in the past 12 months?

	JAPAN	(%)	USA	(%)
0-5	72	(46.5)	79	(91.9)
6-10	30	(19.4)	6	(3.9)
11-20	17	(11.0)	0	
21-30	17	(11.0)	0	
> 30	20	(12.9)	0	

TABLE 3.2.

Which of the following indications for cardiac catheterization apply to your practice? (Multiple answers allowed)

	JAPAN	(%)	USA	(%)
a. All KS patients (pts) regard-less of echo findings	3	(1.9)	2	(2.3)
b. Virtually none of KS pts.	0		25	(29.1)
c. Only those pts suspected of large or multiple coronary aneurysms	101	(65.2)	33	(38.4)
d. Pts with all coronary aneur. large or small	79	(51.0)	30	(34.9)
e. Pts considered to be high risk on the basis of a clinical score (such as Asai-Kusakawa score)	29	(18.7)	8	(9.3)
f. Pts with abnormal LV function by echo	91	(58.7)	23	(26.7)
g. Pts with angina-like symptoms	96	(61.9)	45	(52.3)
h. Pts with peripheral artery aneurysms	58	(37.4)	25	(29.1)
i. Other indications	21	(13.5)	11	(12.8)

TABLE 3.2A.

Other indications for cardiac catheterization:

	JAPAN	USA
Abnormalities noted in other tests (EKG, Thallium scan, Dipyridamole thallium scan, treadmill, etc)	7	6
A-V valve regurgitation	4	0
Myocarditis or pericardial effusion	1	1
Transient coronary dilatation in acute phase	5	0

Continued

Table 3.2A continued

Myocardial infarction	1	1
Clinical cause suggests high risk	1	0
Cholecystitis	1	0
Uncertainty of presence of aneurysm	0	3
2DE not available in acute phase	2	0
Late follow-up of long standing aneurysm	2	3
To look for stenotic lesion	0	1
To confirm regression of aneurysms	3	1
For consideration of aorto-coronary bypass	1	0
Disappearance of previously seen aneurysm	1	0
To comply with family's request	6	0
All patients except those with defined aneurysms	0	1

TABLE 3.3.

Do you visualize coronary arteries mostly with selective arteriography or aortic root injection?

	JAPAN (%)	USA (%)
a. Selective coronary injection	137 (88.4)	34 (39.5)
b. Aortic root injection	23 (14.8)	39 (45.3)

TABLE 3.4.

What is your estimate of risk of major complications or death associated with selective coronary arteriography in children less than 5 years of age?

	JAPAN (%)	USA (%)
a. Less than 1%	139 (89.7)	52 (60.5)
b. 1-5%	5 (3.2)	21 (24.4)
c. 5-10%	0	1 (1.2)

TABLE 3.5.

Have you ever combined cardiac catheterization with any of the following interventional procedures in KS patients?

		JAPAN (%)	USA (%)
a.	Myocardial biopsy	20 (12.9)	1 (1.2)
b.	Streptokinase or urokinase infusion	21 (13.5)	0
c.	Nitroglycerin infusion for research/therapy	17 (11.0)	3 (3.5)
d.	Balloon angioplasty	2 (1.3)	0

TABLE 3.6.

Do you re-catheterize patients with abnormal coronary arteries?

		JAPAN (%)	USA (%)
a.	Yes	115 (74.2)	39 (45.3)
b.	No	39 (25.2)	29 (33.7)

As in other areas related to KS, the Japanese cardiologists have much greater experience in cardiac catheterization. As to the indications of cardiac catheterization (table 3.2), some of the answers reflect individual respondents' own practice as the question was intended, and others appear to be their opinions or future intentions. In both countries relatively few cardiologists (2%) recommend cardiac catheterizations in all KS patients regardless of echo findings. Twenty-nine percent of the responding U.S. cardiologists would recommend it to virtually none of KS patients, while none of the Japanese cardiologists shared that option. In Japan, patients suspected of large or multiple coronary aneurysms (65%), angina-like symptom (61%) and abnormal left ventricular function (59%) lead the list. In the U.S., angina-like symptoms (52%), patients with large or multiple coronary aneurysms (38%) and patients with all coronary aneurysms (regardless of size or number) (35%) lead the list. Thus, the U.S. cardiologists appear uncertain about cardiac catheterization, while the Japanese cardiologists appear to have a consensus about its importance and indications.

In questions related to selective coronary artery in-

jection versus aortic root injections, 88 percent of the
Japanese cardiologists reported using selective coronary arteriography, while only 40 percent of the U.S. cardiologists
chose this technique. This difference is reflected in their
perception of the risk of selective coronary arteriography
(Table 3.4). In addition to routine diagnostic coronary
arteriography, some transcatheter interventions have been
tried in Japan (Table 3.5). More Japanese cardiologists re-
catheterize KS patients after various intervals than do U.S.
cardiologists (Table 3.6). These practices are probably due
to presence of a larger number of patients with chronic coronary artery aneurysms with stenoses and thromboses in Japan
but may also reflect an attitudinal difference between the
two groups.

Other cardiac diagnostic tests

TABLE 4.1.

Do you recommend stress tests in KS patients?

	JAPAN	(%)	USA	(%)
a. None of the patients	26	(16.8)	19	(22.1)
b. All KS patients	61	(37.4)	15	(17.4)
c. Patients with known coronary abnormalities	68	(43.9)	44	(51.2)

TABLE 4.2.

What other cardiac diagnostic tests do you find useful in
KS patients?

	JAPAN	USA
Holter Monitoring	2	2
Thallium-201 scan	35	10
Stress test with Thallium scan	6	4
Dipyridamole scintigraphy	7	1
Radionuclide angiography	9	4
Computerized tomography	0	1
Nuclear magnetic imaging	3	1
Digital subtraction angiography	2	0
Systolic time intervals with amyl nitrate challenge	4	2

More Japanese cardiologists tend to recommend stress tests, Thallium-201 scan and other noninvasive studies on KS patients than the U.S. cardiologists. Value of such tests in predicting functional status of the coronary artery system specifically with respect to this syndrome needs further evaluation.

Treatment --- use of aspirin

Table 5.1.

What do you use to treat patients with residual coronary artery aneurysms or stenosis after the acute phase?

		JAPAN (%)	USA (%)
a.	Aspirin alone	69 (44.5)	62 (72.1)
b.	Aspirin and dipyridamole	77 (49.7)	25 (29.1)
c.	Flurbiprofen	18 (11.6)	0
d.	Warfarin	13 (8.4)	2 (2.3)
e.	Other	23 (14.8)	0

Table 5.2.

Which of the following aspirin dosages do you recommend for a patient with acute KS?

		JAPAN (%)	USA (%)
a.	$\leq$ 5mg/kg/day	0	--
b.	10mg/kg/day	5 (3.2)	10 (11.6)
c.	30mg/kg/day	138 (89.0)	12 (14.0)
d.	100mg/kg/day	9 (5.8)	64 (74.4)

Seventy-two percent of the U.S. cardiologists responded used aspirin alone in patients with residual coronary artery abnormalities, and 29 percent used combination of aspirin and dipyridamole. In Japan physicians using the two regimens are more equally divided. In addition more physicians resort to other drugs.

In regard to aspirin dosage during the acute phase, 89 percent of Japanese cardiologists chose 30 mg per kilogram per day, while 74 percent of U.S. cardiologists preferred 100 mg per kilogram per day. There appears to be a greater concern for hepatotoxicity of aspirin in Japan, causing the physician to limit its dosage.

Treatment --- use of intravenous gammaglobulin

Table 5.3.

Do you believe all KS patients should receive intravenous gamma globulin?

	JAPAN	(%)	USA	(%)
a. Yes	24	(15.5)	55	(64.0)
b. No	129	(83.2)	25	(29.1)
c. No opinion	1	(0.6)	6	(6.9)

Table 5.4.

If your answer is no, what criteria do you recommend for selecting patients who should receive IV gamma globulin?

JAPANESE RESPONSES
N = 67

Not using IVGG	9
No clearcut criteria	17
So-called severe cases	21
Prolonged fever	14
Patients with strong inflammatory reaction	8
Early onset of abnormal echo findings	15
Some specific scoring system (3 mentioned)	11
Shocky state	1
Large gallbladder	1
Other reasons	3

AMERICAN RESPONSES
N = 17

No good criteria available	6
Not using IVGG (no pts with complications)	3
Clinically high risk patients	2
Young patients, high fever, more systemic symptoms	1
Early diagnosis, in acute phase	5

There is a strong majority opinion (83%) among the Japanese cardiologists against universal use of intravenous gammaglobulin (IVGG) in all KS patients during the acute phase. Sixty-four percent of the U.S. cardiologists are in favor of such use. Two strong underlying reasons for the Japanese position are (1) high cost of IVGG in Japan and (2) concerns about adverse effects including immediate anaphylactoid reaction as well as delayed immune paralysis. Both the cost and concerns regarding adverse effects are amplified by a higher prevalence rate of Kawasaki syndrome in Japan. On the other hand, in the U.S. the primary reason for the greater acceptance rate of IVGG therapy is its benefit to the patients in minimizing cardiac sequelae and, secondarily, its potential for saving the cost of both protracted hospital stay in the acute stage and caring for those patients with chronic cardiac problems. The cost of gammaglobulin in the U.S. is becoming lower due primarily to competition among multiple pharmaceutical houses. The cost is approaching $30 per gram as of February, 1987. If IVGG therapy is efficacious in reducing the systemic symptoms rapidly and thus allowing earlier hospital discharge, the cost of IVGG would be easily offset by saving in hospital care cost. In Japan, the cost of nursing and bed occupancy does not figure prominently in estimating the cost/benefit ratio of IVGG therapy.

In response to a question regarding criteria for selecting patients for IVGG therapy, no specific, universally applicable criteria were mentioned by either the Japanese or American cardiologists. At least two scoring systems for this purpose are being tested currently in Japan. Nakano and coworkers have computed a score based on age, C-reactive protein, white cell count, hematocrit and platelet count. (9) Iwasa and coworkers have devised a "Score X" based on age, sex, red cell count, hematocrit and serum albumin. (10) Any such risk factor analysis is under the constraints of having to discriminate high risk patients for coronary aneurysms at a high level of predictivity using readily obtainable clinical data within the first 7-8 days of illness. Depending on where the threshold score is selected, one would be faced with a reciprocal dilemma of either a high predictive value of positive test combined with a low predictive value of negative test or alternately a low predictive value of positive test with a high predictive value of negative test.

For the Japanese physicians the pressing task would be to fine-tune the risk factor analysis and to reach a national consensus regarding selection of patients for gammaglobulin therapy. For the American colleagues, their task is to determine long-term effect of gammaglobulin therapy as applied to all patients of acute Kawasaki syndrome not only in terms of coronary artery outcome but also on its impact on the host immune system. In the meantime, intensifying search for the elusive etiologic agent continues in both countries. Discovery of such an agent may lead to a more specific, less toxic and hopefully less expensive therapy. There will be an ample reason for the two nationals to continue exchanging useful information on this mysterious disease.

REFERENCES

1. Kijima Y, Kamiya T, Suzuki A, Hirose O, Manabe H. A trial procedure to prevent aneurysm formation of the coronary arteries by steroid pulse therapy in Kawasaki disease. Jpn Circ J 1982; 46: 1239-42.
2. Kato H, Ichinose E, Yoshida F, et al. Fate of coronary aneurysms in Kawasaki disease: serial coronary angiography and long-term follow-up study. Am J Cardiol 1982; 49: 1758-66.
3. Takahashi M, Mason W, Lewis AB. Regression of coronary aneurysms in patients with Kawasaki syndrome. Circulation 1987; 75: 387-394.
4. Fujiwara H, Hamashima Y: Pathology of the heart in Kawasaki disease. Pediatrics 1978; 61: 100-107.
5. Report of Subcommittee on Standardization of Diagnostic Criteria and Reporting of Coronary Artery Lesions in Kawasaki Disease, Research Committee on Kawasaki Disease, Ministry of Health and Welfare, Jan. 21, 1984.
6. Arjunan K, Daniels SR, Meyer RA, et al. Coronary artery caliber in normal children and patients with Kawasaki disease but without aneurysms: an echocardiographic and angiographic study. J. Am Coll Cardiol 1986; 8: 1119-24.
7. Personal communications.
8. Nakano H, Ueda K, Saito A, Nojima K: Repeated quantitative angiograms in coronary arterial aneurysm in Kawasaki disease. Am J Cardiol 1985; 56: 846-851.
9. Nakano H, Ueda K, Saito A et al.: Scoring method for identifying patients with Kawasaki disease at high risk of coronary artery aneurysm. Am J Cardiol 1986; 58: 739-742.
10. Iwasa M, Sugiyama K, Kawase A et al. Prevention of coronary artery involvement in Kawasaki disease by early intravenous high-dose gammaglobulin. In Doyle EF, Engle MA, Gersony WM, Rashkind WJ, Talner NS, edit. Pediatric Cardiology Proceedings of the Second World Congress. New York: Springer-Verlag, 1986.

Kawasaki Disease, pages 509–513
© 1987 Alan R. Liss, Inc.

DISCUSSION:

CONCLUSION

The genetic aspects of Kawasaki Disease were first
discussed. Dr. Sasazuki (Fukuoka) asked why Dr. Maclaren
spoke only of risk ratio (RR) rather than Chi square
probability; Dr. Maclaren (Gainesville) responded that this
reflected the small groups studied. Dr. Sasazuki pointed
out that if the dose of the environmental factor that
triggers Kawasaki Disease is extremely low, even genetically predisposed individuals will not develop disease
frequently and a genetic prediposition will be difficult to
detect. Dr. Rauch (Atlanta) reported that CDC has been
notified of 11 sibling pairs concordant for Kawasaki
Disease since 1981, 5 occurring in identical twin pairs
(one Black, 4 Caucasian). Dr. Maclaren emphasized the
problem of ascertainment bias which increases the likelihood of finding concordant twins. Dr. Shulman (Chicago)
reported a Japanese-American boy with Kawasaki Disease who
is one of quintuplets; his four sisters did not develop the
disease. Dr. Melish (Honolulu) noted that the RR is 14 in
Japanese-American children in Hawaii compared to Caucasians
and therefore believes that there is an environmental
trigger in those who are genetically predisposed. The
complication rate did not differ by race in the U.S. IVGG
trial. Dr. Leung (Boston) noted a 9-fold increased risk of
atopic dermatitis in Kawasaki Disease patients and indicated that both atopic dermatitis and Kawasaki Disease have
increased activated helper cells and decreased numbers of
suppressor cells. Dr. Sasazuki pointed out that a genetic
factor that is very common in Japanese but very rare in
Caucasians would require study in Caucasians, and Dr.
Maclaren agreed.

Dr. Brown (New York) asked if coronary endothelial cells express HL-A antigens. Dr. Hansson (Goteberg) indicated that ɤ-interferon treatment of endothelial cells induces DR expression and renders the cells capable of presenting antigen to T cells. It is not known if autopsied coronary endothelial specimens in Kawasaki Disease express DR.

Dr. Leung noted that the association of DR2 with multiple sclerosis is of interest in that MS may be related to a retrovirus and is associated with decreased numbers of T8 cells. He also indicated that Kawasaki sera contain anti-endothelial cell antibodies. No change in titer between Day 1 and 4 is apparent and similar reactivity is present in epidemic and endemic sera. In other vasculitic injury in which there is antibody to interferon-inducible antigens, cyclosporine can produce dramatic improvement. He concluded that immunology has to date offered little of clinical relevance and that only identification of the etiologic agent will be specific. He also suggested that there may be some differences between T cell subsets in endemic and epidemic forms of Kawasaki Disease.

Dr. Kyogoku (Sendai) commented on several unusual pathologic features of Kawasaki Disease. Early on there is diffuse endothelial swelling and granulocytes appear to attack the endothelium. This lasts only about one week, and then there is inflammation within the arterial wall that lasts only about 7-14 days. The repair process seems to start early, and these vessel changes might correlate with changes in interferon levels. Lymph node histology resembles viral attack with decreased numbers of T and B cells and transient rebound hyperplastic changes that include large follicles. He believes that the arteritis does not resemble immune complex-mediated arteritis. The shape of the macrophages is unusual in that they are quite swollen, with an enlarged nucleus and misshapen cytoplasm. Many retroviral animal models (in mice, mink) include arteritis.

Dr. Rauch suggested that the association of Kawasaki Disease with exposure to rug shampoo 13-30 days earlier, with respiratory illnesses 13-30 days earlier, and with other factors could be related to an endogenous retrovirus that has multiple triggers. Dr. Sasazuki asked what could be the means of transmission of a retrovirus, so that in

one-year-old identical twins, for example, there is only
13% concordance for Kawasaki Disease. Dr. Melish emphasized that community-wide epidemics without apparent
person-person transmission suggest that there could be
concordance for infection but discordance for expression of
disease. Drs. Melish and Wiggins (Denver) each reported
one of a set of twins with classic Kawasaki Disease in
which the other member of each set had fever, uveitis,
elevated ESR and platelet count, but no other clinical
findings of Kawasaki Disease. Dr. Evans (New Haven)
suggested that one must use the few available markers
epidemiologically to study contacts and siblings, such as
the ESR or reverse transcriptase activity, to determine if
this is a ubiquitous infection with rare expression, an
unusual disease due to a group of agents, or a disease due
to a unique agent.

Dr. Pachman (Chicago) sought data regarding treatment
of Kawasaki Disease with indomethacin, but there were
none. Dr. Leung pointed out that the improvement seen in a
few very severely ill children treated with exchange
transfusion or plasmaphoresis may support an important role
for inflammatory mediators.

Dr. Bierman (New York) asked whether the variation in
diameter of the coronary arteries during systole and
diastole was significant. Dr. Takahashi (Los Angeles)
indicated that there is about a 10% difference which
approaches the resolution of echo equipment. Dr. Bierman
noted that EKG criteria do not appear to be an indicator
for angiographic study and suggested that results of
procedures such as dipyrimadole stress testing with
thallium should be included as indications for angiogram.
Dr. Suzuki (Tokyo) reported that her studies showed that
dipyrimadole and thallium scanning was not very sensitive
in patients with angiographically proved coronary stenosis
because so many collaterals develop and that thallium
scanning alone was very insensitive. However, Dr. Kato
(Kurume) felt that thallium scanning is sensitive for
stenotic lesions and that 50-60% of stenotic lesions can be
detected by echo using high frequency transducers. Dr.
Wiggins pointed out some problems with dipyrimadole and
thallium studies in acute patients including the facts that
one must change the patient to an upright position during
the infusion and that the sensitivity seems less than with
a stress-thallium study. Dr. Kato noted that dipyrimadole

has been known to precipitate anginal attacks by a "steal" phenomenon and is usually not recommended for those with severe obstructive lesions. Dr. Newberger (Boston) emphasized that because of the risks of catheterization, management decisions should result. Dr. Evans cautioned that the cardiology survey may have included those who haven't seen patients with Kawasaki Disease.

Dr. Melish noted that different IVGG preparations were associated with different incidences of side effects and that pepsin-digested IVGG appears to be ineffective. She emphasized that significant side effects have not been encountered with the product used in the U.S. trial. Dr. Tada (Tokyo) indicated that he is not opposed to the use of IVGG but has certain reservations about using it for all Kawasaki Disease patients: a) there is lot-lot variability in anti-DR titer (in neonatal mice anti-DR can lead to permanent immune deficiency); b) passive GG given to infants with a developing immune system may impair responses to active immunization; and c) IVGG might inter-fere with the developing immune system network that is being formed. He recommended that it be reserved for selected patients. Dr. Usami (Tokyo) objected to the logic of giving IVGG to all patients on the thesis that all Kawasaki Disease patients are undergoing pathological changes in the coronary arteries. Dr. Furusho (Kitakyushu) pointed out that extensive experience with whole blood transfusion of neonates for prevention of kernicterus failed to show evidence of severe immune disturbance that is feared by Dr. Tada. Dr. Usami (Tokyo) reported a recent patient with ITP and Kawasaki Disease who developed a fatal serum sickness-like reaction eight hours after IVGG and another with typical Kawasaki Disease who developed shock during an infusion of IVGG and survived. Dr. Nakano (Shizuoka) noted that he has treated 40 high-risk patients with IVGG (1cc/kg over the first hour) and within two hours 50% developed $\geq 1^\circ$C increased temperature, half accom-panied by chills, including one with temperature >42°C with a tonic-clonic seizure who recovered without sequelae. Dr. Shirai (Juntendo) asked if it was likely that the side effects of IVGG might be mediated by immune complexes and pointed out that in NZ mice, endogenous retroviral antigen is present in serum and that immune complex disease occurs when an immune response to retro-viral antigen develops. Dr. Mason (Los Angeles) found no differences in concentration of circulating immune complexes before and after IVGG and in those treated with aspirin alone. Dr. Shulman stated that IVGG appears to be of unquestioned efficacy but to have theoretical risks with little evidence of definite risks, at least in the U.S.; therefore, continued trials, particularly with long-term follow-up and immune evaluation, are needed. Dr. Brown pointed out that all the speakers reporting risks of IVGG are Japanese and wondered if there was a relation to the preparations used and what the Japanese experience is re side effects of IVGG for ITP. Dr. Yamada (Kanagawa) reported few if any severe side effects in Japan when IVGG is used for ITP and noted that plasma for Japanese products is imported from the U.S. Dr. Newberger reported that one child in the U.S. trial developed chills and itching on the first but not subsequent infusions. Dr. Salo (Finland) reported that IVGG is used in Finland but not in Denmark or Sweden because of fear of adverse reactions. Dr. Rosen (Boston) pointed out that everyone receives a large infusion of gamma globulin in utero, and in 50% there is genetic disparity with respect to the maternal Gm allotype. He agreed that Dr. Tada's concerns were correct for inbred mice but not for man. The small amount of anti-DR in the Immuno AG IVGG is less than received transplacentally, there are no preservatives in this preparation, and chances of an anaphylactic reaction to IgA are very remote. He believes that the Japanese reports of adverse effects reflect the fact that aggregated gamma globulin is present in the Japanese products.

In his closing remarks, Dr. Kawasaki indicated that he had remained quiet during the symposium and thanked Dr. Shulman for his organizational activities for the symposium. He said that he had expected that Kawasaki Disease would not be so mysterious after the symposium, but found that it remains mysterious after this three-day meeting. There are still many unsolved problems, the same questions he has had over the past 20 years. He believes that it is easy to theorize but very difficult to establish the truth, although it is our duty to continue to pursue the truth. He expects to have the Third International Meeting in 1988 in Japan unless all the questions are answered by then. There are a number of candidate sites for the meeting including Kyoto, Tokyo and Hakone, and he hoped as many as possible in the audience in Kauai would attend. He indicated that he is looking forward to seeing further progress to resolve the problems identified at this meeting.

Kawasaki Disease, pages 515–516
© 1987 Alan R. Liss, Inc.

CARDIOVASCULAR INVOLVEMENT IN KAWASAKI DISEASE

Kiyoshi Baba, Kazuo Kitani, Hisahiro Mitomori,
Kazuyo Mitsudo and Mutsuo Tanaka
Division of Pediatrics, Heart Institute,
Kurashiki Central Hospital, Miwa 1-1-1,
Kurashiki City, Okayama Pref., JAPAN

We evaluated the cardiovascular lesions in Kawasaki
Disease using selective coronary cine-angiography and right
ventricular endomyocardial biopsies. Two hundred children
were examined, comprising 131 males and 69 females. Ages
at onset were 2 months to 11 years, and the interval
between onset of disease and the first examination was from
21 days to 12 years. Right ventricular endomyocardial
biopsy specimens were obtained in 143 cases and analyzed
for hypertrophy (Hyp), diarrangement (Dis), degeneration
(Deg) of myocardial fibers, cell infiltration (Inf),
fibrosis (Fib), and vascular changes (Vasc). Thirty-eight
patients were re-examined in order to study the course of
their cardiovascular lesions.

In 80 cases (55 males and 25 females) coronary
involvement was present by angiograms. Both coronary
arteries were involved in 38 cases, the left coronary in 27
cases and the right coronary in 15 cases. Six cases
combined other vessel lesions. Cerebral arterial stenosis
was demonstrated in 2 cases, axillary arterial aneurysms in
2 and iliac arterial aneurysms in 6. Myocardial infarctions due to coronary arterial obstructions were
demonstrated in 6 cases, all of whom appeared to have large
aneurysms. Thirty-eight children were re-examined at
intervals from 5 months to 2 years 8 months. Complete
angiographic regression was recognized in 11 cases,
incomplete regression in 14 cases, development of stenosis
in 3 cases, total obstruction in one case, and no change in
9 cases. In one case with a calcified thrombus in the
coronary artery, "relative stenosis" was demonstrated on

the second examination, because the involved arterial wall did not enlarge as the child grew older.

The endomyocardial histopathological findings could not differentiate clearly between the groups with and without coronary involvement. However, the number of specimens with myocardial hypertrophy and interstitial fibrosis increased on the second examination. Furthermore, findings suggested that obstruction of the small vessels and perivascular fibrosis were important.

We have summarized the course of cardiovascular involvement in Kawasaki Disease and conclude that patients with cardiovascular lesions must be followed throughout their lives, particularly in regard to atherosclerosis, ischemic heart disease and/or cardiomyopathy.

Kawasaki Disease, pages 517–518
© 1987 Alan R. Liss, Inc.

INTRACORONARY STREPTOKINASE IN KAWASAKI DISEASE: ACUTE
AND LATE THROMBOLYSIS

J.P. Cheatham, J.D. Kugler, C.H. Gumbiner,
L.A. Latson and P.J. Hofschire
Department of Pediatrics, University of Nebraska
Medical Center, Omaha, Nebraska

Kawasaki Disease is now recognized as a potentially
life-threatening illness affecting infants and children.
In 20% of patients there is coronary involvement, including
dilatation, aneurysms and thrombosis. The mortality is
2-3% and is secondary to acute myocardial infarction (MI)
from coronary thrombosis. Intravenous and/or intracoronary
streptokinase (Sk) is used in adults with atherosclerotic
coronary occlusive disease with acute ischemia. We report
the use of intracoronary Sk on two separate occasions as
both acute and later thrombolytic therapy in a patient with
Kawasaki Disease.

Intracoronary Sk was administered initially for near-
complete occlusion of the circumflex branch (CFx) with left
anterior descending (LAD) thrombus in a 5-year-old with
Kawasaki Disease who had presented with MI three months
earlier. Echocardiography and angiography confirmed a
large coronary aneurysm with thrombus. Although reperfusion ventricular bigeminy was noted after Sk infusion,
no significant angiographic improvement was seen. Angiogram six months later confirmed recannulization of the CFx
with partial lysis of the LAD thrombus. Subsequent echogram confirmed organization of the thrombus with decreased
aneurysm size of the CFx and LAD.

While receiving aspirin and dipyridamole, the patient
presented 3 1/2 years later with her second major acute
MI, confirmed by elevated MB-CPK, ECG changes and symptoms.
Angiography confirmed complete thrombosis of the LAD, and
emergency intracoronary Sk was given. Immediate relief of

symptoms and improvement of ECG occurred, and reperfusion of the LAD was demonstrated. Subsequent intravenous Sk with systemic heparinization and later therapy with warfarin/dipyridamole for 6 months without aspirin had completely lysed both the recent and 3 1/2-year-old thrombus as confirmed by angiogram and echocardiogram.

Intracoronary Sk may safely and effectively be used for acute and late coronary thrombosis in children with Kawasaki Disease. The mechanism of delayed thrombolysis is unclear, but may be related to "triggered" intrinsic fibrinolysis after Sk/heparin or possibly to interference of this pathway by aspirin.

Kawasaki Disease, pages 519–520
© 1987 Alan R. Liss, Inc.

SIZE OF CORONARY ANEURYSM AS A DETERMINANT FACTOR OF THE
PROGNOSIS IN KAWASAKI DISEASE: CLINICOPATHOLOGIC STUDY OF
CORONARY ANEURYSMS

Takako Fujiwara, M.D., Hisayoshi Fujiwara, M.D.
and Yoshihiro Hamashima, M.D.
Department of Food Science, Kyoto Women's
University, The Third Division, Department of
Internal Medicine and Department of Pathology,
Kyoto University, Kyoto, JAPAN

To assess the prognosis of children with Kawasaki
Disease, the diameter of the largest coronary arterial
aneurysm was examined in 61 autopsied children with
Kawasaki Disease. Of thirty children who died during the
acute stage, the largest diameter of the coronary aneurysm
was ≥ 6 mm in 23 who died of coronary heart disease and
≤ 4.5 mm in 7 who died of myocarditis. Of thirty-one
children who died during the healed stage, the diameter of
the largest coronary aneurysm was ≥ 8 mm in 26, 6-8 mm in 3,
and ≤ 2.5 mm (normal) in 2. The two patients without
coronary aneurysms died of bacterial infections or
accidents. Twenty-nine patients with at least one coronary
aneurysm ≥ 6 mm in diameter died of coronary heart disease.
Of 26 with at least one coronary aneurysm ≥ 8 mm, 23 had
multi-vessel coronary aneurysms ≥ 6 mm in diameter.

Therefore, patients who died during the acute stage of
Kawasaki Disease did not always have large coronary
aneurysms. However, aneurysms ≥ 6 mm in diameter existed in
73%.

In the healed stage (stage IVa&b), only those autopsied
patients with coronary aneurysms ≥ 6 mm in diameter died of
the sequelae of Kawasaki Disease. This indicates that the
prognosis of the patients with coronary aneurysm <6 mm in
diameter is good. The special feature of those who died in
the healed stage was the presence of multi-vessel coronary
aneurysms ≥ 6 mm, at least one of which was ≥ 8 mm in
diameter (Fujiwara et al. 1987).

References

Fujiwara H, Hamashima Y (1978). Pathology of the heart in Kawasaki Disease. Pediatrics 61:100-107.
Fujiwara H, Kawai C, Hamashima Y (1978). Clinicopathological study of conduction systems in 10 patients with Kawasaki Disease (mucocutaneous lymph node syndrome). Am Hear J 96:744-750.
Fujiwara H, Chen CH, Fujiwara T, Nishioka K, Kawai C, Hamashima Y (1980). Clinicopathologic study of abnormal Q waves in Kawasaki Disease (mucocutaneous lymph node syndrome): an infantile cardiac disease with myocarditis and myocardial infarction. Am J Cardiol 45: 797-805.
Fujiwara H, Kao T-C, Shimizu J, Fujiwara T, Oo M-M, Hamashima Y (1983). Microorganism in the heart in Kawasaki Disease. Lancet 10:620-621.
Fujiwara T, Fujiwara H, Ueda T, Nishioka K, Hamashima Y (1986). Comparison among macroscopic, postmortem, angiographic and two dimensional echocardiographic findings of coronary aneurysms in children with Kawasaki Disease. Am J Cardiol 57:761-764.
Fujiwara H, Fujiwara T, Kao T-C, Ohshio G, Hamashima Y (1986). Pathology of Kawasaki Disease in the healed stage--relationships between typical and atypical cases of Kawasaki Disease. Acta Pathol Jpn 36:857-867.
Fujiwara T, Fujiwara H, Hamashima Y (1987). Frequency and size of coronary arterial aneurysm at necropsy in Kawasaki Disease. Am J Cardiol (in press).

Kawasaki Disease, page 521
© 1987 Alan R. Liss, Inc.

INFANTILE POLYARTERITIS AND FATAL CASES OF KAWASAKI
SYNDROME: TWO DISEASES OR ONE?

J.T. Lie

Department of Pathology
Mayo Clinic and Mayo Medical School
Rochester, Minnesota   55905

     The clinical and pathological findings of nine
infants (under 1 year of age) and young children (under 15
years of age) who died of polyarteritis nodosa were studied
in detail. All except the two oldest children died within
10 weeks of the onset of symptoms. The most prominent
clinical features for the entire group included fever
unresponsive to antibiotic therapy; skin rash and maculo-
papular eruption on the trunk and extremities; erythematous oral mucosa and lips; cervical lymphadenopathy;
arthralgia; leukocytosis; thrombocytosis; proteinuria and
signs of cardiac or renal failure. The two infants under
one year of age died of cardiac failure, whereas renal and
neurological involvement were the common cause of death in
the older children. A consistent finding at autopsy was
arteritis and aneurysmal disease of the coronary arteries,
completely indistinguishable from that of fatal cases of
Kawasaki Syndrome.

Kawasaki Disease, page 523
© 1987 Alan R. Liss, Inc.

EXPERIMENTAL CANDIDA-INDUCED ARTERITIS IN MICE--RELATION TO
ARTERITIS IN KAWASAKI DISEASE

Hisao Murata and Shiro Naoe

Departments of Public Health and Research
Laboratory of Pathology, Toho University School
of Medicine, Tokyo, Japan

We have found in previous experiments that when Candida
albicans isolated from children with Kawasaki Disease is
injected into mice under certain conditions, systemic vasculitis, mainly involving the coronary artery, is produced. We
showed that this experimentally produced vasculitis is similar to the vascular lesion found upon autopsy in cases of
Kawasaki Disease both in regard to the histopathological
findings and the site of the lesions. This experimental
procedure has very high reproducibility, and we are presently
attempting to establish an animal model for systemic vascu-
litits, particularly as related to Kawasaki Disease.

We obtained the following results so far:

1) Some immunological disorder, especially IgE antibody may
    be related to the incidence of arteritis.
2) Predomine may prevent the development of the arteritis
    rather than aspirin.
3) No difference of pathogenicity exists among the different
    strains of C. albicans isolated from clinical sources.
4) Polysaccharide fraction of C. albicans may be related
    to the incidence of arteritis and it is confirmed that
    polysaccharide fraction has cardiotonic and coronary
    vasodilatatory activities on Langendorff's preparation
    pharmacologically.
5) It is confirmed that polysaccharide of C. albicans
    contains digitoxoses by use of thin-layer chromatography,
    gas chromatography and gas-mass spectrometry methods. It
    is strongly suspected that C. albicans polysaccharide may
    contain cardiac glycosides such as digitoxin or digoxin.

Kawasaki Disease, page 525
© 1987 Alan R. Liss, Inc.

ON MORPHOGENESIS OF ARTERITIS AND ANEURYSM OF THE CORONARY
ARTERY IN KAWASAKI DISEASE

Shiro Naoe, Noburu Tanaka, Hirotake Masuda and
Toshihiko Atobe
Research Laboratory of Pathology
Ohashi Hospital, Toho University
2-17-6 Ohashi Meguroku, Tokyo, Japan   153

The earliest instance of coronary artery aneurysms in
Kawasaki Disease was seen in the case where death occurred
on the twelfth day from onset. By the tenth day, dissociation and disruption of the internal elastic lamina were
seen along with a panangiitis. All of this suggests that
the formation of coronary artery aneurysms begins about the
tenth day from onset and is completed by about the twelfth
day. The coronary artery aneurysms arise from symmetrical
dilatations which result from the dissociation and
destruction of the internal elastic lamina. This resembles
the process by which a balloon expands with an increase in
internal pressure. The formation of the aneurysms is
offset by the tendency toward self-healing which results in
fibrosis. The shape of the aneurysm depends on the degree
of scarring. When fibrosis is marked, the aneurysm is
generally elliptical. When fibrous formation is slightly
delayed, however, the weakened arterial walls fail because
they cannot withstand the pressure, and the aneurysm
expands to become spherical. Turbulence occurs more easily
within the lumen of spherical aneurysms than in the lumen
of elliptical ones, and in such a setting, thrombi are
formed, and there is the danger of sudden death. These
observations confirm morphologically the coronary artery
angiographic findings.

Kawasaki Disease, pages 527–528
© 1987 Alan R. Liss, Inc.

EARLY OCCLUSION OF SAPHENOUS VEIN GRAFTS DUE TO MARKED
INTIMAL PROLIFERATION IN KAWASAKI DISEASE

Hiroshi Nishida, Masahiro Endo, Hisae Hayashi,
Hitoshi Koyanagi and Atuyoshi Takao*
Heart Institute of Japan
Tokyo Women's Medical College
Department of Cardiovascular Surgery and
Pediatric Cardiology*

From 1977 to 1986, nine children aged 4 to 11 years
underwent coronary artery bypass grafting (CABG) for coronary arterial lesions associated with Kawasaki Disease.
Seven children had CABG alone (single CABG: 3; double CABG:
4), and the other two children received single CABG with
mitral valve replacement and double CABG with mitral valvu-
loplasty, respectively. Autologous saphenous vein grafts
(SVG) were used in six cases, homologous SVG from the
mother was employed in one case, and in the other two cases
bilateral internal mammary arteries were used for the left
anterior descending and right coronary arteries. There
were no operative deaths. Early graft patency rate confirmed by selective angiography one month after the operation was 100%. Despite these excellent early operative
results, three patients who had SVG died suddenly 4 months,
6 months and 3 years after operation, respectively. All
three were 6 years or younger, weighing less than 20 kg at
operation. Postmortem examinations showed total occlusion
of the SVG due to marked intimal proliferation along the
total length of the grafts. In these cases postoperative
angiography revealed that the stenosis of the engrafted
native coronary arteries progressed to total occlusion. On
the other hand, four patients older than 7 years and the
two children who had bilateral internal mammary artery
grafts are now in good condition.

These results showed that in children 6 years or
younger, SVG tend to occlude too early to allow development
of adequate collateral circulation, and occlusion of SVG
causes sudden death under the situation of totally occluded

native coronary arteries by progression. CABG with
internal mammary artery is technically difficult in these
small children. We conclude that if the condition of the
patients allows, the operation should be delayed at least
until 7 years of age or older even if CABG with SVG is
possible.

Kawasaki Disease, pages 529–530
© 1987 Alan R. Liss, Inc.

COMPARATIVE STUDY OF THE CORONARY ARTERIAL INVOLVEMENT IN
INFANT AND ADULT RABBITS WITH EXPERIMENTAL ALLERGIC
ANGIITIS

Z. Onouchi,* H. Tamiya,* Y. Sakakibara,*
T. Fujimoto,* K. Ikuta,** N. Nagamatsu,**
N. Kiyosawa,*** and T. Minaga****
The Department of Pediatrics* and Pathology,**
Aichi Medical University, The Department of
Pediatrics,*** Kyoto Prefectural University of
Medicine, Cutter Japan Ltd.****

Various diseases involve the coronary arteries in the
inflammatory process. Smaller branches are invariably
involved, but the main trunks rarely. The term "arteritis"
suggests a definitive change of the vessel wall resulting
in stenosis or aneurysm. Arteritis of the main coronary
arteries in adults tends to result in stenosis, while that
in infants and children in aneurysm. This study seeks to
clarify the pathogenesis of aneurysm formation in infants
and children with coronary arteritis such as Kawasaki
Disease, infantile polyarteritis nodosa and rheumatic
fever.

Albino rabbits formed the experimental series,
comprised of three groups: group A, male adults weighing
about 3 kg; group B, young males weighing about 2 kg; and
group C, weanlings 3-4 weeks of age. Horse serum (10mg/kg
body weight) was administered intravenously twice 2 weeks
apart. Animals were sacrificed 3 hours to 2 weeks (acute
stage) and 4-5 months (chronic stage) after the last
injection and prepared for histologic study. Heart
sections were stained with H & E and also according to van
Gieson's technique and immunoperoxidase method for horse
serum and IgG.

(Acute stage) Coronary lesions in all groups were
segmental. In adults, coronary lesions were uniformly
severe, involving all three arterial layers. However, the
elastica interna and externa were almost intact despite
extensive proliferation of fibroblasts. In children,

coronary lesions were the most severe in all three layers
and were characterized by fibroblastic proliferation and
collagen formation accompanied, in some cases, by the
formation of endothelial buds and capillaries, giving them
a granulomatous appearance. There was striking thickening
of the intimal coat with extensive destruction of the
internal elastic membrane. In weanlings, coronary lesions
generally were mild with much variation in the grade of
involvement. From 24 to 72 hours, coronary trunks showed
severe edema, degeneration and deposition of immune
complexes without cell infiltrations throughout all three
layers, resulting in segmental or diffuse dilatation of
the vessels. Intimal hyperplasia was slight, but elastic
layers were quite destroyed, accompanied by thinning of
the media in the most active stage. The striking feature
was rapid disappearance of the inflammatory process and
repair of the structural change.

(Chronic stage) Even in weanlings, there was mild
thickening of the intimal coat accompanied, in some cases,
by elastosis in all three layers.

Conclusion: Histologic findings in weanling rabbits
revealed weakening of the coronary arterial wall and
dilatation, with the striking feature that the inflammatory
change was rapidly repaired with few sequelae. Those in
older but not adult animals showed intense tissue reaction
with destruction of the vessel wall, resulting in formation
of persistent aneurysms when dilatation occurred.

Kawasaki Disease, pages 531–533
© 1987 Alan R. Liss, Inc.

A STUDY OF PSYCHO-SOCIAL EFFECTS OF CHRONIC MCLS UPON
MOTHERS

Shizen Ishikawa,* Yoshinari Inaba,*
Kazuo Okuyama,* Takashi Asakura,**
Yoo Sook Kim,*** and Setsuko Sasa***
*Department of Pediatrics, Showa University
**Department of Health Sociology, School of Health
    Sciences, Faculty of Medicine, Tokyo University
***Department of Mental Health, School of Health
    Sciences, Faculty of Medicine, Tokyo University

A survey of chronic MCLS children and their mothers was
conducted by the authors. 113 mothers responded to a
questionnaire and the collection rate was 75.3%. First, we
defined the actual degree of maternal anxiety and
childrens' life restriction. After analyzing the data, the
psycho-social characteristics of mothers and their children
were examined statistically, particularly in those cases in
which the mothers had more worries and the children's lives
were more restricted by them.

The main findings were as follows:

1) 89.4% of mothers worried about their children, with the
    main worries relapse (62.8%), aneurysm (59.3%), unable
    to participate fully in sports (26.5%).

2) We found 7 characteristics of those mothers and their
    children who were much more worried about children.
    Their children: a) went to the hospital frequently, and
    b) took medicine. Mothers: c) hoped that long-term
    follow-up for MCLS could be held periodically; d) asked
    many persons to help them to deal with the children's
    disease; f) had some other family members to be cared
    for; g) felt that their daily lives were more stressful
    compared with same aged women; and h) had more
    complaints of their mental and physical condition.

3) Only 6.2% of mothers were thought to require counsel-
    ling, as evaluated by the Cattell Anxiety Scale (CAS).

4) 28.3% of mothers were restricting their children's daily activities. The main subjects of restriction were vaccination (12.4%), playing sports (10.6%) and sitting up late at night (10.6%).

5) The characteristics of such mothers and children were as follows: a) Time passed <6 months or > 5 years since children were diagnosed MCLS; b) Children went to the hospital more frequently than once every three months; c) Took medicine. Mothers' characteristics were: d) have been helped or wanted to ask other mothers with MCLS children for some advice; e) took great responsibility for rearing children as is typical in mother-and-child families; and f) experienced some stressful life events other than the children's disease in the past.

Degree of mother's Anxiety

Duration after KAWASAKI disease	Degree of Anxiety based on CAS			
	Stable	Average	Slightly Anxietic	Anxietic
	1 ~ 3	4 ~ 6	7	8
> 6 Mos	5	7	0	1
> 1 yr	6	6	0	0
> 3 yrs	22	27	5	1
> 5 yrs	12	5	0	0
>10yrs	9	6	0	0
<10yrs	1	0	0	0
Total	55 (49)	51 (45)	5 (4)	2 (2)

Age of children	Degree of Anxiety based on CAS			
	Stable	Average	Slightly Anxietic	Anxietic
	1 ~ 3	4 ~ 6	7	8
> 6 Mos	3	3	0	1
> 4 yrs	15	21	2	1
> 7 yrs	16	16	2	0
>10yrs	15	8	1	0
>13yrs	4	3	0	0
<13yrs	2	0	0	0
Total	55 (49)	51 (45)	5 (4)	2 (2)

Figure 1

Comparison with mother's anxiety of handicapped children

	Degree of Anxiety based on CAS			
	Stable	Average	Slightly Anxietic	Anxietic
	1 ~ 3	4 ~ 6	7	8
mother with KAWASAKI disease	55 (49)	51 (45)	5 (4)	2 (2)
mother with handicapped children	31 (40)	35 (45)	7 (9)	5 (6)

Figure 2.

Kawasaki Disease, pages 535–537
© 1987 Alan R. Liss, Inc.

PREDICTIVE FACTORS OF CORONARY ANEURYSM IN KAWASAKI
DISEASE--CORRELATION BETWEEN CORONARY ARTERIAL LESIONS AND
SERUM ALBUMIN, CHOLINESTERASE ACTIVITY, PREALBUMIN,
RETINOL-BINDING PROTEIN AND IMMATURE NEUTROPHILS

Masao Nakano
Department of Pediatrics
Gifu Prefectural Tajimi Hospital

Kawasaki Disease (MCLS) is thought to be systemic
angiitis from the pathophysiological point of view. It has
been reported that excessive production of the hydroxyl
radical (OH^-) and singlet oxygen ($^1O_2$) in neutrophils
(PMN), and decreased serum concentration of vitamin E
nicotinate (VEN) as the quencher for activated oxygens are
seen in the early stage of MCLS. I have also found that
the serum albumin (AL) concentration decreased to <3g/dl
and the serum cholinesterase activity (ChE) decreases to
<0.50 Δ PH in the early stage of MCLS in some cases. Those
findings seem to reflect the severity of MCLS angiitis. It
is suggested that there is a strong correlation between
hypoalbuminemia <3g/dl and the ChE <0.50 Δ PH and coronary
aneurysm formation at the early stage of MCLS.

It is very important to know how to predict coronary
aneurysm formation in the acute phase of Kawasaki Disease
in order to prevent coronary aneurysm formation. We
studied the correlation between coronary arterial lesions
found by 2 dimensional echocardiography (2 DE) and serum
albumin (AL), cholinesterase activity (ChE), prealbumin
(PA), retinol binding protein (RBP) and immature
neutrophils (IN).

Twenty two cases with typical Kawasaki Disease within 7
days of onset were evaluated. 2 DE was done daily until we
recognized improvement of fever and of findings of coronary
artery by 2 DE. Thereafter it was done two times a week
for one month of illness. We defined abnormal findings of
the coronary artery by 2 DE to be very mild coronary

arterial dilatation <3mm diameter with echo-enhanced
lesion. AL, ChE, PA, RBP and IN were examined more than
two times per week until one month of illness. We studied
the daily changes of values of AL, ChE, PA, RBP and IN of
each group. The 22 cases were divided into two groups, 8
cases with coronary arterial lesions and 14 cases without.
The minimal level of ChE was seen at 7.90+2.26 (M+SD) days
of illness, the lowest level of AL was seen at 8.29+2.15
(M+SD) days of illness, and very mild coronary arterial
dilatation by 2 DE was first observed at 8.50+1.93 (M+SD)
days of illness. All findings were seen at almost the same
time in the illness. ChE values <0.50 Δ PH and AL <3g/dl
correlated well and were good predictors of coronary
arterial lesions. Both PA and RBP decreased within 6 days
of illness and continued to decrease in 7 to 12 days of
illness in cases with coronary arterial lesions. However,
in cases with normal coronary arteries, the values tended
to normalize after 7 to 12 days of illness. The number of
immature neutrophils (myelocytes, metamyelocytes and bands)
is also a good index to predict coronary arterial lesions.
In cases with coronary arterial lesions, the number of
immature neutrophils continued to increase at 6 to 9 days
of illness, but in cases with no coronary arterial lesions,
tended to decrease after 6 to 9 days of illness. In the
group that was given intact gamma globulin (I γ -Gl), the
number of immature neutrophils decreased more quickly than
in Co-Aneu. group (non-1 γ -Gl group). The number of
immature neutrophils in the I γ -Gl group was almost the
same with that of non Co-Aneu. group at 5 to 50 days of
illness.

We studied combination therapy for Kawasaki Disease
with VEN and I γ -Gl. 100mg/kg/day of VEN was administered
p.o. to all patients as soon as possible. The patients who
had the findings a or b listed below were additionally
given 400mg/kg of I γ -Gl DIV one or five times. The number
of times of I γ -Gl administration was reduced to the
minimum when we recognized improvement of findings by 2 DE
and of physiological findings, and decreased immature
neutrophils.
a) Cases with hypoalbuminemia <3g/dl and/or decreased
   cholinesterase activity <0.50 Δ PH checked every 24 to
   48 hours.
b) Cases with echo-enhanced lesions and very mild dilatation of coronary arteries examined by daily 2 DE.
The mean initial date of I γ -Gl administration was 8.1 days

of illness. The mean number of doses of Iγ-G1 was 2.97, and the mean total administered dose of Iγ-G1 was 1,188mg/kg. The indicated rate for Iγ-G1 was 39/77 (50.1%). The number of cases with no coronary arterial lesion was 75/77 (97.4%), while 2/77 (2.6%) had transient coronary arterial dilatation (4mm in diameter, regressed in 4 months). Transient high fever 39°C up to 41°C was seen about 50% with the initial Iγ-G1 administration.

It is thought that the combination therapy of VEN and Iγ-G1 for Kawasaki Disease might regulate the excessive production of activated oxygens in PMN and result in the prompt improvement of systemic angiitis.

Kawasaki Disease, pages 539–540

THE ENHANCEMENT OF ANTI-MYOSIN ANTIBODY IN MUCOCUTANEOUS
LYMPH NODE SYNDROME

A. Arimura and T. Shimbo

Department of Pediatrics, Mizonokuchi Hospital,
Teikyo University School of Medicine,
Kawasaki, Japan

Since mucocutaneous lymph node syndrome (MCLS) was
first reported in 1967, therapeutic results have been
satisfactory, but the etiology of MCLS remains unknown.
Myocarditis complicates MCLS. Therefore, we examined the
presence of serum antibodies to myosin, which is the main
antigen in the myocardium.

Patients: Sera from sixteen patients (11 boys, 5
girls) with MCLS, aged from 5 months to 4 years old, were
compared with sera from 16 age-matched healthy controls.

Methods: Anti-myosin antibodies were measured by
enzyme-linked immunosorbent assay (ELISA). Anti-myosin
IgM and IgG antibody titers examined twice at intervals of
about 10 days in healthy controls did not differ between
the two determinations. These results established the
normal range. No IgA anti-myosin antibody was detected in
the sera of controls or patients with MCLS. Elevated
anti-myosin IgM antibody titers were observed in MCLS as
early as 2 or 3 days after the onset of the disease, and
then declined in the early convalescent stage.

Anti-myosin IgG-antibody titers were within the normal
limit in the early acute stage of MCLS, but became
increased between Day 20 and 30 of the disease, thereafter
returning to the normal range.

Since myocardial myosin was reported to share cross-
reactive antigens with group A streptococci, we examined
titers of ASO, anti-streptokinase and ADNse B in the sera

of patients with MCLS. These titers did not correlate with anti-myosin antibodies. Moreover, anti-myosin antibody titers were not correlated with serum CPK levels, abnormalities of the electrocardiogram, or the presence of coronary aneurysm detected by echocardiography.

Our results are summarized as follows:
(1) Anti-myosin IgM and IgG antibodies were detected in the sera of both MCLS patients and normal children.
(2) An increase of IgM antibody levels was observed in the acute stage of MCLS. However, IgG antibody titers were normal in the early acute stage of the disease, and an increase was observed in the early convalescent stage.
(3) The fluctuations in anti-myosin antibody levels resembled those of a primary antibody response to an antigen in vivo. We speculate that this immune response begins one or two weeks before the clinical onset of MCLS.

Kawasaki Disease, page 541
© 1987 Alan R. Liss, Inc.

ANALYTICAL STUDIES ON IMMUNOSUPPRESSIVE FACTOR(S) IN SERA
FROM PATIENTS WITH KAWASAKI DISEASE USING MONOCLONAL
ANTIBODIES

J. Hirao,* N. Yoshimura,*** N. Homma,** and
K. Kano***
The First Department of Pediatrics, Dokkyo
University School of Medicine,* Dokkyo
University School of Medicine,** Department of
Immunology, Institute of Medical Science,
University of Tokyo***

We have previously reported that acute phase sera
from patients with Kawasaki Disease contained suppressive
factor(s) which inhibit concanavalin A-induced lymphocyte
proliferation. In this report, we show the procedure for
the purification of this factor(s) from sera and for the
production of murine monoclonal antibodies to this
factor(s). We also present the results detected regarding
this factor(s) in sera from patients or from control
children by using these antibodies.

Suppressive factor(s) purified from patient serum was
used to immunize Balb/c mice. Spleen cells from the
immunized mice were fused with NS-1 (murine myeloma cell
line) using polyethylene glycol. Hybridomas secreting
antibodies (screened by enzyme-linked immunosorbent assay)
were selected and cloned by the limiting dilution method.
Detection of the suppressive factor(s) in sera was carried
out by Western blot analysis using biotinylated monoclonal
antibodies and avidin-peroxidase.

Four monoclonal antibodies were produced, and they
reacted equally with the serum factor with M.W. = 140,000
daltons. This factor was present in 78% and 29% of sera
from acute phase patients and control children,
respectively. These antibodies may be useful for analysis
of the pathogenesis of Kawasaki Disease.

Kawasaki Disease, pages 543-544
© 1987 Alan R. Liss, Inc.

SELECTION OF HIGH-RISK CHILDREN FOR IMMUNOGLOBULIN THERAPY IN KAWASAKI DISEASE

M. Iwasa, K. Sugiyama, T. Ando, H. Nomura,
T. Katoh and Y. Wada
Department of Pediatrics, Nagoya Daini Red Cross
Hospital, Nagoya Higashi Shimin Hospital, and
Nagoya City University Hospital

Because some children with Kawasaki Disease do not
need to receive immunoglobulin, we studied the selection
of high-risk children with Kawasaki Disease and the effect
of immunoglobulin on high-risk children. From November,
1981, to June, 1986, 222 eligible children with Kawasaki
Disease admitted to three hospitals before the eighth
illness day and given treatment with aspirin and/or immunoglobulin before the ninth day were studied. The risk score
previously reported was calculated from the formula: risk
score = -1.537×10^{-2} x age (months) + 1.004 x sex (male = 1,
female = 0) - 1.501×10^{-2} x RBC ($\#/10^4/mm^3$) + 1.129×10^{-1} x
hematocrit (%) - 1.965 x serum albumin (g/dl) + 8.462.
Children whose risk score exceeded 0 were considered high
risk, and those ≤ 0 low risk.

After hospitalization, all children received aspirin
30 mg/kg/d; this was decreased to 10 mg/kg/d when fever
resolved. Low-risk children (122) received aspirin alone,
while 100 high-risk children were divided into groups
receiving aspirin alone, IV immunoglobulin 200+40 mg/kg/d
x 5 days, and IV immunoglobulin 400+50 mg/kg/d x 5 days.
Two-dimensional echocardiography was performed twice
weekly during the febrile period prior to Day 29, at Days
30, 60, 90, and 6 months and one year, with an abnormality
defined as lumen at least 3 mm diameter or 1.5 times the
adjacent segment, with three grades: I, < 4 mm; II, > 4 mm
to 8 mm; and III, > 8 mm.

The incidence of coronary artery abnormalities was
significantly greater at all times of assessment among

high-risk aspirin alone recipients compared to low-risk aspirin alone recipients. When initiated before the ninth day of illness, 400 mg/kg/day immunoglobulin x 5 days was highly effective in reducing the prevalence of coronary artery abnormalities, while the 200 mg/kg/day dose x 5 days was only partially effective. There was no relation between the duration of illness prior to immunoglobulin therapy and the incidence of coronary artery abnormalities. The mean durations of fever and of positive C-reactive protein were shorter in the gamma globulin groups than in the aspirin alone group.

The incidence of development of coronary abnormalities was low when immunoglobulin was begun immediately upon determination of a score indicating a high risk, as compared to those starting therapy one or more days after determination of a high-risk score. We conclude that early administration of immunoglobulin is necessary to treat high-risk children with Kawasaki Disease most effectively.

Kawasaki Disease, pages 545–546
© 1987 Alan R. Liss, Inc.

T-CELL SUBSETS IN KAWASAKI SYNDROME

N.J. Marchette, M.E. Melish, S. Kihara,
F. Caplan, D. Ching
Department of Tropical Medicine (N.J.M., S.K.,
F.C.) and Pediatrics (M.E.M., D.C.)
John A. Burns School of Medicine, University of
Hawaii, Honolulu, Hawaii   96816

Peripheral blood mononuclear cells were obtained from heparinized blood by standard Ficoll-Hypaque sedimentation. Adherent cells were removed by incubation on plastic. Becton-Dickinson monoclonal antibodies with the following specificities were used: total T cells (anti-Leu-1); T cytotoxic/suppressor cells (anti-Leu-2a); T helper/ inducer cells (anti-Leu-3a); lymphoblasts (anti-transferrin receptor); activated T cells (anti-HLA-DR). Direct immunofluorescent assays were done using fluorescein or phycoerythrin-labelled antibodies, and the cells were counted with a Zeiss fluorescent microscope fitted with epi-illumination.

Lymphocyte subset analyses on 45 KS patients in Hawaii suggest that there is an alteration in the Th/Ts ratio due to an absolute decrease in the number of T suppressor cells. The magnitude of the T suppressor cell depression varied within rather wide limits, and in approximately one third of those tested, the Th/Ts ratio was two or more standard deviations above the published normal value (1.8 + 0.6) at some time during the acute phase or early convalescence. The T suppressor cells recovered and the Th/Ts ratio generally returned to normal during convalescence. When tested one or more years after the illness, both suppressor cells and Th/Ts ratios were within normal limits in most cases.

Two scarlet fever patients included in the febrile controls had depressed Th/Ts ratios of less than 1.0 whereas two measles patients had ratios that were essentially normal (1.3 and 1.9) on the days tested. Unfortunately, these patients were tested during the acute phase of illness only.

There was an increase in activated (transferrin+) T-cells in the acute phase of illness, but there was no consistent increase in Dr+ T-cells or Dr+ T-helper cells.

Treatment with gamma globulin resulted in rapid recovery of T-suppressor cells and a concomitant decrease in Th/Ts ratio in most cases. Gamma globulin appeared to decrease the activated (transferrin+) T-cells, but had little effect on the number of Dr+ T-cells or T-helper cells.

One KS patient (M.K.) recovered clinically after aspirin therapy but relapsed four months later, at which time he was treated with gamma globulin. In retrospect, it appears that aspirin alone did not completely resolve the initial episode; Ts cells remained depressed and the Th/Ts ratio was elevated 44 days after onset. It is unknown if T suppressors recovered before the relapse, but the Th/Ts ratio was elevated to about the same level as during the initial convalescence. After gamma globulin, Ts cells rapidly recovered and the Th/Ts ratio normalized and remained normal during convalescence. The number of Dr+ T-cells increased during late acute and early convalescence phases of both episodes and subsequently fell to low levels in late convalescence. Gamma globulin for the recurrent illness had no apparent effect on the number of Dr+ T-cells.

Changes in absolute number of T-cells or alteration of T-cell subset ratios are commonly observed in a variety of infectious diseases and often are part of the normal immune response to a foreign agent. These changes are usually transient and may not be of great magnitude, but a decrease in Th/Ts ratio appears a general phenomenon in viral infections. In those well studied (herpes viruses, hepatitis B, measles, respiratory viruses), the decreased Th/Ts ratio is due to increased Ts cells with either no change or decreased Th cells. Increased Th/Ts ratios are rare except in autoimmune disease (e.g., rheumatoid arthritis) and possibly some bacterial infections.

Kawasaki Disease, page 547
© 1987 Alan R. Liss, Inc.

KAWASAKI SYNDROME EPIDEMIOLOGY - HAWAII 1971-1986

Marian E. Melish, M.D. and D. Ching

Kapiolani-Children's Medical Center and
John A. Burns School of Medicine
Honolulu

Kawasaki syndrome has been recognized in the state of Hawaii since 1971. Active surveillance since 1973 demonstrated a pattern of rising annual incidence until approximately 1980 when an apparent plateau was achieved. Sharply defined epidemics during winter and spring months have occurred at 2-3 year intervals since 1978. Epidemics have been community-wide with no evidence of geographic progression from one contiguous residential area to another and no evidence of direct person-to-person spread nor a common source exposure. On the island of Oahu, where case finding is nearly complete, analysis of the geographic distribution of cases demonstrates that the 4 areas with the highest incidence share an urban-suburban character, above average socioeconomic status, and multi-ethnic population. Average monthly incidence shows that during epidemic periods the months of January through May have the highest incidence but that in non-epidemic years cases occur evenly throughout the year. Case control studies show no significantly increased frequency of exposure to carpet or carpet shampooing in cases. Other factors evaluated in age-, sex- and race-matched case-control studies show no significant differences in family income, exposure to pets, diet, exposure to products from Japan, exposure to tourists, exposure to other small children and attendance at day care centers. Recurrent disease was encountered as were cases in siblings of previously diagnosed patients. The most striking feature of the epidemiology of Kawasaki syndrome in Hawaii is the difference in incidence among children belonging to different ethnic groups. Children of Japanese and Korean ancestry showed the highest race-specific incidence rates while Caucasians were underrepresented.

Kawasaki Disease, pages 549–551
© 1987 Alan R. Liss, Inc.

EPIDEMIOLOGICAL FEATURES OF AN OUTBREAK OF KAWASAKI DISEASE IN YOKOHAMA

M. Minowa, H. Mori, N. Kubo and H. Satomi

Department of Epidemiology
The Institute of Public Health
Tokyo

Epidemiological features of Kawasaki Disease in Yokohama during the period of February, 1985, to March, 1986, were investigated. Subjects were 566 cases of Kawasaki Disease which occurred during the study period and notified to the Yokohama City Health Bureau. Four hundred eighty cases were concentrated between November, 1985, and February, 1986, as part of a nationwide epidemic.

The incidence rate of the disease was 14.6 per 100,000 population under the age of 10. The proportion of the cases under the age of one year was 32.5% and that under the age of two years 71.2%. The male to female ratio was 1.48. The epidemic moved from the north to the south with an increasing attack rate. Mild time-space clustering was observed as assessed by Knox's method.

In a case-control study, a questionnaire was mailed to cases and to sex-and-age-matched (within 1 month) neighborhood controls. Out of 566, 483 cases (85.3% and 416 (73.5%) controls responded to the questionnaire. The results of preliminary analyses of the data were as follows:

(1) The DPT vaccination rate was somewhat lower among cases than controls (Table 1).
(2) Bottle feeding in infancy was more common, and less breast feeding and use of home made juice were observed in the cases (Table 2).

(3) The cases lived on lower floors than controls (data not shown).
(4) No differences were observed in employment status and income of the father between cases and controls (Table 3).

Table 1

Vaccination Rate of Cases of Kawasaki Disease (MCLS) and Controls

Vaccination		N	Vaccin (+)	%
BCG	MCLS	478	422	88.3
	Cont.	410	374	91.2
DPT 1	MCLS	428	120	28.0*
	Cont.	366	127	34.7
Polio 1	MCLS	470	416	88.5
	Cont.	404	365	90.4
Polio 2	MCLS	451	295	65.4
	Cont.	382	269	70.4
JEV	MCLS	418	38	9.1
	Cont.	345	36	10.4
Measles	MCLS	430	141	32.8
	Cont.	361	140	38.8

*P<.05

Table 2

Use of Feeding in Infancy
by Cases of Kawasaki Disease (MCLS) and Controls

Feeding		N	Yes	%
Breast Feeding	MCLS	467	404	86.5*
Within 1 Month	Cont.	414	384	92.5
Bottle Feeding	MCLS	447	396	88.6**
	Cont.	396	322	81.3
Cow Milk	MCLS	453	364	80.4**
	Cont.	410	385	93.9
Home Made Juice	MCLS	483	284	58.8**
	Cont.	416	304	73.1
Instant Juice	MCLS	483	245	50.7
	Cont.	416	196	47.1
Canned Juice	MCLS	483	48	9.9**
	Cont.	416	21	5.1
Bottled Juice	MCLS	483	190	39.3
	Cont.	416	157	37.7

*.05> P>.01
**P<.01

Table 3

Employment Status of Parents

Employment Status	Father				Mother			
	MCLS(%)		Control(%)		MCLS(%)		Control(%)	
Employees	411	(86.7)	353	(86.1)	28	(5.9)	35	(8.6)
Directors	27	(5.7)	27	(6.6)	2	(0.4)	0	(0.0)
Self-Employed,								
Employing Others	14	(3.0)	13	(3.2)	3	(0.6)	1	(0.2)
Not Employing Others	17	(3.6)	10	(2.4)	1	(0.2)	1	(0.2)
Family Workers	3	(0.6)	5	(1.2)	10	(2.1)	12	(2.9)
Pay Job at Home	0	(0.0)	0	(0.0)	7	(1.5)	1	(0.2)
Not in Labor Force	1	(0.2)	0	(0.0)	4	(0.8)	2	(0.5)
Unemployed	1	(0.2)	2	(0.5)	2	(0.4)	1	(0.2)
Housewife					422	(88.1)	356	(87.0)
TOTAL	474	(100.0)	410	(100.0)	479	(100.0)	409	(100.0)

Kawasaki Disease, pages 553–554
© 1987 Alan R. Liss, Inc.

TWO-COLOR FLOW CYTOMETRIC ANALYSIS OF PERIPHERAL
LYMPHOCYTES IN KAWASAKI DISEASE

Shigeaki Nonoyama, Kozo Takase, Yoshiko Matsuoka,
and Junichi Yata
Department of Pediatrics, School of Medicine,
Tokyo Medical and Dental University

The lymphocyte subsets in Kawasaki Disease (KD) were
analyzed using two-color flow cytometry. Twenty one
patients (11 male, 10 female) with KD and 15 age-matched
normal controls (8 male, 7 female) were included in this
study. Specimens were obtained three times from each KD
patient at various stages: Acute phase (mean 4.7 days);
early convalescent phase (13.8 days); late convalescent
phase (28 days). The first specimens were obtained before
intravenous gammaglobulin (IVGG) therapy. Five patients
were treated with aspirin (ASA) alone and 15 patients were
treated with ASA and IVGG.

We found that B1(+) cells were increased during the
acute phase of KD (KD: 18.5%$\pm$4.0%, control: 10.4%$\pm$3.6%,
p<0.005), and values subsequently decreased to the normal
level by the late convalescent phase. This result was
consistent with the transient hyperglobulinemia of KD.
B1(+)B2(-) cells, which are suggested to be activated B
cells, were not increased, but another activation marker
must be chosen to clarify the activation of B cells in
marker analysis. Leu1(+)B1(+) cells, which were reported
to be increased in some autoimmune diseases, were not
increased in KD.

T8(+) cells were decreased during the acute phase (KD:
12.4%$\pm$2.7%, control: 19.7%$\pm$5.3%, p<0.005), and T8(+)Mo1(+)
cells, which are known as suppressor subsets of T8(+)
cells, were also decreased. But the number of T8(+) cells
and T8(+)Mo1(+) cells returned to normal by the late
convalescent phase. This transient reduction of suppressor

T cells may have some role in the activation of B cells in KD.

Although percentages of T4(+) cells were normal in KD, the ratio of T4(+)2H4(+)/T4(+)2H4(-) (suppressor inducer/ helper) was high during the acute phase (KD: 5.8±2.7, control: 3.3±1.9, p<0.005) and returned to normal level by the early convalescent phase.

There was one KD patient whose course was complicated by coronary aneurysms in this study. T8(+)Ia(+) cells and T4(+)Ia(+) cells in this patient were increased, while they were not increased in any of the patients without coronary artery aneurysm. Therefore, some relation between Ia expression of T cells and complication of coronary artery aneurysm was suggested. Further study is needed.

Kawasaki Disease, pages 555–556
© 1987 Alan R. Liss, Inc.

CLINICAL EVALUATION OF GAMMAGLOBULIN PREPARATIONS FOR THE
TREATMENT OF KAWASAKI DISEASE

Osaka Kawasaki Syndrome Study Group
Hirotaro Ogino,* Minoru Ogawa, Yoshikazu Harima,
Shuzo Kono, Hidekazu Ohkuni, Masaru Nishida,
Yohnosuke Kobayashi and Hyakuji Yabuuchi
*Department of Pediatrics
 Kansai Medical University
 Fumizonocho-1, Moriguchi, Osaka 570 Japan

A multicenter prospective controlled study was
conducted in an attempt to prevent the coronary arterial
lesions (CAL) of Kawasaki Syndrome with high-dose intravenous gammaglobulin plus aspirin (GG-ASA) versus aspirin
alone (ASA). Patients randomly assigned to the GG-ASA
group received intravenous gammaglobulin (S-sulfonated
gammaglobulin, GGS), 200mg/kg/day (STUDY-I, from May 1984
to April 1985) or 400mg/kg/day (STUDY-II, from July 1985 to
June 1986), for three consecutive days; both treatment
groups received aspirin, 30 mg/kg/day until CRP became
negative, after which it was reduced to 10mg/kg/day. The
development of CAL was monitored by two-dimensional
echocardiography. Patients in the ASA and GG-ASA groups
were similar in age distribution, sex ratio and duration of
illness when treatment was started. In all patients,
treatment was started within seven days after the onset of
disease both in STUDY-I and -II.

In STUDY-I (GGS 200mg/kg/day for 3 days), patients were
allocated to the ASA group (Asp-I, 42 cases) or GG-ASA
group (GGS-200, 50 cases). No significant difference in
the occurrence of CAL during the acute phase (11-25 days),
at 30 days, 60 days and one year after the onset of
disease, respectively, was found between the two groups
(Figure 1). The extent of coronary aneurysms and the time
course of regression of these lesions were not different
between the two groups.

In STUDY-II (GGS 400mg/kg/day for 3 days), patients
were allocated to the ASA group (Asp-II, 54 cases) or

GG-ASA group (GGS-400, 63 cases). During the acute phase,
CAL were present in 17 of 51 cases (33.3%) in the ASA
group, as compared with 11 of 62 cases (17.7%) in the
GG-ASA group (p<0.05 by Fisher's exact test). At 30 days
and 60 days, CAL were present in 17.6% and 13.5% in the ASA
group, as compared with 9.5% and 4.8% in the GG-ASA group,
respectively (Figure 1). When patients whose admission
echocardiograms indicated coronary abnormalities were
excluded, CAL were present in 15 of 49 cases (30.6%) in the
ASA group, as compared with 6 of 57 cases (10.5%) in the
GG-ASA group during the acute phase (p<0.01) (Figure 1,
lower panel). When we considered the degree of CAL and the
time course of regression in STUDY-II, middle-sized
aneurysms (ANm) were present in 3 of 51 cases (5.9%) in the
ASA group, as compared with 2 of 62 cases (3.2%) in the
GG-ASA group during the acute phase. At 30 and 60 days,
ANm were present in 2 of 51 (3.9%) and 1 of 52 (1.9%) in
the ASA group, as compared with none of 63 (0%) and none of
62 (0%) in the GG-ASA group, respectively.

We conclude that high-dose intravenous gammaglobulin
therapy for Kawasaki Syndrome was effective in reducing the
frequency and degree of CAL and in improving the time
course of regression. However, the effective gammaglobulin
dosage was at least 400mg/kg/day for at least three
consecutive days.

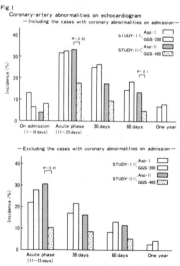

Fig.1
Coronary-artery abnormalities on echocardiogram
— Including the cases with coronary abnormalities on admission —

Kawasaki Disease, pages 557–558
© 1987 Alan R. Liss, Inc.

ENZYME RELEASE AND O_2 PRODUCTION OF NEUTROPHILS AND
VASCULAR LESIONS IN GAMMA GLOBULIN THERAPY OF KAWASAKI
DISEASE

Tomio Okazaki, M.D.,[1]
Tatsuichiro Sakatani, M.D.,[2],
Sumiko Sasagawa, Ph.D.,[3] Hiromi Ohta, B.S.,[4]
Hisashi Ohnishi, B.S.[3] Kazuo Suzuki, Ph.D.[5]
[1]Hiroshima City Hospital
[2] Fukushima Seikyo Hospital
[3] Radiation Effects Research Foundation
[4]Hiroshima University 5 NIH in Japan
7-33 Motomachi Naka-Ku Hiroshima Japan 730

Platelet aggregation, adhering neutrophils and damage
of endothelial cells of vascular lesions are all thought to
be possibly related to Kawasaki Disease. High doses of
intact gamma globulin has been proven clinically effective
in treating this disease.

At Hiroshima City Hospital pediatrics department, we
compared the effects of aspirin and gamma globulin on
neutrophil function in 25 patients with Kawasaki Disease.
In both the group treated with intact gamma globulin
(440-500mg/kg/day for 3-5 days) and the group treated with
aspirin (30-50mg/kg/day during the febrile period, thereafter 10mg/kg/day P.O.), we conducted 44 neutrophil
function tests. Those patients in whom ectasia or coronary
aneurysm were detected are referred to as the 2DE(+) group.

We measured release of lysosomal enzymes, myeloperoxidase (MPO), B-glucuronidase (BGL) and lysozyme (LYS) as
well as O_2 production from adhering and non-adhering
neutrophils stimulated with N-formyl-methionyl-leucyl-
phenylalanine (FMLP) and cytochalasine B (CB).

We found a slight increase of lysosomal enzyme release
from adhering neutrophils in the second phase of the
disease. In all phases of the disease, both adhering and
non-adhering neutrophils from 2DE(+) patients showed a
great tendency to release myeloperoxidase and B-glucuronidase. Since the most severe coronary lesions appeared
during the second phase of the disease, the results in the

present study suggest a good correlation between increased release of lysosomal enzymes from both adhering and non-adhering neutrophils and coronary artery abnormalities. In the gamma globulin therapy group, release of myeloperoxidase decreased. Lysosomal release showed a high level of sensitivity to FMLP. High levels of O_2 production were also observed.

In conclusion, the differences in neutrophil function found between the gamma globulin therapy group and the aspirin therapy group are thought to have great significance regarding the healing mechanism, as well as the effectiveness of treatment of Kawasaki Disease.

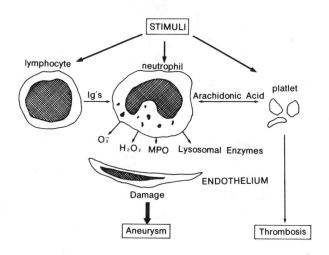

Figure 1. A scheme for role of neutrophils in aneurysm formation of Kawasaki Disease.

REFERENCES

Suzuki K et al (1983). Age-related decline in lysosomal enzyme release from polymorphonuclear leukocytes after N-formyl-methionyl-leucyl-phenylalanine stimulation. Exp Hematol 11:1005-1013.
Suzuki K et al (1983). Assay method for myeloperoxidase in human polymorphonuclear leukocytes. Anal Biochem 132: 345-352.

Kawasaki Disease, pages 559–561

CYTOTOXICITY OF SERA FROM KAWASAKI DISEASE TO RAT AORTIC
SMOOTH MUSCLE CELLS

Tsutomu Saji, Tetsuro Umezawa, Norio Matsuo,
Reiko Hashiguchi and Hiroyuki Matsuura
Department of Pediatrics, Toho University,
School of Medicine

Kawasaki Disease (KD) is characterized by aneurysms of
coronary arteries. Histopathology of structural changes of
the coronary artery exhibit interruption of the lamina
elastica interna and hydrophobic changes of smooth muscle
cells in the media. Cell-mediated and humoral immunological abnormalities contributing to the pathogenesis of KD
have been observed. In this study, we attempted to examine
the possible effect of sera from KD against vascular smooth
muscle cells.

Serum was obtained from patients with KD in the acute
phase, on the 5.2±1.8 day of illness, and from the same
patients in the convalescent phase, 60±22.7 day of
illness. The serum was heat-inactivated at 57°C for 45
minutes and filter sterilized. Rat embryonic aortic smooth
muscle cells (ATCC CRL-1476) and K562 cells (ATCC CCL-243)
were cultured in MEM Eagle Earl's Salt with 10% heat-
inactivated fetal calf serum for utilization as target
cells and control cells. 1×10^4 cells were cultured in 96
flat-bottomed micro titer wells for 24 hours. Monolayers
were labeled with ^{51}Cr (10uCi/well) for 90 minutes and
the supernatant removed. After addition of 0.18ml medium
and 0.02ml treated serum (diluted 1:10), cells were
cultured for 24 hours and ^{51}Cr release was measured.

The % cytotoxicity was calculated as follows:
(cpm experiment release - cpm spontaneous release/
cpm complete release - cpm spontaneous release).
Comparison of cytotoxicity between patient and control sera
was carried out using the Student's t test.

The % cytotoxicity of acute phase KD sera diluted 1:3
to SMC increased to 74+23.8%, as compared with 54.9+21.4%
(0.05<p<0.1, n=7) with sera from other acute infectious
diseases. The % cytotoxicity of 1:10 KD sera increased to
15.5+18.7% in the acute phase and to 12.9+23.5% in the
convalescent phase, compared to sera from age-matched
healthy controls (p<0.01, n=22). The % cytotoxicity to
K562 cells were not increased and sera fractionated to a
molecular weight of 30,000 were not increased. Sera from
patients with coronary arterial lesions revealed 11.7+25.3%
and sera from those without lesions was 9.0+23.8% (N.S.).
Sera positive for anti SMC-antibody (SMA) was 22.9+26.9%
and negative sera was 5.4+18.5% (0.05<p<0.1).

Coronary arterial SMC involvement was reported in
vascular lesions in KD. Specific enhanced endothelial cell
proliferation by sera in acute KD was reported[1] . It is
possible that a cytotoxic factor may be present in the KD
serum. Leung reported that cytotoxic antibodies against
γ-INF-treated human umbilical vein endothelial cells are
present in acute KD[2] . SMA, which is detected using rat
gastric SMC, was positive in 36% (9/25 KD cases) in our
previous studies[3] . In that observation, the presence of
coronary artery lesion was significantly more frequent in
SMA positive than negative patients (22% vs 6.3%, p<0.05).
But SMA is a non-specific antibody, belonging to the IgG
and IgM class. We did not detect a direct effect of sera
upon formation of aneurysms in the coronary artery.
However, the sera had cytotoxic effects on rat embryonic
aortic SMC. Masuda et al[4] observed an intercostal
arterial lesion characterized by reactive proliferative
change of the medial smooth-muscle cells and frequent
aneurysmal dilatation, similar to those in the coronary
arteries except for some delay in the occurrence. It is
suggested that the proliferation of medial smooth muscle
cells after their degeneration is a key feature of the
arterial lesion in KD.

Therefore, we suggest that sera from KD in the acute
phase possibly has cytotoxic effects, and if so, this
activity may play an important role in the pathogenesis of
the SMC injury of arterial lesions associated with KD.

REFERENCES

Hashimoto Y, Yoshimoya S, Aikawa T, Mitamura T, Miyoshi Y, Muranaka M, Miyamoto T, Yanase Y, Kawasaki T (1986). Enhanced endothelial cell proliferation in acute Kawasaki Disease (mucocutaneous lymph node syndrome). Ped Res 20:943-946.

Leung DYM, Collins T, Lapierre LA, Geha RS, Pober JS (1986). Immunoglobulin M antibodies present in the acute phase of Kawasaki Syndrome lyse cultured vascular endothelial cells stimulated by gamma interferon. J Clin Invest 77:1428-1435.

Saji T, Umezawa T, Hashiguchi R, Matsuo N (1983). Auto-antibodies in patients with mucocutaneous lymph node syndrome (Kawasaki Disease). Jap J Allergol 32:1129-1133 (English abstract).

Masuda H, Shozawa T, Naoe S, Tanaka N (1986). The inter-costal artery in Kawasaki Disease. Arch Pathol Lab Med 110:1136-1142.

KAWASAKI DISEASE: CIRCULATING IMMUNE COMPLEXES MONITORED
DURING THE DISEASE

E. Salo,* P. Pelkonen,* R. Kekomaki,**
O. Ruuskanen,*** M. Viander,**** O. Wager*****
*Children's Hospital, Helsinki University Central
  Hospital
**The Finnish Red Cross Blood Service Department
***Department of Pediatrics
****Department of Microbiology, University of Turku
*****Laboratory of Clinical Immunology, Helsinki

We followed the levels of circulating immune complexes
(IC) in 27 patients with Kawasaki Disease from their acute
stage of the disease through convalescence, using the tests
for platelet-reactive IgG-IC (PIPA), and Clq-binding (Clg)
and conglutinin-binding (KgB) enzyme immunoassays.
Circulating IC were detected by one or more techniques in
all but one patient. The PIPA test was the one that gave
positive results most often (24 of 27 patients), and the
blood platelet count correlated directly with the IC
level. 15/27 patients had positive KgB tests and 10/27
positive Clq tests. CIC could be detected even during the
first week of the disease, but the levels were highest
during the 3rd to 7th weeks.

The results support the possibility of immune complex-
mediated mechanisms in Kawasaki Disease.

Kawasaki Disease, pages 565–566
© 1987 Alan R. Liss, Inc.

THE METABOLISM OF THE ARACHIDONIC ACID CASCADE IN PATIENTS
WITH KAWASAKI DISEASE

Keiko Sasai, Susuma Furukawa and Keijiro Yabuta

Department of Pediatrics, Juntendo University
School of Medicine
2-1-1 Hongo, Bunkyo-ku, Tokyo, 113, JAPAN

Recently, the metabolites of the arachidonic acid
cascade have been reported to be important mediators of
inflammation. We investigated the arachidonic acid
metabolism in Kawasaki Disease.

We measured several metabolites of the arachidonic acid
cascade including plasma levels of prostaglandin E_2
(PGE_2), thromboxane B_2 (TXB_2), 6-keto $PGF_{1\alpha}$ and
immunoreactive Leukotriene C_4 (i-LTC_4) by
radioimmunoassay. PGE_2, TXB_2 and 6-keto $PGF_{1\alpha}$ are
formed during arachidonic acid metabolism via the
cyclooxygenase pathway. LTC_4 is one of the metabolites
of the arachidonic acid cascade via the lipoxygenase
pathway.

The results were as follows:

1) Plasma PGE_2, TXB_2, and 6-keto $PGF_{1\alpha}$ levels in
   patients with Kawasaki Disease were significantly
   elevated in the acute stage (P<0.015 for each compared
   to control values) and returned to the normal range in
   the convalescent stage. There was correlation among
   the levels of the three mediators in plasma.

2) Plasma i-LTC_4 levels were significantly elevated in
   the acute stage (P<0.015) and decreased gradually during
   favourable progress. LTC_4, LTD_4 and LTE_4 analyzed
   by the HPLC method were detected in plasma of Kawasaki
   Disease patients.

We suggest that there is activation of the arachidonic acid cascade both via the cyclooxygenase and via the lipoxygenase pathways in children with Kawasaki Disease. The metabolites of the arachidonic acid cascade may play an important role in the pathogenesis of Kawasaki Disease.

Kawasaki Disease, pages 567–568
© 1987 Alan R. Liss, Inc.

KAWASAKI DISEASE WITH ATYPICAL PRESENTATION

S. Schuh, R.M. Laxer, J. Smallhorn,
R.I. Hilliard and R.D. Rowe
Department of Pediatrics, The Hospital for Sick
Children, Toronto, Canada

Kawasaki Disease is a clinical diagnosis based on the presence of 5 of 6 criteria, and exclusion of other diseases with similar presentations. Recently it has been accepted that patients with 4 criteria and coronary aneurysms can also be diagnosed as having Kawasaki Disease. Cases which do not fulfill the suggested criteria can only be diagnosed by abnormal coronary echocardiography or suspected when desquamation later appears. Unfortunately, desquamation tends to occur in the subacute phase when the coronary abnormalities are already established.

We present two children with incomplete criteria at presentation in whom the diagnosis of Kawasaki Disease was confirmed by abnormal echocardiography. The purpose of this report is to de-emphasize rigid adherence to the usual criteria.

The first patient was a 7-month-old Vietnamese boy who had 13 days of fever, conjunctivitis and an erythematous rash, i.e., only 3 criteria at presentation late in the febrile phase of the illness. The WBC was 20,000/mm^3 with 50% PMN's, platelet count = 835,000/mm^3, and ESR was 54 mm/hr. On the 16th day of illness, the RCA was 2.3 mm (normal $\leq$1.7 mm) and the LCA was 2.7 mm (normal $\leq$2.4 mm) by echocardiogram. On the same day the fingertips began to desquamate. The child was treated with aspirin alone and then with aspirin and dipyridimole. Follow-up echocardiogram 11 months after onset showed RCA = 3.3 mm and LCA = 3.5 mm.

The second patient was a 15 1/2-year-old Caucasian male who presented with 10 days of fever (40°C) and red lips, strawberry tongue, conjunctivitis and mild diarrhea. The WBC = 27,000/mm^3 with 80% PMN's, platelet count = 474,000/mm^3 and ESR = 44 mm/hr. Echocardiogram on Day 12 of illness was normal. Desquamation was present on Day 14. Repeat echocardiogram on Day 31 showed LCA = 5.6 mm (normal $\leq$3.8 mm) and RCA = 3.5 mm (normal $\leq$3.1 mm). This child had only three criteria and is unusual because of his age.

Most patients with Kawasaki Disease present within the first seven days of illness with characteristic features allowing a prompt clinical diagnosis. A small proportion do not fulfill diagnostic criteria. Since such cases may result in omission or delay of initiation of appropriate therapy, it is important to maintain a high index of suspicion in patients with atypical features. Where there is doubt it may be advisable to initiate treatment pending clarification of the diagnosis by echocardiography and exclusion of other illnesses. Additionally, coronary dimensions based on a large number of normal children need to be firmly established.

Kawasaki Disease, pages 569–570
© 1987 Alan R. Liss, Inc.

EPSTEIN-BARR VIRUS-SPECIFIC CYTOTOXIC T LYMPHOCYTE
(EBV-CTL) ACTIVITIES IN PATIENTS WITH KAWASAKI SYNDROME

K. Shinohara, T. Katsuki and M. Koike

Department of Pediatrics, Wakayama Medical
College, Japan, and Department of Microbiology,
Kumamoto University Medical School

We studied EBV-CTL activity in patients with Kawasaki
Syndrome to understand the role of EBV infection-immunity.

Sera and peripheral lymphocytes were collected from
14 patients with Kawasaki Syndrome and 28 age-matched
controls. EBV-CTL activity was determined by using the
method described by Moss et al. (1978) termed the
regression assay method. Antibodies to EB virus capsid
antigen (VCA) and early antigen (EA) were determined by
the indirect immunofluorescence technique. Antibody to
EBV-associated nuclear antigen (EBNA) was determined by
the anticomplement immunofluorescence technique.

Data are presented in Table 1. Results are as
follows:

(1) Seronegative and seropositive control groups showed
    values of $\geq$ 112.8 and 2.5 to 56.6 $IR_{50} \times 10^4$ cells/ml,
    respectively.
(2) In the acute or subacute stage of Kawasaki Syndrome,
    CTL activities were lower.
(3) Case 1 had EBV-CTL activity with EBNA antibody negative
    on the 109th day after onset but not on the 10th or
    64th day. Case 2 did not have EBV-CTL activity but was
    EBNA antibody positive on the 64th day and had EBV-CTL
    activity with VCA-IgG antibody positive on the 107th
    day. Case 3 did not have EBV-CTL activity but was EBNA
    antibody positive on the 119th day. Case 9 did not
    have EBV-CTL activity on days 3 and 30 but had VCA-IgG
    and EBNA antibodies positive on the 30th day. This

patient had EBV-CTL activity with EBNA antibody negative and positive VCA-IgG on the 79th day. Case 14 was seronegative for VCA-IgG antibody on the 5th day. Although VCA-IgG and EBNA antibodies of Case 14 became seropositive on the 19th day (after IV gamma globulin therapy), the patient did not demonstrate EBV-CTL activity.

Table 1. EBV-CTL Activities and EBV Antibody Titers in 14 Children with Kawasaki Syndrome

Case	Age (Yr) at Onset	Sex	No. of Days After Onset	Titers of EBV Antibody To				IR_{50}x10^4 Cells/ml*
				VCA-IgG	VCA-IgM	EA-IgG	EBNA	
1	1	M	10	<5	<5	<5	<5	≥112.8
			64	<5	<5	<5	<5	≥112.8
			109	40	ND+	<5	<5	11.9
2	7/12	F	9	<5	<5	<5	<5	≥112.8
			64	<5	<5	<5	10	≥112.8
			107	40	ND	<5	10	40.0
3	6	M	21	<5	<5	<5	10	≥112.8
			70	<5	<5	<5	10	≥112.8
			119	<5	<5	<5	10	≥112.8
4	8/12	M	16	<5	<5	<5	<5	≥112.8
			54	<5	<5	<5	<5	≥112.8
			105	<5	<5	<5	<5	≥112.8
5	1	M	15	<5	<5	<5	<5	≥112.8
			46	<5	<5	<5	<5	≥112.8
			90	<5	<5	<5	<5	≥112.8
6	4	F	5	<5	<5	<5	<5	≥112.8
			30	<5	<5	<5	<5	>112.8
7	2	M	7	10	<5	<5	5	>112.8
8	2	M	4	10	<5	<5	5	>112.8
9	1	M	3	<5	<5	<5	<5	≥112.8
			30**	20	<5	<5	20	≥112.8
			79**	20	<5	<5	<5	28.4
10	5/12	F	26**	80	ND	20	20	>112.8
11	1	M	16**	320	ND	20	40	>112.8
12	1	M	13**	40	ND	<5	20	≥112.8
			30**	20	ND	<5	10	>112.8
13	4	F	13**	40	ND	<5	10	≥112.8
			27**	10	ND	<5	<5	≥112.8
14	8/12	F	5**	<5	ND	<5	<5	≥112.8
			19**	20	ND	<5	10	>112.8
Controls++	(A)	(n=10)		<5				>112.8
	(B)	(n=18)		>5				56.6-2.5

NOTE: *Minimum number cells/ml for 50% incidence of regression in EBV infected cells.

+ Not Determined
** After IVGG Treatment
++ Age-Matched (A) Seronegative Healthy
            (B) Seropositive Healthy

Kawasaki Disease, pages 571–572
© 1987 Alan R. Liss, Inc.

VARIANT STREPTOCOCCUS SANGUIS AS AN ETIOLOGICAL AGENT OF KAWASAKI DISEASE

N. Shinomiya, T. Takeda, T. Kuratsuji,
K. Takagi, T. Kosaka, O. Tatsuzawa,[1]
T. Tsurumizu,[2] T. Hashimoto,[2] and N. Kobayashi
National Children's Medical Research Center,[1]
National Children's Hospital,[2] The Kitazato
Research Institute, Tokyo, Japan

Clinical findings and laboratory data strongly suggested that a bacterial infection or toxin might be
associated with the cause of Kawasaki Disease (K.D.).
Streptococcus sanguis (St. sanguis) with a specific serotype has been predominantly isolated from K.D. patients.
We examined whether these strains were related to the
pathogenic mechanisms of K.D.

We measured Interleukin-1 (IL-1) activity induced from
peripheral blood mononuclear cells (PBMNCs) of K.D.
patients cultured with or without stimulation by both
phorbol-myristate acetate (PMA) and lipopolysaccharide
(LPS). Each culture supernatant (50 μl) was co-cultured
with mouse thymic cells with PHA for 3 days and ^{3}H-thymi-
dine incorporation was measured.

K.D. PBMNCs spontaneously
produced increased IL-1
compared to controls
(Figure 1).

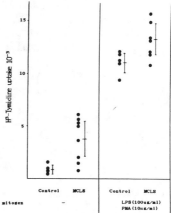

We assessed IL-1 induction in control PBMNCs by supernatants of various bacteria, including St. sanguis with K.D.-specific serotype, Y. pseudotuberculosis, St. sanguis type III (not related to K.D.), Y. enterocolitica and St. pyogenes. Each supernatant was concentrated by ammonium sulfate. PBMNCs (5×10^5/250 μl) were cultured with 20 μl supernatant. IL-1 inducing activity of PBMNCs supernatant was measured as above and was found only with K.D.-associated St. sanguis (Figure 2).

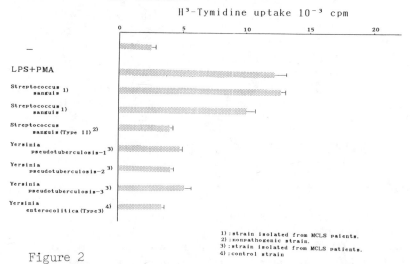

H^3-Tymidine uptake 10^{-3} cpm

1): strain isolated from MCLS paients.
2): nonpathogenic strain.
3): strain isolated from MCLS patients.
4): control strain

Figure 2

Supernatant from a K.D. strain of St. sanguis was precipitated with 80% ammonium sulfate and fractioned by Sephadex-G-100. IL-1 inducing activity was found in the 30K dalton fraction. T cells from controls were cultured for 6 days with 1 unit/ml of IL-1. Autologous B cells (3×10^5/250 μl) were then added and cultured for 3 days with 1 μg/ml pokeweed mitogen (PWM). After 7 additional days of culture, supernatant IgE was measured by ELISA. IgE production by B cells was enhanced by IL-1-activated T cells.

The effect of IL-1 on granulocyte function was assessed by measuring aggregation and O_2 production by cypridinaluciferin analog-inducer chemiluminescence. IL-1 enhanced granulocyte aggregation and O_2 production.

These results suggest that IL-1 is associated with K.D. and that K.D.-associated St. sanguis might be one of the causative agents of K.D.

Kawasaki Disease, pages 573–575
© 1987 Alan R. Liss, Inc.

EFFECT OF LIPOSOMAL ENCAPSULATED SUPEROXIDE DISMUTASE ON PATIENTS WITH KAWASAKI DISEASE

Kyoichi Somiya,[1] Yukie Niwa,[2]
Shigeko Fukami[3] and A. Michael Michelson[4]
[1]Department of Pediatrics, Hamamatsu Medical
Center; [2]Niwa Institute for Immunology;
[3]Department of Pediatrics, Hamamatsu Red-Cross
Hospital; [4]Institute de Biologie Physico
Chimique, 13, rue Pierre et Marie Curie,
75005 Paris, France

The cause and the pathogenesis of Kawasaki disease (KD) has remained unclear despite intensive studies.

We speculated that the pathogenesis of this disease may be related to oxygen radicals that induce tissue damage. Therefore, oxygen intermediate generation by polymorpho-nuclear leukocytes (PMNs) were assessed in these patients. Previously we showed that their PMNs showed a marked increase in oxygen radical generation within five days after onset of this disease. Furthermore, the patients who developed coronary aneurysms had elevated generation of hydroxyl radical, which is considered the most potent oxygen radical in the induction of tissue damage. In this regard, the clinical efficiency of liposomal encapsulated superoxide dismutase (L-SOD) was investigated in the treatment of KD patients.

L-SOD (100-300ug/kg) was administered to nineteen patients with KD two or three times a week by intravenous or intramuscular injection until cardinal clinical signs disappeared. Among the patients receiving L-SOD, 7/19 cases had been given a single injection of intravenous ¥-globulin (200mg/kg) prior to L-SOD administration.

As a control study, 20 age- and sex-matched KD cases receiving aspirin (50-90mg/kg per day) were studied, in comparison with the L-SOD group.

Examination of the coronary arteries was performed by two-dimensional echocardiography three times/week for 30 days after onset of the disease and diagnosed according to the criteria of the Kawasaki Disease Research Committee.

In most of the patients treated with L-SOD, fever disappeared within three days after administration. Bilateral hyperemia of the bulbar conjunctivae, non-purulent swelling of cervical lymph nodes, and skin rash subsided within four days after injection.

Coronary aneurysm was demonstrated in 6 (30%) patients of the aspirin group but in only 1 (8%) of the L-SOD group 30 days after onset of the disease (Tables 1 and 2).

TABLE 1. COMPARISON OF CLINICAL EFFECT BETWEEN ASPIRIN GROUP AND L-SOD GROUP

	Aspirin Group	L-SOD Group
Number of Patients	20	12
Age (Months)	22.9+16.2	29.3+19.1
Sex (Male/Female)	13/7	7/5
Cardinal Symptoms*		
Fever	6.7+4.6	2.5+1.5*
Exanthema	4.9+3.4	2.4+1.5*
Conjunctival injection	6.9+4.1	3.3+1.2*
Oropharyngeal change	8.3+3.4	5.1+1.3**
Cervical lymphadenopathy	6.8+4.5	4.0+1.2*
Indurative edema	5.5+3.5	3.3+1.8**
Elevated CRP Levels (Above 0.5mg/dl)	17.7+7.9	10.8+3.9
Coronary Artery Damage	6/20 (30%)	1/12 (8%)*

The duration of cardinal clinical symptoms and elevated CRP level in each group were expressed as mean+SD.
*p<0.01 vs Aspirin Group
**0.01<P<0.05 vs Aspirin Group

TABLE 2. THE DURATION (DAYS) OF CLINICAL SIGNS AND ELEVATED CRP LEVELS IN THE PATIENTS RECEIVING COMBINATION THERAPY OF L-SOD WITH ɣ -GLOBULIN

Cases	7
Age (Months)	20.9+15.2
Sex (Male/Female)	6/1
Cardinal Symptoms	
Fever	1.6+0.5
Exanthema	2.3+1.4
Conjunctival injection	1.7+0.5
Orophayrngeal change	3.4+1.5
Cervical lymphadenopathy	3.4+0.8
Indurative edema	3.6+1.3
Elevated CRP Levels (Above 0.5mg/dl)	6.1+3.2
Coronary Artery Damage	0/7 (0%)

The duration of cardinal clinical symptoms and elevated CRP level were expressed as mean+SD.

L-SOD treatment in KD patients was effective and showed significant improvement compared with aspirin therapy. The combination therapy of L-SOD with γ-globulin seems to be more beneficial and is recommended for the treatment of seriously ill patients with the disease.

Although more patients are required to be studied, our clinical research suggests that the use of L-SOD can be recommended not only because of its efficiency and prevention of coronary aneurysm, but also its lack of toxicity.

Kawasaki Disease, pages 577–578
© 1987 Alan R. Liss, Inc.

CAN EARLY TREATMENT PROVIDE BETTER PROGNOSIS IN KAWASAKI
DISEASE? A RETROSPECTIVE STUDY ON 616 CHILDREN

Hitoshi Usami, M.D., Kensuke Harada, M.D. and
Masahiko Okuni, M.D.
Department of Pediatrics, Nihon University School
of Medicine

A retrospective analysis of 616 children with Kawasaki
Disease was performed concerning the relationship between
the prevalence of coronary abnormality (CA) and timing of
the initiation of specific therapy. The subjects consisted
of 360 boys and 256 girls (male/female ratio = 1.25) from
five hospitals in or around Tokyo. Age at the onset of
disease ranged from 1 month to 13 years (25.6 ± 20.1 months;
m$\pm$SD). Information concerning medications, dose and the
day of illness at the initiation of therapy were obtained
from individual clinical records. The coronary arteries
were evaluated by angiography and/or 2-dimensional
echocardiography during or shortly after the acute stage in
all patients. A coronary artery of "beady" or "spindle-
like" appearance was diagnosed as abnormal. A CA was
detected in 155 children (25.2%) in at least one examination during their course. The initial therapeutic agent
was aspirin (30-50mg/kg) in 500 cases, aspirin plus
intravenous gamma globulin (small dose) in 44, and
flurbiprofen (3-5mg/kg/day) in 47. The rest of the
patients received dypiridamole, corticosteroid or
combination of 2 or more agents.

The mean time from the onset of the illness to the
initiation of therapy was significantly shorter in the
normal coronary artery group than in the abnormal group
(6.2 ± 3.0 vs. 7.1 ± 3.6 days, p<.01). Subjects were divided
into three subgroups (1st, 2nd and 3rd week groups) based
on the week of illness duration at the initiation of the
therapy. The percentage of patients with CA in the 1st,
2nd and 3rd week groups were 22.5, 31.9 and 40.0%,

respectively. The difference between the 1st and 2nd week group was significant by Chi-square (p<.01). The male/female ratio did not differ among these three groups; however, mean age at the onset of disease was signficantly lower in the 1st week group than that in the 2nd week group.

These results suggest the presence of a positive correlation between early therapy and lower prevalence of CA in children with Kawasaki Disease. In the early therapy group (initiation of therapy during the 1st week of illness), mean age was lower and male/female ratio was similar, as compared with those whose initiation of therapy was later than 1 week of illness. Therefore, the relationship between early therapy and low CA incidence appears to be independent from the influence of sex and age distribution. It cannot be concluded from this retrospective analysis that early therapy actually decreases the prevalence of CA in Kawasaki Disease because there may be some unidentified factor(s) correlating with both high prevalence of CA and late initiation of therapy. However, it seems a reasonable assumption that earlier therapy is better than late therapy in Kawasaki Disease, as seen in many other diseases. The time from the onset of illness to the initiation of therapy may be one of the possible prognostic determinants in Kawasaki Disease.

Kawasaki Disease, page 579
© 1987 Alan R. Liss, Inc.

LONG TERM PROGNOSIS OF GIANT CORONARY ANEURYSMS IN
KAWASAKI DISEASE

K. Tatara and S. Kusakawa

Department of Pediatrics
Tokyo Women's Medical College
Daini Hospital, Tokyo

The incidence of coronary obstruction subsequent to
giant aneurysm formation in Kawasaki Disease was studied.
In 20 cases, giant aneurysms with a maximal diameter
greater than 8 mm were identified by coronary angiography
at 2 to 120 months (mean = 16.9 months) after onset of
Kawasaki Disease. All of the cases with giant aneurysms
were followed up with repeat coronary angiograms performed
between 12 months and 134 months (mean = 31.7 months) after
initial angiographic study.

In every case, combination treatment with aspirin,
10 mg/kg/d, and dipyridamole, 5 mg/kg/d, was started after
the initial angiogram. Coronary obstruction occurred in
six of 20 cases (30%), all within four years of disease
onset. One of these patients developed symptomatic
myocardial infarction, and two had abnormal ECG findings
suggesting myocardial infarction. In five cases, persistent
perfusion defects were found by myocardial imaging.

On the other hand, there were two cases in which giant
aneurysms persisted for more than 10 years without development of obstructive changes. In both cases, obstruction of
the right coronary artery was found at initial examination.

These results indicate the limitation of antiplatelet
therapy for Kawasaki disease, and suggest that giant
aneurysms will likely progress with development of
obstruction within a few years even if antiplatelet therapy
has been administered.

Index